This book is to be returned on or before
the last date stamped below.

15. FEB 1999

22. APR 1996   15. FEB 1999

- 4. DEC. 1996

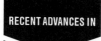

RECENT ADVANCES IN

Urology/Andrology

RECENT ADVANCES IN UROLOGY/ANDROLOGY

Contents of Number 5
Edited by W. F. Hendry

ISBN 0 443 04354X

You can place your order by contacting your local medical bookseller or the Sales
Promotion Department, Robert Stevenson House, 1–3 Baxter's Place, Leith Walk,
Edinburgh EH1 3AF, UK
Tel: (031) 556 2424; Telex: 727511 LONGMN G; Fax: (031) 558 1278

Look out for *Recent Advances in Urology/Andrology* 7 in September 1995

RECENT ADVANCES IN

Urology/Andrology

Edited by

W. F. Hendry MD ChM FRCS
Consultant Urologist, St Bartholomew's and Royal Marsden Hospitals, London, UK;
Civilian Consultant in Urology to the Royal Navy

R. S. Kirby MA MD FRCS
Consultant Urologist, St Bartholomew's Hospital, London, UK

NUMBER SIX

CHURCHILL LIVINGSTONE
EDINBURGH LONDON MADRID MELBOURNE MILAN NEW YORK AND TOKYO 1993

CHURCHILL LIVINGSTONE
Medical Division of Longman Group UK Limited

Distributed in the United States of America by
Churchill Livingstone Inc., 650 Avenue of the Americas,
New York, N.Y. 10011, and by associated companies,
branches and representatives throughout the world.

First published 1993

ISBN 0-443-04868-1
ISSN 0309 2739

British Library of Cataloguing in Publication Data
A catalogue record for this book is available from The British Library

Library of Congress Cataloging in Publication Data
is available

The
publisher's
policy is to use
**paper manufactured
from sustainable forests**

Produced by Longman Singapore Pte Ltd
Printed in Singapore

Contents

Preface

The sum of human knowledge is said to be doubling every five years. Certainly within Urology the pace of change has been breathtaking, hence the production of this sixth issue of *Recent Advances in Urology* only two years after its predecessor instead of after the usual five years. Concepts that were regarded as fundamental a few years ago are now being challenged, and it has never been more important for the urologist to stay up to date: with more and more patients better informed, the specialist must be able to discuss in a balanced way the relative benefits of operative and non-operative treatment, present alternative viewpoints and respect the patient's fundamental right to take an active and informed part in planning his or her management.

Nowhere have these advances been more spectacular than in laparoscopic surgery, where in the course of a few years open surgery has been challenged by keyhole specialists who are now doing more and more operations through smaller and smaller holes, using the most delicate techniques and helped by instruments of increasing sophistication. Increased patient satisfaction and rapid recovery periods more than repay the extended time needed to learn and carry out these elegant procedures.

Hardly a patient appears with prostatism nowadays without a series of questions: Is it cancer? Can you be sure? Do you have to operate? Can't you shrink it with drugs? What about microwaves or laser, doctor? The urologist who is unable to answer these questions reasonably and knowledgeably can expect the patient to go elsewhere. Some of the answers to these and other all-too-common questions are provided in this issue.

Transrectal ultrasound produces such clear images that early carcinoma can be recognized and its extent defined, and the diagnosis is firmly established by accurately guided biopsy. Magnetic resonance offers superb imaging, reflecting not only the anatomy but also the pathophysiological nature of the tissues. But does screening for early disease improve disease-specific survival? This is a most topical issue which will be debated for a considerable time yet. For the patient with advanced prostatic cancer, carefully conducted clinical trials have recently provided clear guidance on optimum treatment regimens.

Also for those affected by bladder cancer, there is new hope. Bladder reconstruction is now a reality, with experience gained in hundreds of patients available to encourage the urological trainee. Chemotherapy continues to promise much yet delivers little of lasting benefit, though once again carefully controlled clinical trials are distinguishing regimens of true value from those of passing fancy. Immunological therapy has always fascinated the oncologist and the urologist, and now provides some promise of response in patients with renal carcinomas. Most testicular tumours are now curable but at what cost to the patient and his loved ones? Reducing toxicity whilst maintaining efficacy is truly an art, and there are clear signs that this approach is now producing valid and long-lasting results.

Reconstruction of the genitourinary tract provides a continuing challenge for the urologist concerned with acceptable functional results of surgery. Bladder exstrophy, that most challenging of urological conditions, is now successfully corrected where urinary diversion was the norm, and urethral reconstructive surgery is undergoing major re-evaluation with the merits and demerits of the perineal, as opposed to the abdominoperineal, approach being the subject of critical scrutiny. Similarly, penile revascularization is put under the microscope literally and figuratively to establish how and when this elaborate procedure provides worthwhile benefit. All surgery of this magnitude of course needs adequate bacteriological cover, and the pernicious role of anaerobes is recognized and countered.

The urologist has had the privilege of seeing the specialty grow and grow in recent years: it is his or her responsibility to keep up to date as techniques and technology change at a pace that has never been faster.

London 1993   W.F.H.
                                                                         R.S.K.

Contributors

Freda E. Alexander BA MSc PhD
Deputy Director, Leukaemia Research Fund Centre for Clinical
Epidemiology, Universities of Leeds and Southampton, UK

Peter Boyle PhD
Director, Division of Epidemiology and Biostatistics, European Institute
of Oncology, Milan, Italy

E. David Crawford MD
Professor and Chairman, Division of Urology, University of Colorado,
Denver, Colorado, USA

Louis J. Denis MD
Professor of Urology, Department of Urology, A.Z. Middelheim, Antwerp,
Belgium

Susannah J. Eykyn MB BS MRCP FRCS FRCPath
Reader, and Honorary Consultant, in Clinical Microbiology, St Thomas's
Hospital, London, UK

John P. Gearhart MD FACS FAAP
Associate Professor of Pediatric Urology and Pediatrics, and Director of
Pediatric Urology, James Buchanan Brady Urological Institute, The Johns
Hopkins Hospital, Baltimore, Maryland, USA

Mohamed A. Ghoneim MD MD (Hon)
Professor of Urology, University of Mansoura; Director, Urology and
Nephrology Center, Mansoura, Egypt

Martin Gore MB BS PhD MRCP
Consultant Medical Oncologist, Royal Marsden Hospital, London; Honorary
Senior Lecturer, Institute of Cancer Research, London, UK

W. F. Hendry MD ChM FRCS
Consultant Urologist, St Bartholomew's and Royal Marsden Hospitals,
London, UK

Alan Horwich MB BS MRCP FRCR PhD
Professor of Radiotherapy, Institute of Cancer Research, Sutton, Surrey;
Consultant in Clinical Oncology, Royal Marsden Hospital, Sutton, Surrey,
UK

J. E. Husband FRCP FRCR
Consultant Radiologist, and Co-Director, Cancer Research Campaign
Clinical Magnetic Research Unit, Royal Marsden Hospital, Sutton, Surrey,
UK

R. S. Kirby MA MD FRCS
Consultant Urologist, St Bartholomew's Hospital, London, UK

J. S. P. Lumley MS FRCS
Professor of Vascular Surgery, St Bartholomew's Hospital, London, UK

Scott A. MacDiarmid MD
Fellow, Reconstructive Urology and Urodynamics, Division of Urology,
Duke University Medical Center, Durham, North Carolina, USA

David MacVicar MA MRCP FRCR
Senior Lecturer, Department of Radiology, Royal Marsden Hospital, Sutton,
Surrey, UK

Frank J. Mayer MD
Instructor in Urology and Urologic Oncology, University of Colorado Health
Sciences Center,
Denver, Colorado, USA

Dennis S. Peppas MD
Instructor in Urology and Pediatric Urology, James Buchanan Brady
Urological Institute, The Johns Hopkins Hospital, Baltimore, Maryland, USA

David Rickards FRCR FFRDSA
Consultant Uroradiologist, The Middlesex Hospital, London, UK

Baudouin Standaert MD
Director, Provincial Institute of Hygiene, Antwerp, Belgium

Harpreet S. Wasan MB BS MRCP
Senior Registrar, Department of Clinical Oncology, Royal Postgraduate
Medical School, Hammersmith Hospital, London, UK

J. Waxman BSc MD FRCP
Reader in Oncology, Royal Postgraduate Medical School, Hammersmith
Hospital, London, UK

George D. Webster MD ChB FRCS
Professor of Surgery, Division of Urology, Duke University Medical Center,
Durham, North Carolina, USA

J. E. A. Wickham MS MB BSc FRCS
Director, Academic Unit, Institute of Urology, University of London;
Senior Research Fellow and Surgeon, United Medical Schools of Guy's
and St Thomas's Hospitals, London, UK

1

MRI in urology

J. E. Husband   D. MacVicar

Magnetic resonance imaging (MRI) is now becoming recognized as an important method of imaging the pelvis and is likely to be increasingly used by urologists in the investigation of bladder and prostate cancer. In the abdomen the technique has not yet gained such wide acceptance, largely because movement artefacts due to long scanning times have degraded image quality. However, these technical difficulties are rapidly being overcome by the introduction of fast scanning techniques, thus opening the way to successful renal and adrenal imaging. The future of MRI in the management of lower urinary tract disease seems secure and in the long term, MRI may even supersede the use of computed tomography (CT) as the investigation of choice for many urological problems.

BASIC PHYSICS

The complexity of magnetic resonance is such that a comprehensive account of the basic physics is beyond the scope of this review and interested readers are therefore referred to some of the excellent texts on this subject.[1,2] It is essential however, to explain a few key principles to facilitate understanding of the images obtained and to appreciate some of the advantages of the system when compared with the more established methods of imaging such as ultrasound and CT.

Clinical MRI is made possible by the presence of countless hydrogen nuclei (protons) in the human body. Protons carry a positive charge and therefore possess electrical and magnetic properties. When placed in a powerful magnet, the patient's protons align in the direction of the magnetic field and spin in a way which is analogous to the oscillation of a compass needle in the earth's magnetic field. This phenomenon is known as precession and continues while the patient remains in the magnet. If a pulse of energy in the radiofrequency range is applied, two things happen. Firstly, the protons absorb the energy, and continue to precess with an increased angular momentum; secondly, the protons spin in phase. When the pulse is switched off, the protons emit energy, also in the radiofrequency range, as they revert to their previous state. This radiosignal is detected by a receiver coil. The time taken to reach the equilibrium precession energy is known as the T1 relaxation time, and the time taken for the protons to lose phase with each other is the T2 relaxation time, and these parameters determine the intensity of the signal emitted. T1 and T2 are influenced by the immediate environment of the protons; relaxation times are much longer in fluid than they are in, for example, muscle or bone, so that different tissues return distinguishable signal intensities. In general, T1 and T2 relaxation times are longer if the protons are relatively free to spin, which is the case if there is abundant water in the tissues. If protons are tightly bound, as in bone, relaxation times will be so short that virtually no signal is returned. Tumours have an abnormally high water content, giving longer relaxation times and signal characteristics which are distinct from normal tissues. In the early days of MRI it was hoped that MRI would differentiate benign from malignant tissue. This has not been possible owing to the degree of overlap in the signal characteristics of inflammatory and neoplastic conditions. However, the tissue contrast available with MRI is unrivalled, and this allows very accurate assessment of disease extent, although histological proof of its exact nature remains necessary.

TECHNICAL CONSIDERATIONS

A wide range of MRI scanners are now available. Most machines operate at 0.5–1.5 T, employing a superconducting copper coil magnet. A computer of bewildering complexity is required to quantify the received radiofrequency signals and reconstruct an anatomical image. Technical advances are continually being made, and are aimed at increasing tissue contrast, improving spatial resolution and reducing scan times and artefacts. Most MRI of the abdomen and pelvis still utilizes a radio transmitter and receiver coil which is housed in the magnet tunnel. Multiple body surface coils and endorectal coils, which are just becoming available for routine clinical use, will improve image quality as their proximity to the tissues will result in better reception of the signal.

The development of intravenous contrast medium (gadolinium-diethylenetriaminepentaacetic acid (DTPA), Schering Health Care), has made a major impact on the MRI of the central nervous system, but its value in body imaging is less clear. This contrast agent acts in a similar manner to intravenous iodinated radiographic contrast medium, having vascular, parenchymal and excretory phases. During the parenchymal phase, gadolinium DTPA shortens T1 relaxation time, thereby increasing the signal of enhancing tissue on T1-weighted imaging.

Another important advance in body MRI has been the recent development of bowel contrast agents which are likely to make a profound impact on the ability to detect lesions within the abdominal cavity. These should be available commercially within the next 2–3 years.[3,4]

Since MRI utilizes high field magnetism, there are a small group of patients in whom the technique is absolutely contraindicated. These include patients with pacemakers, those with intracranial aneurysm clips and patients with metal fragments within the orbit. Occasionally patients are claustrophobic and the examination cannot be undertaken or completed, but with the help of sedation, this problem can usually be overcome without too much difficulty.

PULSE SEQUENCE SELECTION AND IMAGE INTERPRETATION

MRI has some important advantages over other imaging techniques, particularly CT scanning. Firstly, the technique has superior contrast resolution to CT so that tumours and other masses in certain sites can be demonstrated with greater clarity than with CT. MRI also has the facility to obtain images in multiple planes but, even more important, it has the ability to provide greater detail with regard to the inherent characteristics of tissues, based on their relaxation parameters.

T1- and T2-weighted spin-echo images provide a standard MRI examination. Proton density images (which are the images produced from the first echo of a T2-weighted sequence) may be also be included in the study. Fat suppression techniques are sometimes employed, or contrast enhancement may be used, in which case the T1-weighted sequence is repeated following intravenous injection.

Sequences are selected according to the clinical problem. Sometimes T1 information is more important than T2, or vice versa. The exact relaxation times are rarely measured, but the sequence is weighted towards one of the parameters. The orientation of the scan plane is likewise selected to give the maximum clinically useful information. Acquisition of data for each sequence can take several minutes. Although scan times are being reduced, the number of sequences used is limited predominantly by time.

T1-weighted images provide an elegant anatomical display. Fat has a high signal, which appears white on the MR image and fluid, for example urine within the bladder, has a very low signal, which appears black. Other soft tissue structures such as muscle have an intermediate signal between fat and fluid. T2-weighted images are more prone to artefacts than T1-weighted images and are therefore less pleasing to view, but are equally informative, giving high tissue contrast. On T2-weighted images, the internal anatomy of an organ can be visualized due to the high sensitivity of the system in depicting small differences in the water content of different tissues. For example, the central zone of the prostate can be readily distinguished from the peripheral zone, which returns a higher signal intensity (Fig. 1.1). The seminal vesicles have a very high signal intensity due to their high fluid content and are also well-demonstrated. On T2-weighted sequences, urine within the bladder has a high signal and muscle has a low signal. Fat has a lower signal than on T1-weighted images.

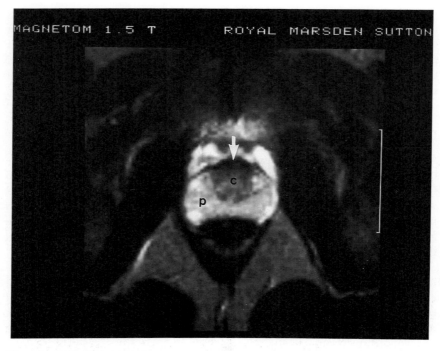

Fig. 1.1 Axial T2-weighted image of normal prostate. The peripheral zone (p) is a horseshoe of high signal (white) surrounding the central zone (c). The fibromuscular septum (arrow) is of very low signal. Anterior to this is a very high signal returned from slow-flowing blood in periprostatic vessels. (Reproduced with permission from Imaging in the management of prostatic carcinoma, MacVicar et al 1993 *Imaging* 5 (1).

THE PELVIS

Over the last 20 years there have been major advances in imaging of the pelvis. The most important of these have been the introduction of CT, the development of transrectal ultrasound and, most recently, the advent of MRI. MRI is still in its infancy, but already the technique is making a valuable contribution to staging pelvic tumours. To date, most information has been obtained using body coil images from equipment that has now been superseded by scanners with much faster scanning times and superior image quality. There seems little doubt therefore that as technology progresses even further, the results of MRI compared with CT and ultrasound will continue to improve during the coming years.

Bladder cancer

Although CT has made a tremendous contribution to the staging of invasive bladder tumours, the technique has many well-known disadvantages. The most significant of these is the inability to stage early tumours confined to the

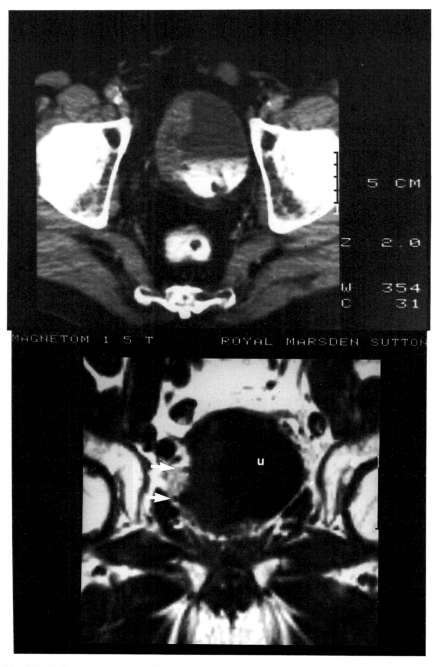

Fig. 1.2 **A** Contrast-enhanced CT scan of a large right-sided bladder tumour. Extravesical spread was suspected. **B** Coronal T1-weighted image confirms extravesical spread. High contrast between tumour and extravesical fat enables a clear demonstration of the extent of tumour spread (arrows). Urine (u) returns low signal on this sequence.

bladder wall and the difficulty of diagnosing early organ invasion. These limitations result from an inherent lack of contrast between tumours and adjacent normal tissue as well as limitations imposed by the single cross-sectional axial plane of imaging.

Since the mid 1980s, there have been several studies reported which have evaluated the accuracy of CT and MRI for staging bladder cancer.[5-8] Taking into account the variety of equipment used for both CT and MRI, as well as the developing experience in MRI, there is general agreement on several major issues. Advanced extravesical tumour spread, into the perivesical fat or even as far as the pelvic side wall, is clearly demonstrated by both MRI and CT, and there is no significant difference in the accuracy of both techniques. Although early extravesical invasion can be demonstrated on CT, particularly if intravenous contrast medium is given, such early disease is often better appreciated on MRI. Futhermore, MRI may demonstrate extravesical spread in the sagittal or coronal plane which cannot be so readily appreciated on axial plane CT images (Fig. 1.2). On balance, MRI appears to have a small but significant advantage over CT in the assessment of early extravesical disease, although in advanced disease MRI provides similar information. Early extravesical tumour spread is best appreciated on a T1-weighted sequence, as a result of the natural contrast between tumour and perivesical fat. If infiltration of pelvic muscles is suspected then this will be shown best on a T2-weighted sequence, which gives greater contrast between tumour and muscle. In addition, multiplanar imaging may provide the optimal method of confirming tumour within a diverticulum, which can be a singularly difficult clinical problem (Fig. 1.3).

T2-weighted images are valuable for assessing adjacent organ invasion such as spread of tumours at the bladder base into the prostate or seminal vesicles in the male, or into the vagina and cervix in the female. The presence of invasion is inferred when tumour signal replaces the normal signal of the adjacent structure. Early studies suggested that MRI was highly accurate for diagnosing seminal vesicle invasion, but further experience has revealed that low signal within the seminal vesicles does not always represent tumour.[9] Nevertheless, in many patients in whom CT interpretation is difficult, MR provides additional useful information with respect to the presence or absence of adjacent organ invasion.

On T2-weighted images, the bladder wall may be identified as a low signal line, separating the high signal urine from the surrounding perivesical fat. There is now substantial evidence to support the view that disruption of this black line indicates invasion of the deep muscle layer of the bladder wall (T3A), whereas integrity of the black line implies that tumour is limited to the superficial layers (T1 and T2). Thus it appears that MRI can provide some information on early tumour staging which is not available with CT.[5,10]

In the studies reported to date, the overall accuracy of MRI compared with CT is not significantly different since the accuracies for MRI range from 72 to 96% and those for CT from 40 to 92%.[5,8,10-12] However, when staging is

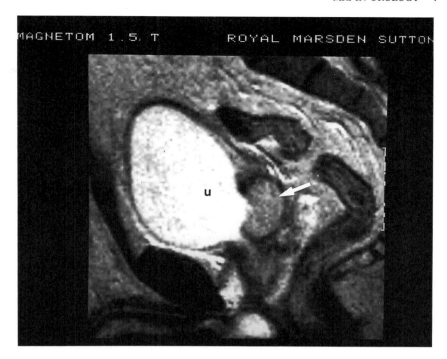

Fig. 1.3 Sagittal T2-weighted image of bladder. Urine (u) returns high signal on this sequence. There is tumour of intermediate signal within a diverticulum (arrow). The neck of the diverticulum could not be appreciated on axial computed tomography scans, and cystoscopy had failed to detect the tumour.

carried out using both techniques in the same patient, MRI sometimes provides additional information which may upstage the disease. In the light of these encouraging results and the dramatic advances taking place in technology, there is little doubt that MRI will eventually supersede CT in the evaluation of bladder cancer. The technique does however have important limitations which should be recognized. For example, it is not possible to distinguish oedema and fibrosis of the bladder wall from active tumour, which therefore leads to errors of overstaging following treatment with radiotherapy. As with all imaging techniques, microscopic spread beyond the bladder wall cannot be appreciated. Even though information regarding adjacent organ invasion may be superior to CT, there still remain some patients in whom the MRI findings are confusing. The current lack of a suitable bowel contrast agent sometimes leads to difficulties in interpretation, but this disadvantage is likely to be short-lived.

The prostate

Since MRI was first introduced into clinical practice there has been great enthusiasm for imaging of the prostate gland and many studies have been undertaken to determine the role of MRI for staging prostatic cancer. In this field, MRI is only rivalled by transrectal ultrasound because CT has proved inadequate for staging prostate tumours unless disease is grossly advanced.[13] On T2-weighted MRI, tumours of the prostate appear as areas of comparatively low signal which usually arise within the high-signal peripheral zone (Fig. 1.4). Small tumours arising in the central zone can be difficult to identify; tumour signal is often close to that of the normal tissues of the central zone. Tumours within the gland are best demonstrated on T2-weighted sequences, but advanced spread beyond the gland is often best appreciated on a T1-weighted image when tumour–fat contrast is accentuated. Following injection of intravenous contrast medium, prostatic tumours enhance and this may be valuable for defining the intraprostatic extent of tumour as well as spread beyond the gland.

The most useful imaging planes for evaluating prostatic cancer are the axial image in which the relationship of the tumour to the various components of the prostate can readily be appreciated, and the sagittal plane where invasion of tumour into the bladder anteriorly, or rectum posteriorly, can also be detected. Spread of tumour into the seminal vesicle is best demonstrated on

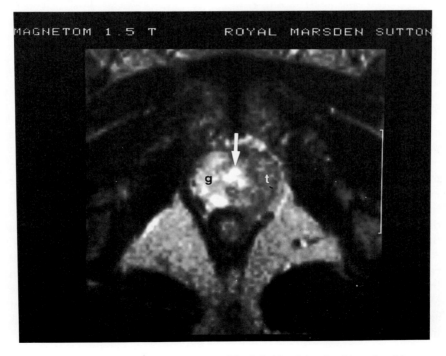

Fig. 1.4 Axial T2-weighted image of prostate. The left side of the gland is replaced by tumour (t), which returns a lower signal than the normal glandular tissue (g). Note the high signal of urine in the transurethral resection of the prostate defect centrally (arrow). (Reproduced with permission from Imaging in the management of prostatic carcinoma, MacVicar et al 1993 *Imaging* 5 (1).

a T2-weighted sequence and is easiest to depict in the axial plane. Tumour spread from the gland is seen as relatively low-signal tumour extending from the prostate into the adjacent seminal vesicles. However, if the prostate is grossly enlarged the proximity of the gland to the seminal vesicles may lead to errors in interpretation. In the late 1980s several studies were reported evaluating the accuracy of MRI for staging prostate cancer: these revealed a range of accuracies from 78 to 89%.[14-16] A large multi-institutional study in 260 patients compared the results of body coil MRI with those of transrectal ultrasound in detection of extracapsular spread in patients who had been selected for radical prostatectomy.[17] The results of MRI were better than those for ultrasound, with an overall accuracy for detection of early extraprostatic spread of 69% (sensitivity 77%, specificity 57%) compared with an accuracy of 57% for transrectal ultrasound (sensitivity 66%, specificity 46%). These studies have also shown that MRI has significant limitations, a major one being the inability to distinguish benign focal lesions within the prostate gland from early cancers. Further improvements with MRI can now be achieved using an endorectal coil and early results using this coil have shown MRI staging may be improved by as much as 16% when compared with conventional body coil imaging to an overall accuracy of over 80%.[18]

An important application of MRI in the evaluation of patients with prostatic cancer is the diagnosis of spinal cord compression due to metastatic bone involvement. MRI obviates the need for myelography and provides superior information by demonstrating the presence of spinal cord compression, the sites of involvement and the full extent of disease. In addition, the identification of small extradural lesions offers the potential for treating small foci of tumour before neurological damage has occurred.

KIDNEYS

While the signal of most soft tissue tumours on T2-weighted sequences is obviously different from normal fat and muscle tissue, the signal of many renal tumours is unfortunately very similar to that of surrounding renal parenchyma on both T1- and T2-weighted images.[19] Discovery of renal lesions therefore depends upon recognizable alterations of renal morphological characteristics. For small tumours which do not distort the anatomy of the kidney, MRI is relatively insensitive. Therefore most authors agree that MRI should not be used for detection of renal tumours, but should be reserved for evaluation of tumours which have been discovered by other means. Extra-renal extension of tumours may be seen well on MRI. Tendrils of tumour invading the perirenal space appear as low-intensity tissue invading the perirenal fat which is of high signal on T1-weighted imaging. Unfortunately, the renal capsule cannot be seen directly and it may thus be difficult to distinguish tumours which merely abut and distort the capsule from those which have truly breached the capsule. The criterion used for diagnosing invasion of the perirenal space and adjacent organs is similar on MRI and

CT–the obliteration of perirenal fat. MRI has the advantage of multiplanar imaging, which will enable minor degrees of extrarenal extension to be detected at the upper and lower renal poles. These areas are difficult to image on CT, because the axial scan plane is parallel to the interface of the tumour with adjacent areas of invasion.[20]

MRI is capable of demonstrating tumour invasion of vascular structures. Large vessels containing flowing blood appear as signal voids on spin-echo sequences. The spatial resolution of MRI does not permit the diagnosis of tumour in renal vein branches, but a thrombus extending into the renal vein, inferior vena cava or right atrium will be clearly visible. Care must be taken to avoid misinterpretation of flow artefacts within the vessels as tumour. Special pulse sequences or computer software packages dedicated to vascular imaging are frequently employed for optimum demonstration of tumour thrombi.

In paediatric patients, MRI is often employed in preference to CT. The technique avoids ionizing radiation, and the multiplanar capacity is helpful in the differential diagnosis of upper pole Wilms' tumours from adrenal neuroblastomas. Wilms' tumour is demonstrable on MRI, but like renal cell carcinomas, may have a signal intensity close to that of renal parenchyma, and often contains regions with a wide and unpredictable range of signal intensities.[21]

Angiomyolipomas may have a distinctive appearance on MRI. If sufficient fat is present within the lesion, the signal intensity will be high on both T1- and T2-weighted images. However, if there is little fat within the lesion, they may be indistinguishable from other renal neoplasms, and no definite advantage of MRI over CT has been demonstrated in the differential diagnosis of these tumours. Other unusual tumours of the kidney, such as medullary fibroma and oncocytoma, have been detected by MRI. However there are no reliable diagnostic features, and histological confirmation remains necessary.[20,22,23]

Observation of signal change allows diagnosis of diffuse renal parenchymal disease in both native and transplanted kidneys. In the normal kidney, good quality T1-weighted spin-echo images will reveal a differentiation between cortex and medulla.[24] The medulla, which has a longer T1 relaxation time than the cortex, will return a lower signal. This distinction is lost in a wide range of conditions, including acute oliguric renal failure, glomerulonephritis, collagen vascular diseases, chronic ureteral obstruction, and end-stage renal failure from any cause. This abnormal sign has a high specificity and positive predictive value for the presence of renal disease, although the differential diagnosis is wide. In transplanted kidneys, the distinction may be lost in rejection, particularly if it is severe or chronic. Acute tubular necrosis and cyclosporin toxicity are usually associated with preservation of the corticomedullary distinction. However, the expense and relative inconvenience of MRI have prevented it from replacing ultrasound and isotope studies for investigation of the transplant kidney. MRI angiography is capable of detecting stenosis of a renal transplant artery; refinement of the MRI techniques and evaluation in a clinical setting are underway, but for the present, conventional or digital subtraction intra-arterial angiography should remain the investigation of choice for diagnosis of transplant artery stenosis.

ADRENAL GLANDS

The sensitivity of MRI in detection of morphological abnormalities of the adrenal gland is similar to that of CT.[25] With modern equipment, all adrenal masses of 1.5 cm or more in diameter should be visible. Most normal adrenal glands are demonstrable on T1-weighted imaging and appear as low signal intensity organs outlined by the high signal intensity of the surrounding fat. Differential diagnosis of adrenal masses relies on information from both T1- and T2-weighted images. Adenomas of the adrenal gland have a higher lipid content than malignant tumours. As a result, primary and secondary carcinomas of the adrenals have longer T1 and T2 relaxation times, and return a discernibly different signal. Unfortunately some 20% of cases return an intermediate signal, and such cases should be regarded as indeterminate. However, when allied to clinical and biochemical information, MRI appearances may be sufficiently characteristic to make adrenal biopsy unnecessary in a significant number of cases.

Neuroblastoma is of low signal on T1-weighted images and of a mixed high signal on T2-weighted images. In young children, neuroblastoma rarely presents a problem of differential diagnosis, but the multiplanar capacity of MRI may assist in the distinction of adrenal from upper pole renal masses, and large neuroblastomas may be displayed in multiple planes to demonstrate the relationship of the tumour to vascular structures and neural foramina (Fig. 1.5). The technique is useful for following tumour response to systemic therapy and planning surgery.

SCROTUM

MRI is capable of producing images of scrotal contents with exquisite anatomical detail, and appears to be a sensitive technique for detecting focal lesions of the testis. However, ultrasound remains the investigation of choice as it is less expensive and time-consuming. Neither technique correlates well with histological findings for local staging of primary testicular neoplasms.[26] Infiltration of the testis by leukaemia or lymphoma may be difficult to identify by ultrasonography, and an asymmetry of MRI signal between the testes may help to confirm unilateral involvement in this clinical setting.[27]

Hydroceles and varicoceles have a characteristic appearance on MRI. The twisted stalk of the testis and a thickened proximal spermatic cord may be seen in testicular torsion. In torsion, epididymitis and orchitis, MRI may be used in preference to ultrasonography, as the latter requires manipulation of

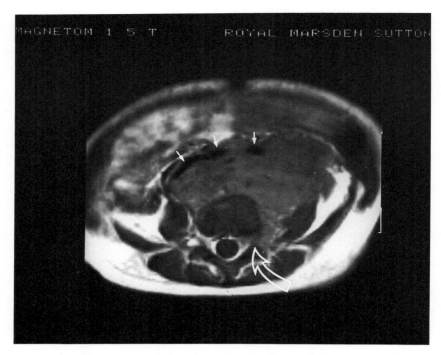

Fig. 1.5 Axial proton density image of a child aged 30 months. A large retroperitoneal neuroblastoma is shown enveloping the iliac vessels, which are shown as signal voids (small arrows). Tumour signal obliterates the normal fat planes as it invades the left-side neural foramen (curved arrow).

the scrotum, which may be extremely painful. Following testicular trauma, lacerations and haematomas are easily identified. MRI clearly demonstrates the tunica albuginea and its integrity, and may therefore help in determining whether surgical therapy is necessary.

Fears that scrotal heating engendered by deposition of radio frequency energy is sufficient to cause male infertility have been allayed by a recent publication.[28]

LYMPH NODES

Lymph node masses in the retroperitoneum are demonstrable by MRI but CT remains the most frequently used method for detection of retroperitoneal nodes in malignancies of the testis, pelvic tumours and lymphoma. In the evaluation of testicular tumour metastases, MRI enables clear demonstration of cystic components within masses, and requires no intravenous contrast to distinguish nodes from adjacent vessels. The multiplanar capability demonstrates the relationship of residual nodal masses to vessels (Fig. 1.6), and artefacts from surgical clips are rarely as troublesome as they are on CT.

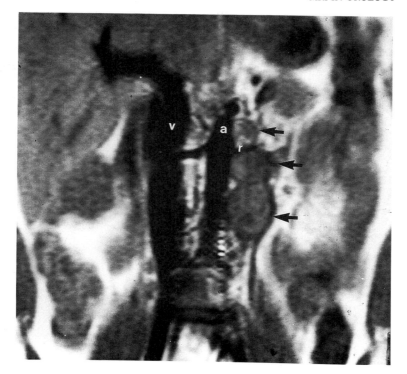

Fig. 1.6   Coronal T1-weighted image of residual retroperitoneal nodal masses following systemic chemotherapy for metastatic testicular teratoma. Aorta (a) and inferior vena cava (v) are shown as signal voids. The nodal masses (arrows) extend above the renal arteries (r).

Retroperitoneal fibrosis usually appears as low signal intensity on both T1- and T2-weighted images. However, the technique is not reliable for distinguishing malignant from non-malignant fibrosis.

Pelvic lymph node imaging is usually performed in the axial plane but coronal images may also provide useful confirmatory evidence of lymphadenopathy. MRI will clearly identify enlarged pelvic lymph nodes. Malignant nodes return low signal on T1-weighted images, and relatively high signal on T2-weighted images. Once again, MRI cannot reliably discern benign from malignant causes of lymph node enlargement, but if the signal intensity in nodes is similar to that of the primary tumour, the diagnosis can be made with some confidence. Most studies of pelvic tumour staging quote similar false-negative rates for CT and MRI. A major advantage of MRI over CT is that enlarged lymph nodes can easily be distinguished from pelvic side-wall vessels, which appear as signal voids. With CT, even when intravenous contrast medium is given, such distinction may be difficult because minimally enlarged lymph nodes may enhance with contrast medium to the same degree as adjacent vessels.[29]

KEY POINTS FOR CLINICAL PRACTICE

- The physics and technology of MRI are radically different from any other imaging technique.
- The tissue contrast available with MRI is unrivalled, but it does not permit tissue characterization of benign from malignant disease.
- High tissue contrast and multiplanar anatomical display can give additional information in local tumour staging.
- Increased availability and further technical advance will result in MRI replacing CT as a staging investigation for many urological tumours.

ACKNOWLEDGEMENTS

The authors would like to thank Pippa Johnston and Pauline Kennedy for assistance in preparation of the manuscript, and Janet MacDonald and Jackie Seckel for help in preparation of the illustrations. We are also grateful to the Cancer Research Campaign and Daniel Marks Fund for continuing financial support to the Unit.

REFERENCES

1   Kean DM, Smith MA. Magnetic resonance imaging; principles and applications. London: William Heinemann 1986
2   Wehrli FW. Principles of magnetic resonance. In: Stark DD, Bradley WG, eds. Magnetic resonance imaging. St. Louis: CV Mosby. 1988
3   Rinck PA, Smevick O, Nilsen G et al. Oral magnetic particles in MR imaging of the abdomen and pelvis. Radiology 1991; 178: 775–779
4   MacVicar D, Jacobsen TF, Guy R, Husband JE. Phase III trial of oral magnetic particles in magnetic resonance imaging of abdomen and pelvis. Clin Radiol 1993; 47 (3): 183–188
5   Husband JE, Olliff JFC, Williams MP, Heron CW, Cherryman GR. Bladder cancer: staging with CT and MR imaging. Radiology 1989; 173: 435–440
6   Bryan PJ, Butler HE, Li Puma JP et al. CT and MR imaging in staging bladder neoplasms. J Comput Assist Tomogr 1987; 11: 96–101
7   Johnson RJ, Charrington BM, Jenkins JPR et al. Accuracy in staging carcinoma of the bladder by magnetic resonance imaging. Clin Radiol 1990; 41: 258–261
8   Buy J-N, Moss AA, Guinet C et al. MR staging of bladder carcinoma; correlation with pathologic findings. Radiology 1988; 169: 695–700
9   Secaf E, Nuruddin RN, Hricak H et al. MR imaging of the seminal vesicles. Am J Roentgenol 1991; 156: 989–994
10   Rholl KS, Lee JKT, Heiken JP et al. Primary bladder carcinoma: evaluation with MR imaging. Radiology 1987; 163: 117–121
11   Amendola MA, Glazer GM, Grossman HB et al. Staging of bladder carcinoma: MRI-CT-surgical correlation. Am J Roentgenol 1986; 146: 1179–1183
12   Morgan CL, Calkins RF, Cavalcanti EJ. Computed tomography in the evaluation, staging and therapy of carcinoma of the bladder and prostate. Radiology 1981; 140: 751–761
13   Platt JF, Bree RL, Schwab RE. The accuracy of CT in the staging of the prostate. Am J Roentgenol 1987; 149: 315–318
14   Bezzi M, Kressel HY, Allen KS et al. Prostatic carcinoma: staging with MR imaging at 1.5T. Radiology 1988; 169: 339–346
15   Biondetti PR, Lee JKT, Ling D et al. Clinical stage B prostate carcinoma: staging with MR imaging. Radiology 1987; 162: 325–329

16 Hricak H, Dooms GC, Jeffrey RB et al. Prostatic carcinoma: staging by clinical assessment, CT and MR imaging. Radiology 1987; 162: 321–336

17 Rifkin MD, Zerhouni EA, Gatsonis CA et al. Comparison of magnetic resonance imaging and ultrasonography in staging early prostate cancer. N Engl J Med 1990; 323: 621–626

18 Schnall MD, Imai Y, Tomaszewski J et al. Prostate cancer: local staging with endorectal surface coil MR imaging. Radiology 1991; 178: 797–802

19 Hricak H, Demar BE, Williams RD et al. Magnetic resonance imaging in the diagnosis and staging of renal and perirenal neoplasms. Radiology 1985; 154: 709–714

20 Fein AV, Lee JKT, Balfe DM et al. Diagnosis and staging of renal cell carcinoma: a comparison of MR imaging and CT. Am J Roentgenol 1987; 148: 749–754

21 Boechat MI, Kangarloo H. MR imaging of the abdomen in children. Am J Roentgenol 1989; 152: 1245–1249

22 Dooms GC, Hricak H, Solitto RA et al. Lipomatous tumours and tumours with fatty components: MR imaging potential and comparison of MR and CT results. Radiology 1985; 157: 479–482

23 Sohn HK, Kim SY, Seo HS. MR imaging of a renal oncocytoma. J Comput Assist Tomogr 1987; 11: 1085–1087

24 Demas BE, Stafford SA, Hricak H. Kidneys. In: Stark DD, Bradley WG, eds. Magnetic resonance imaging. St. Louis: CV Mosby. 1988

25 Dunnick NR. CT and MRI of adrenal lesions. Urol Radiol 1988; 10: 12–20

26 Thurnher S, Hricak H, Carroll PR et al. Imaging in the testis: comparison between MR imaging and ultrasound. Radiology 1988; 167: 631–634

27 Klein EA, Kay R, Norris DG et al. Non-invasive testicular screening in childhood leukaemia. J Urol 1986; 136: 864–868

28 Schellock FG, Rothman B, Sarti D. Heating of the scrotum by high field strength MR imaging. Am J Roentgenol 1990; 154: 1229–1232

29 Husband JE, Robinson L, Thomas G. Contrast enhancing lymph nodes in bladder cancer: a potential pitfall of CT. Clin Radiol 1992; 45: 395–398

2

Recent advances in ultrasound

D. Rickards

ULTRASOUND AND PROSTATE STENTS

The use of metallic stents in the treatment of outflow obstruction offers one of many alternatives to transurethral prostatectomy. The stents are either temporary or permanent: the former are intraluminal, and if left in situ long enough will encrust with phosphatic debris and become infected, whilst the latter become completely covered with urothelium and are not intraluminal. Two permanent stents are currently available. The (ASI) titanium stent (Advanced Surgical Intervention) is introduced in a collapsed state on a balloon catheter which is inflated once the stent is in position, expanding the stent within the posterior urethral lumen. The AMS Urolume stent (American Medical Systems) is made of a fine mesh of corrosion-resistant superalloy which is available is varying lengths and diameters. It was initially inserted into the posterior urethra under linear array transrectal ultrasound (TRUS) control, mounted on a 9F catheter whilst held in its compressed state under a plastic membrane which when pressurized to 3 atm would shorten, allowing the stent to assume its unconstrained configuration. It is now inserted under direct vision at cystoscopy using a dedicated introducer upon which the stent is mounted and which comes presterilized from the manufacturers. Stents with an unconstrained diameter of 14 mm are used, allowing for subsequent cystoscopy.[1,2] Pre- and postoperative assessment of these stents can be achieved by cystoscopic review, TRUS, pelvic ultrasound and urethrography. Of these modalities, TRUS in non-invasive, uncomplicated, quick to perform and provides the following information:

1. Preoperative: urethral length and prostate pathology
2. Postoperative:

   a. stent position
   b. stent dimensions
   c. urothelial covering of the stent
   d. complications.

Preoperative TRUS

The only preoperative imaging needed is TRUS which can image the urethral walls and the verumontanum, allowing posterior urethral length from bladder neck to verumontanum to be measured. In those patients who present in retention with urethral catheters in situ, such measurements are much easier, but catheters can alter the configuration of the prostate and distort measurements of urethral length. Although the length of the posterior urethra is assessed using graduated catheters at cystoscopy, preoperative measurements are useful in order that the correct-length stents are available for insertion in the operating theatre and as a back-up to correlate with the intraoperative measurements. The relationship of the prostate to the bladder base, the presence of a median lobe and coexistent pathology are also assessed (Fig. 2.1). Any areas suspicious of malignancy can be biopsied under TRUS control.

Postoperative TRUS

Position of the stent

Temporary stents have a closely woven mesh that attenuates the ultrasound beam to such an extent that it is not possible to image the intrastent lumen

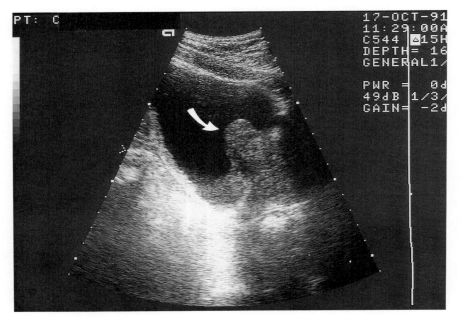

Fig. 2.1 Suprapubic transabdominal ultrasound of the full bladder. There is considerable invagination of the bladder base by an enlarged prostate (arrow). This might be difficult to gauge by transrectal ultrasound.

or the relationship of the stent to the bladder neck—not that it is important to do so as the stents extend into the bladder by design. The position of permanent stents is clearly defined by TRUS. For accurate scanning, the bladder needs to be partially full so that the relationship of the stent to the bladder neck can be seen (Figs. 2.2 and 2.3). The position of the distal end of the stent and its relationship to the distal sphincter and apical prostatic tissue are then assessed (Fig. 2.4). Postoperative incontinence may be due to pre-existing instability, instability as a result of instrumentation or compromise of distal sphincter function because the stent is partly or wholly covering it. TRUS will help to differentiate between poor positioning and a functional abnormality.

Stent dimensions

When deployed, the stent should assume its unconstrained diameter of 14 mm, the dimension recommended for the prostate, allowing for both adequate relief of obstruction and subsequent cystoscopy. Should the stent not fully open, it will necessarily be longer. If, for example, pre- and intraoperative measurements of prostate length indicate that a 4 cm stent is needed to cover the entire posterior urethra which when positioned does not fully open,

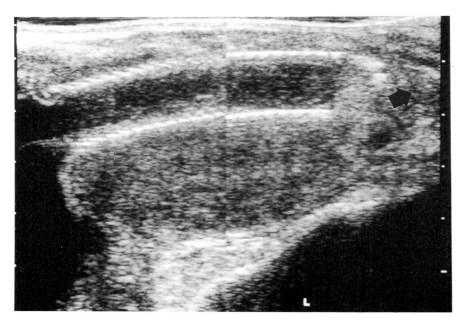

Fig. 2.2 Transrectal ultrasound showing the stent covering nearly all the prostatic urethra. The stent is positioned exactly at the bladder neck and is short of the apex of the gland (arrow).

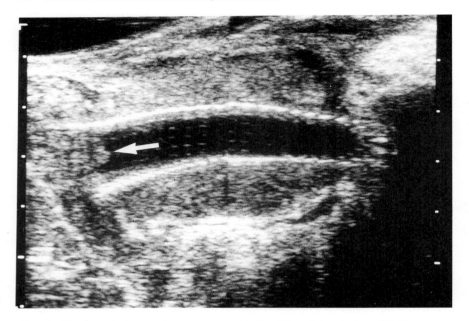

Fig. 2.3 Transrectal ultrasound with an empty bladder. There is herniation of bladder mucosa into the proximal end of the stent (arrow). This makes it difficult to determine the relationship of the stent to the bladder neck.

part of the stent will either cover the distal sphincter or project into the bladder. Although immediate cystoscopic review may show the stent to be in an ideal position, if it hasn't fully opened, it tends to shorten from its distal end, which will leave apical prostatic tissue uncovered, potentially compromising a satisfactory result. Stent dimensions are measured 24 hours after insertion, by which time shortening will have occurred if it is going to happen. The length of the anterior and posterior stent margins is measured, as is the diameter at the distal and proximal ends and in the mid-stent area. This ensures that there has been uniform opening of the stent.[3] In some cases, the stent never assumes its correct dimensions, presumably because the prostate is not compliant enough to allow the expansile forces inherent in the stent to exert sufficient pressure on the prostate. To measure such compliance is difficult, but is the subject of current research.

Urothelial covering of the stent

In the first few months following insertion, permanent stents invoke a hyperplastic reaction which is difficult to image by TRUS, but this settles within 6 months to leave a smooth urothelial covering of the stent (Fig. 2.5). The extent and uniformity of urothelium can easily be assessed by TRUS. Usually, the stent is covered by a uniform thickness of 1–2 mm of urothelium,

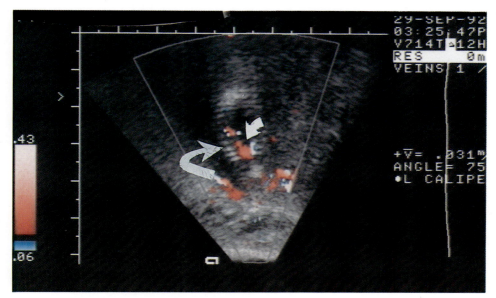

Plate 1 Colour Doppler imaging of a stent complicated by recurrent haematuria. Large vessels (small arrow) can be seen within the lumen of the stent (large arrow); these vessels were confirmed at cystoscopy to be reposonsible for the heamaturia.

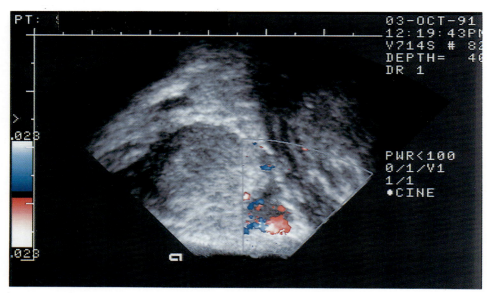

Plate 2 High-resolution transverse axial colour Doppler scan of the prostate shown in Figure 2.7. There is an echopoor area in the prostate which is vascular on Doppler. Guided biopsy proved malignancy.

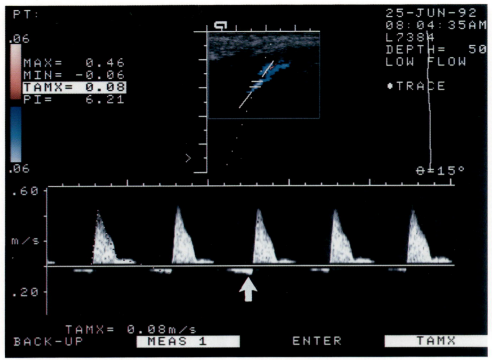

Plate 3 Normal parameters seen on colour Doppler imaging with a grade 3 erection. Flow in systole is 46 cm/s (or 0.46 m/s) and there is reversal of flow in diastole (arrow).

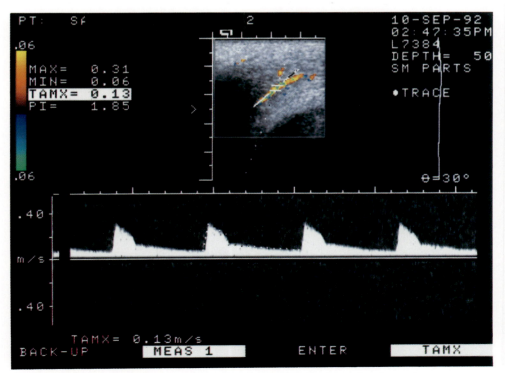

Plate 4 Arterial insufficiency seen on colour Doppler imaging. Maximum flow in systole was recorded at 31 cm/s (or 0.31 m/s) with no reversal of flow in diastole.

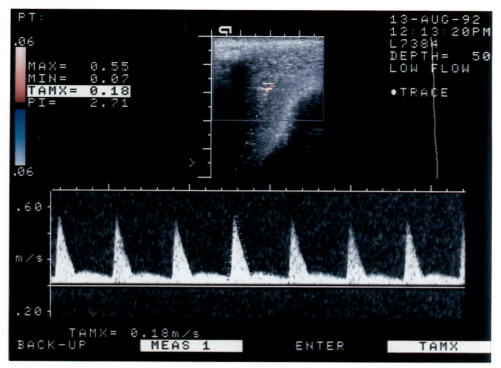

Plate 5 Venous leakage on colour Doppler imaging. Flow in systole is high at 55 cm/s (or 0.55 m/s), indicating good arterial inflow. Despite this, flow in diastole never went below 7 cm/s (or 0.07 m/s). There was no reversal of flow in diastole.

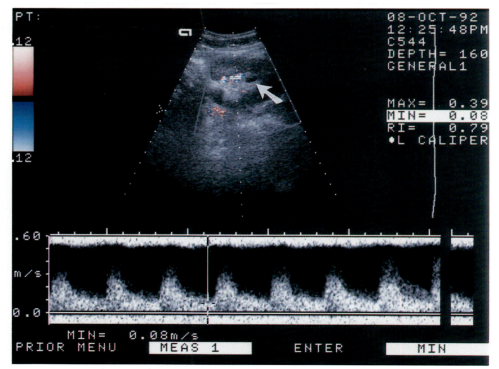

Plate 6 There is minimal dilatation of the collecting system (arrow). The resistive index (RI) calculated from the spectral waveform was 0.79, suggesting that the dilatation is due to true obstruction.

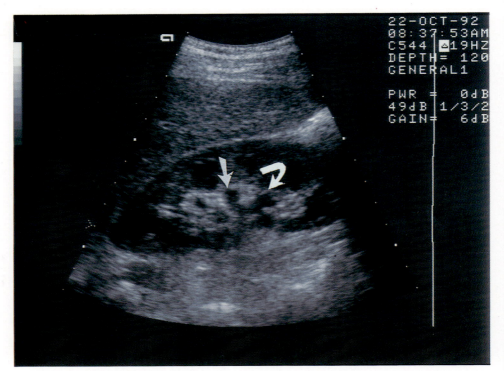

Plate 7 **A** There is apparent mild dilatation of the collecting system suggesting obstruction (arrows).

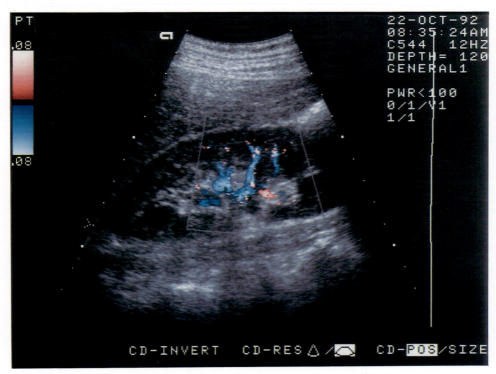

Plate 7 **B** Colour Doppler imaging shows that the dilatation is due to vessels.

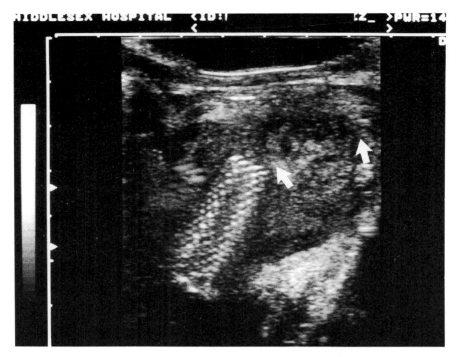

Fig. 2.4 Transrectal ultrasound of a stent in a patient with a prostate cancer. The stent is too short and not covering the inferior half of the prostatic urethra (between arrows).

leaving an adequate intrastent lumen. Occasionally focal areas of overgrowth are seen. Colour Doppler imaging (CDI) in the transverse axial or forward-looking sagittal planes allows for definition of the vascularity of the neourothelium.

Complications of stent insertion

Misplacement of the stent at the bladder neck with free wires not in contact with urothelium is likely to lead to encrusting. TRUS will demonstrate such free wires and show if small stones are forming on them (Fig. 2.6). This complication occurred commonly when the stents were inserted under TRUS control. It has proved rare if they are put in under direct vision. In no case in the author's experience has the distal sphincter been compromised by stent insertion, but TRUS would define that. Perineal pain following stent insertion may be due to the development of prostatic inflammatory disease, prostate abscess or blockage to the prostatic and ejaculatory ducts. TRUS will differentiate between these entities and point towards appropriate therapy. Prolonged haematuria following stent insertion may be due to prominent

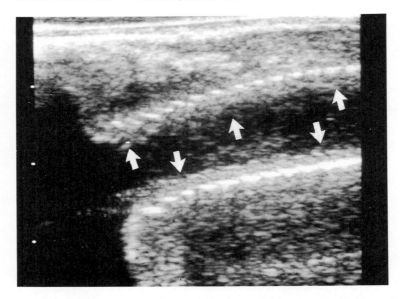

Fig. 2.5 Transrectal ultrasound showing good placement of the stent at the bladder neck and smooth urothelial lining of the stent (arrows).

vessels supplying the urothelial covering. TRUS combined with CDI will demonstrate such vessels (Plate 1).

ULTRASOUND IN PROSTATE CANCER

Technique and biopsy methods

Transverse axial sections of the prostate (like computed tomography images) provide anatomical detail of the gland symmetry, the seminal vesicles and zonal anatomy. Sagittal sections are essential for imaging the urethra and its surrounding tissues and the configuration of the prostate to the bladder base.

Early ultrasound transducers allowed imaging in only one plane and it is clear that multiplane imaging is now essential for complete evaluation of the prostate.[4] This can be achieved with a variety of probes. Biplane probes allow for transverse axial and sagittal imaging using two transducers housed at the end of the same probe. The resolution afforded by each transducer is presently limited by probe diameter and, whilst good spatial resolution is achieved with 7 MHz linear array transducers providing sagittal sections, the axial images are less good and in general use 5 MHz transducers. Guided biopsy is by the perineal route. Monoplane probes scan in one dimension only and to assess the prostate at least two probes will be needed, but each will operate at 7 MHz, providing excellent spatial resolution and CDI is available on the curved array probes. Multiplane probes have a single transducer which can be electronically oriented in any plane and can operate at varying

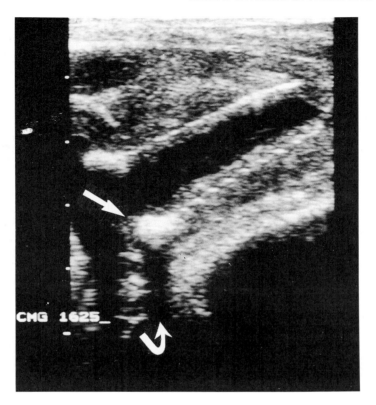

Fig. 2.6   Transrectal ultrasound showing small stones (arrow) encrusted on free wires of the stent. Note the acoustic shadowing because of the stones (curved arrow).

frequencies from 5 to 7 MHz, but cannot run CDI. Both mono- and multiplane probes allow transrectal guided biopsy, which requires an end-viewing transducer in which the scan plane is centred along the long axis of the transducer and is altered by rotating the housing of the probe. Any suspicious area can be readily scanned in three dimensions.

With advancing probe technology, transrectal as opposed to perineal biopsy is emerging as the most accurate method. It permits all areas of the gland and the periglandular tissues to be biopsied—this is difficult via the perineal route. No local anaesthesia is used; it is done on an outpatient basis; it is almost painless as long as the anal sphincter is avoided and it is not associated with significant complications, but prophylactic antibiotics should be given immediately before and for 2 days after the procedure.[5] The risk of faecal contamination is reduced by a cleansing enema before biopsy.

Perineal biopsy is a safe and perfectly acceptable option for biopsy, does not necessitate prophylactic antibiotics, is not associated with significant complications and is just as quick. It does require the extensive use of local anaesthesia to the skin, subcutaneous tissues and pericapsular area, typically 15 ml of 1% lignocaine. It is the preferred route if prostate abscess or inflammatory disease is suspected. Core biopsy using an automatic triggering device and 18-gauge needles has replaced aspiration cytology. Such triggering devices take a 2 cm core so the biopsy needle tip must be placed well proximal to a suspicious lesion. There is no doubt that TRUS-guided biopsy is more accurate than digitally guided procedures, even when malignancies are palpable.

The appearances of prostate cancer

The diagnosis of malignancy on digital examination depends upon its size, location and consistency as well as the ability of the examiner, whose findings are subjective. TRUS can and does detect non-palpable malignancies.[6] TRUS cannot detect microscopic spread of malignancy either within the gland or into the prostate capsule. Prostate cancer's malignant potential correlates with tumour volume,[7] histological grade[8] and stage. Tumour size is important in determining the natural history of prostate cancer and can be utilized to predict capsular infiltration, diferentiation and metastatic spread.[9]

Prostate cancer was first described as echogenic.[10,11] It is now recognized that cancer is predominantly echo poor, although isoechoic cancers are common, and mixed echogenic and hyperechoic ones do rarely occur. The relationship of tumour morphology and echogenicity is proportional to the amount of normal tissue present in a malignant area. More malignant than normal tissue lowers the echogenicity. However, only 20% of peripherally situated hypoechoic lesions are malignant.[12] Small cancers are more hypo-echoic than larger ones and the majority of large tumours are not hypoechoic as they are associated with stromal fibrosis which renders their echogenicity more like normal prostatic tissue. Cancers have an irregular outline and capsular distortion is suggestive of invasion.

Not all carcinomas can be detected by grey-scale TRUS alone. Up to 25% are isoechoic with normal prostate tissue.[13,14] Apparent echogenic malignancies are due to those involving calcified corpora amylacea and in some high-grade tumours due to comedonecrosis, centrally necrotic tumours with calcification that appears on TRUS as fine and stippled.[15] Recent work suggests that specific patterns of increased blood flow in patients with prostate cancer and inflammatory disease are seen on CDI. TRUS alone has a high sensitivity, but a low specificity in diagnosing cancer, because most echopoor lesions are benign. Those echopoor lesions that are associated with increased vascularity as seen on CDI (Fig. 2.7 and Plate 2) are more likely to be malignant. In a series of 100 biopsy-proven cases in which cancer prevalence was 55%, TRUS alone had a specificity of 22%: when combined with CDI, this improved to 77%. Clearly, CDI has an important role in the diagnosis of prostate cancer.

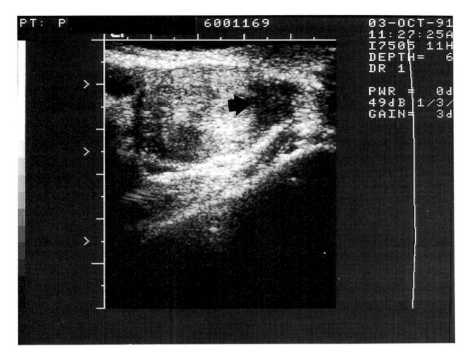

Fig. 2.7   Sagittal transrectal ultrasound showing an echopoor lesion at the apex of the prostate gland (arrow).

A crucial factor in staging prostate cancer is determining whether the tumour is confined to the gland and potentially amenable to radical prostatectomy.[16] On TRUS, localized deformity of the capsule or an interruption in the normally bright capsular echoes (formed by the interface of prostate with periprostatic fat) suggests involvement. Such criteria only apply to the peripheral zone and using them correctly can correctly stage 70% of tumours that could be seen on TRUS.[14] There is considerable overlap in the appearance of benign and malignant disease in the rest of the gland; TRUS does not provide good definition of the anterior capsule of the gland, especially when there is prostatomegaly,and TRUS has little role to play in staging isoechoic tumours. So, staging is only potentially possible in the 75% of hypoechoic tumours that arise in the peripheral zone (70% of tumours).

There are many conditions that simulate prostate cancer. Malakoplakia,[15] nodules of benign hypertrophy, cysts, infarcts, inflammatory processes, cystic atrophy, blood vessels and muscular tissue count amongst them.

Following radiotherapy for localized cancer, the prostate becomes small and echogenic. Persistent tumour is difficult to detect, but TRUS is emerging as an effective modality in some cases. Persistent tumour maintains its pretreatment echo characteristics—it is mainly an echopoor lesion—and lesions over 5 mm in diameter persisting for 12 months following radiotherapy are specifically suspicious of malignancy and should be biopsied.[16,17] A decrease of total prostate volume is not a reliable indicator of prognosis.[18,19] This is not surprising as coexistent normal and hypertrophied prostatic tissue will shrink in response to radiotherapy.

ULTRASOUND AND IMPOTENCE

Duplex ultrasound and CDI have provided a non-invasive method of assessing patients with suspected vasculogenic impotence. Once psychogenic, endocrinological, neurological or pharmacological factors have been investigated, further studies to evaluate the penile vasculature and classify the aetiology of the impotence into one of four clinically useful groups can be performed as long as the patient is willing to undergo surgery on the potential findings of:

1. Normal penile vasculature
2. Arterial insufficiency
3. Venous leakage
4. A combination of arterial and venous disease.

All tests of erectile function are performed before and after the injection of vasoactive agents into the corpora. The most commonly used is papaverine hydrochloride, which can be used in combination with phentolamine. Prostaglandin E1 may be effective where others fail. All vasoactive agents carry the risk of priapism and the dose administered to an individual patient should take account of the clinical picture and age. Ultrasound is performed using high-frequency linear array probes (7–7.5 MHz) utilizing the low-flow programme and with the wall filter at its lowest setting to ensure that frequency shifts of 125 Hz are not recorded. CDI is capable of visualizing blood flow over the entire field of the ultrasound image and encoding the blood flow velocity pixel by pixel according to a colour scale. It can document the number of cavernosal arteries, their tortuosity and the presence of abnormal collateral vessels. CDI assists the identification of the origin of the cavernosal arteries and allows for accurate angle correction from the colour Doppler signal, yielding a true velocity value on duplex imaging. This test will provide the following information:

1. Erectile grade
2. Grade 0 = no response
3. Grade 1 = tumescence but no deviation from the vertical
4. Grade 2 = tumescence but less than 90° deviation
5. Grade 3 = normal response, suitable for penetration
6. Flow in cm/s in both cavernosal arteries in systole
7. Flow in cm/s in both cavernosal arteries in diastole
8. Flow in cm/s in the dorsal vein
9. Diameter of both cavernosal arteries.

Normal penile vasculature

Initially, the flaccid penis is scanned to determine if there are any structural abnormalities of the corpora or plaques. The diameter of the cavernosal arteries can be measured, but this is difficult, subjective and time-consuming. In response to erection, the cavernosal arteries may dilate up to 75% indicating good vessel compliance, but correlation with other parameters is poor.[20,21] In practice, such measurements are of little clinical relevance. In the flaccid state, monophasic flow in the cavernosal arteries is seen with minimum flow in diastole. With the onset of erection, flow in systole and diastole increases and as the intracavernosal pressure rises, flow in diastole decreases to zero and then flow in diastole reverses, indicative of high intercavernosal resistance (Plate 3). With a firm erection, diastolic flow may disappear completely. Dorsal vein flow may also increase as erection occurs and may occasionally become retrograde with a firm erection. The significance of this is not known. There is a wide variation between investigators as to when to sample flow. It is important to measure flow up to 20 min after injection of vasoactive drugs; to sample flow every 5 min up to then is probably sufficient. If flow is continuing to increase at 20 min, delayed sampling must be done.[22,23] Normal parameters are:

1. Grade 3 erection
2. Cavernosal artery flow in systole <35 cm/s
3. Cavernosal artery flow in diastole >5 cm/s.

Arterial insufficiency

Arterial insufficiency is diagnosed if the peak cavernosal arterial flow in systole does not exceed 35 cm/s (Plate 4).[24] Some investigators take a lower figure based on angiographic correlation that a flow of 25 cm/s has a 92% accuracy in the diagnosis of arterial disease.[25] A difference of more than 12 cm/s between the cavernosal arteries, failure of the cavernosal arteries to dilate and focal stenoses or occlusions are further evidence of arterial disease. Flow in diastole may be normal, but the veno-occlusive mechanism may not engage with low flows in systole.

Parameters for arterial insufficiency are:

1. Grade 0–1 erection
2. Cavernosal artery flow in systole >35 cm/s
3. A difference of more than 12 cm/s in the cavernosal arteries.

Venous leakage

If there is persistence of flow in diastole with elevated end-diastolic velocities in the presence of normal arterial flow, a failure of the veno-occlusive mechanism is diagnosed. The absolute velocities required to make this diagnosis are under debate. Some investigators take a persistent forward flow throughout the cardiac cycle of 8 cm/s to be diagnostic,[26] whilst others take the lower figure of 5 cm/s (Plate 5).[27] Persistent dorsal vein flow may also indicate veno-occlusive failure, but measuring dorsal vein flow velocities has not proved to be useful in the diagnosis of a venous leak.[28] In practice, pharmacocavernosometry provides a more complete assessment of venous integrity, especially in patients who have coexistent arterial insufficiency. Such studies provide quantification of the degree of leak in ml/min by measuring the maintenance flow required to maintain a cavernosal pressure of 100 cm H_2O. Upon such figures and the venous anatomy demonstrated with cavernography, decisions as to whether venous ligation surgery are likely to be successful can be based. Diagnostic parameters are:

1. Grade 0–1 erection
2. Cavernosal artery flow in systole <35 cm/s
3. Cavernosal artery flow in diastole <5–8 cm/s.

Mixed arterial and venous disease

This is difficult to diagnose because venous leakage can only be accurately reported in the presence of normal arterial inflow. In practice, when flow rates in diastole and systole are borderline, mixed disease is suspected. Further imaging with cavernosometry will be required.

ULTRASOUND AND UPPER TRACT OBSTRUCTION

The demonstration of dilatation of the collecting system with ultrasound does not necessarily imply obstruction,[29] which may be due to:

1. Extrarenal pelvis
2. Prominent vasculature
3. Increased urine production, e.g. diabetes insipidus, diuretic therapy
4. Renal cystic disease, e.g. polycystic disease, parapelvic cysts
5. Postobstructive atrophy
6. Vesicoureteric reflux
7. Congenital megacalyces.

With obstruction, there is an increase in renal vascular resistance which falls when the obstruction is relieved.[30] The spectral waveform produced by Doppler ultrasound changes with obstruction with a reduction of diastolic flow when compared to flow in systole. From waveform patterns, the resistive index (RI) can be measured (RI = peak systolic flow – diastolic flow/peak systolic flow). In studies performed on obstructed kidneys that were subsequently unobstructed by percutaneous nephrostomy, an RI above 0.7 should be considered suspicious of obstruction (Plate 6).[31,32] CDI is also useful in the diagnosis of pseudohydronephrosis caused by vessels within the renal sinus which mimic early degrees of dilatation of the upper tract. In one study of 100 patients with minimal hydronephrosis, CDI proved that the apparent hydronephrosis was vascular (Plate 7).[33] Such a distinction is clearly important.

ACKNOWLEDGEMENT

The author is grateful to the Acuson Corporation who have generously provided the funding for printing the colour plate section in this chapter.

REFERENCES

1   Chapple CR, Rickards D, Milroy EJG. Permanently implanted urethral stent for prostatic obstruction in the unfit patient: preliminary report. Br J Urol 1990; 66: 58–65
2   Williams G, Jager R, McLoughlin J et al. Use of stents for treating obstruction of the urinary outflow in patients unfit for surgery. Br Med J 1989; 298: 1429
3   Chapple CR, Rickards D, Milroy EJG. Stents in benign prostatic hyperplasia. Semin Int Radiol 1991; 8: 273–283
4   Rifkin MD. Transrectal prostatic untrasonography: comparison of linear array and radial scanners. J Ultrasound Med 1985; 4: 1–5
5   Torp-Pedersen ST, Lee F. Transrectal biopsy of the prostate guided by transrectal ultrasound. Urol Clin North Am 1989; 6: 703–712
6   Lee F, Bronson JP, Lee F et al. Nonpalpable cancer of the prostate: assessment with transrectal US. Radiology 1991; 178: 197–199
7   Stamey TA, McNeal JE, Freiha FS. Morphometric and clinical studies on 68 consecutive radical prostatectomies. J Urol 1988; 139: 1235–1241
8   Gleason DF. Histological grading and clinical staging of prostate carcinoma. In: Tannenbaum M, ed. Urologic pathology: the prostate. Philadelphia: Lea & Febiger 1977: pp 171–198
9   McNeal JE. Regional morphology and pathology of the prostate. Am J Clin Pathol 1968; 49: 347–357
10 Resnick MI, Willard JW, Boyce WH. Transrectal sonography in the evaluation of patients with prostatic carcinoma. J Urol 1980; 124: 482
11 Brooman PJC, Griffiths GJ, Roberts EE et al. Per rectal ultrasound in the investigation of prostatic disease, Clin Radiol 1981; 32: 669–676
12 Rifkin MD, Choi H. Implications of small, peripheral hypoechoic lesions in endorectal US of the prostate. Radiology 1989; 166: 619–622
13 Salo JO, Ranniko S, Makinen J, Lehtonen T. Echogenic structure of prostatic cancer imaged on radical prostatectomy specimens. Prostate 1987; 10: 1–9
14 Hamper UM, Sheth S, Walsh PC et al. Capsular transgression of prostatic carcinoma: evaluation with transrectal ultrasound with pathologic correlation. Radiology 1991; 178: 791–795
15 Chantelois AE, Parker SH, Sims JE et al. Malakoplakia of the prostate sonographically mimicking carcinoma. Radiology 1990; 77: 193–195
16 Hamper UM, Sheth S, Walsh PC et al. Bright echogenic foci in early prostatic carcinoma: sonographic and pathologecal correlation. Radiology 1990; 176: 3390–3343
17 Egawa S, Carter SS, Wheeler TM et al. Ultrasonographic changes in the normal and malignant prostate after definitive radiotherapy. Urol Clin North Am 1989; 16: 741–749
18 Walsh PC, Jewiett HJ. Radical surgery for prostate cancer. Cancer 1980; 45: 1906–1911
19 Clements R, Griffiths GJ, Peeling WB et al. Transrectal ultrasound in monitoring response to treatment of prostate disease. Urol Clin North Am 1989; 16: 735–740
20 Collins JP, Lewandowski BJ. Experience with intracorporeal injection of papaverine with duplex ultraound scanning for the assessment of arteriogenic impotence. Br J Urol 1987; 59: 84–88

21   Lue TF, Hriack H, Marich KW et al. Vasculogenic impotence evaluated by high scale resolution ultrasonography and pulsed Doppler spectrum analysis. Radiology 1985; 155: 777–781
22   Quam JP, King BF, James EM et al. Duplex and color doppler sonographic evaluation of vasculogenic impotence. Am J Radiol 1989; 153: 1141–1147
23   Krysewicz S, Mellinger BC. The role of imaging in the diagnostic evaluation of impotence. Am J Radiol 1989; 153: 1133–1139
24   Benson CB, Vickers MA. Sexual impotence caused by vascular disease: diagnosis with duplex sonography. Am J Radiol 1989; 152: 1149–1153
25   Paushter DM. Role of duplex sonography in the evaluation of sexual impotence. Am J Radiol 1989; 153: 1161–1163
26   Hattery RR, King FK, Lewis WR et al. Vasculogenic impotence: duplex and color Doppler imaging. Radiol Clin North Am 1991; 29: 629–645
27   Fitzgerald SW, Erikson SJ, Foley WD et al. Color Doppler ultrsound in the evaluation of erectile dysfunction: prediction of venous imcompetence. Radiology 1990; 177 (suppl): 129–130
28   King BF, Charboneau JW, Hattery RR et al. Color Doppler imaging evaluation of the dorsal penile vein in vasculogenic impotence. Radiology 1989; 173(P): 371
29   Amis ES, Cronan JJ, Pfister RC et al. Ultrasonic inaccuracies in diagnosing renal obstruction. Urology 1982; 19: 101–105
30   Murphy GP, Scott WW. The renal haemodynamic response to acute and chronic ureteral occlusions. J Urol 1966; 95: 636–657
31   Platt JF, Rubin JM. Ellis JH, DiPietro MA. Duplex Doppler US of the kidney: differentiation of obstructive from nonobstructive dilatation. Radiology 1989; 171: 515–517
32   Rodgers PM, Bates JA, Irving HC. Intrarenal Doppler ultrasound studies in normal and acutely obstructed kidneys. Br J Radiol 1992; 65: 207–212
33   Scola FH, Cronan JJ, Schepps B. Grade 1 hydronephrosis: pulsed Doppler US evaluation. Radiology 1989; 171: 519–520

3

Anaerobic infection in urological practice

(Based on the Winsbury-White Lecture, 23 January 1992)

S. J. Eykyn

Any tissue or organ in the body may be affected by these organisms [anaerobes], and all clinicians, regardless of specialty, must deal with them.[1]

Thus wrote Dr Finegold, doyen of American infectious disease physicians, in the first edition of his book, *Anaerobic Bacteria in Human Disease*, and urologists are no exception, even if not all are familiar with these microbes and the infections that they cause.

Anaerobic infections are not new, nor are anaerobes new organisms, but a good deal of rediscovery of their importance has taken place, particularly during the 1970s, a period that is often referred to—with good reason—as the anaerobic renaissance. Anaerobes were first recognized by Van Leeuwenhoek in the late 17th century, and then some 200 years later, described by Pasteur during his studies on fermentation. Clinicians have long been familiar with the toxin-mediated clostridial anaerobic infections, gas gangrene and tetanus, but in the developed world at least these diseases have become increasing rarities, such that many surgeons practising in the UK today will never have seen them.

The anaerobic infections that I shall consider in this chapter are those not mediated by toxin, whose distinctive feature is the putrid pus that is often produced. Over 100 years ago, French and German workers wrote of the 'fetid suppuration' so characteristic of these organisms, but then these anaerobic infections slipped again into obscurity. Apart from a few enlightened visionaries who were aware of their importance in clinical medicine, most doctors were oblivious to the existence of anaerobes, and surgeons attributed putrid pus to an organism they addressed as *Bacillus coli*. Microbiologists were of little help to their surgical colleagues since few anaerobes were ever isolated from specimens sent to hospital laboratories. All this was to change in the early 1970s: technological advances made the isolation of anaerobes a routine procedure for all laboratories, and microbiologists at last realized how common anaerobic infections were. At the same time, serendipitously, the manufacturers of the supremely active antianaerobic drug metronidazole realized its true potential for the prevention and treatment of anaerobic infection. Remarkably, oral metronidazole had already been on the market for more than a decade for the treatment of trichomoniasis,

31

amoebic infection and giardiasis. The oral preparation was unsuitable for very sick patients and for use perioperatively, and metronidazole was soon supplied as suppositories and then as an intravenous formulation. This antibiotic was to make a major impact on surgical practice, particularly as a prophylactic agent, and it is largely responsible for the demise of the severe anaerobic infections that used to occur after gastrointestinal surgery.

Since virtually all anaerobic infections are of endogenous origin, that is to say the normal anaerobic commensals act as pathogens, it is useful to define briefly the extent and nature of normal human anaerobic flora before consideration of its pathogenic role. Unfortunately, anaerobes, perhaps more than other bacteria, have undergone considerable recent taxonomic change; in this chapter, I shall use the new nomenclature, where necessary relating this to the old, to try and avoid confusion.

NORMAL HUMAN ANAEROBIC FLORA

Human beings, in common with all other animals, are hosts to vast numbers of anaerobic bacteria, bacteria that can grow and reproduce without oxygen. They constitute the predominant flora of all mucosal surfaces, including those of the genitourinary tract. The composition of this flora varies according to its site; for example that of the gastrointestinal tract differs from that of the upper respiratory tract and the genitourinary tract. The gastrointestinal anaerobes have been subjected to the most extensive studies and several hundred different species of bacteria isolated; the anaerobes of the upper respiratory tract and the vaginal anaerobes have received less attention, and the urethral anaerobes least of all, perhaps partly because such investigations are unlikely to appeal to normal volunteers. A simplified version of normal human anaerobic flora is shown in Table 3.1. From this it can be seen that the gastrointestinal tract uniquely supports *Bacteroides fragilis* (and other *fragilis*-like *Bacteroides* spp.) and *Clostridium* spp. The other anaerobes such as *Prevotella* spp. (previously the *B. melaninogenicus–oralis* group), *Porphyromonas* (previously *Bacteroides*) *asaccharolytica*, the fusobacteria and the peptostreptococci are common to all sites. The urethra supports only small

Table 3.1 Simplified version of normal human anaerobic flora

Organism	Gut	Respiratory tract	Urethra
Bacteroides fragilis	+ + +	–	–
Prevotella spp.*	+ +	+ +	+
Porphyromonas sp.*	+ +	+ +	+
Fusobacterium spp.	+ +	+ +	+
Peptostreptococcus spp.	+ + +	+ +	+
Clostridium spp.	+ + +	–	–

*Previously *Bacteroides* spp.

numbers of anaerobes in addition to small numbers of aerobic organisms such as coagulase-negative staphylococci.

ANAEROBIC INFECTIONS

Urinary infection

Genuine urinary infection caused by anaerobes is very rare, and seems only to occur when there are abnormalities within the urinary tract such as vesicocolic fistulae, tumours, pyonephrosis, and perinephric abscess etc. Studies on very large numbers of specimens of urine have shown that anaerobes can be isolated from urine, albeit rarely, but only in exceptional cases can they be considered of any significance. Headington & Beyerlein isolated anaerobes from 147 (1%) of 15 250 midstream or catheter urines, but they inoculated the urine into thioglycollate broth, thus enabling the recovery of even a few organisms.[2] Lactobacilli accounted for over half the anaerobic isolates, followed by *Clostridium* spp. (29.3%) and *Bacteroides* that were not speciated (7.3%). In only a third of cases were the anaerobes present in pure culture, a combination of aerobes and anaerobes was usual. Only 7 of their patients with anaerobic bacteriuria from whom a single species was isolated were symptomatic, and most of these had known urinary tract abnormalities. On the basis of these findings they concluded that urine should not be routinely cultured anaerobically, and few would disagree with this dictum. A few years later, Segura et al investigated 5781 midstream urine specimens by Gram stain and aerobic culture, and detected bacteria in significant numbers on the Gram stain in 795 (13.8%).[3] Aerobic culture confirmed the presence of the bacteria seen on the Gram stain in all but 25 specimens. Suprapubic bladder aspirations were then done on 17 of these cases and the urine was inoculated into a prereduced enrichment broth; anaerobes were isolated from 10 specimens, thus giving an incidence of anaerobic bacteriuria of 0.2%. As in Headington & Beyerlein's study, the urine was inoculated into an enrichment broth thus rendering quantitation of the actual number of anaerobes originally present in the specimen impossible. The commonest anaerobes isolated were *Bacteroides* spp., but in only 1 case did the anaerobe grow in pure culture: aerobes were present in the others. All but one patient had obstructive uropathy.

Anaerobes and other fastidious bacteria have been frequently sought in women with dysuria and frequency from whom no conventional urinary pathogens are isolated. There is no convincing evidence that they are relevant pathogens in such patients. The dissolved oxygen level in urine may well discourage the growth of anaerobes. Urine inoculated with bacteria under laboratory conditions allows *Escherichia coli* to multiply significantly more rapidly than anaerobes.

Routine anaerobic culture of urine is unnecessary, indeed would be a waste of time and money. A more reasonable approach is to confine anaerobic cultures to those urine specimens that contain large numbers of pus cells on microscopy but from which conventional cultures fail to isolate an organism in the absence of detectable antimicrobial activity in the specimen. Some would argue that only specimens obtained by suprapubic aspiration warrant anaerobic culture, and it is hard to disagree.

Secondary infection/colonization of genital lesions

Any genital ulcer or other lesion is likely to become colonized or secondarily infected with bacteria, including anaerobes. There is no evidence that anaerobes are involved in the pathogenesis of such lesions, nor that specific treatment for these organisms, once isolated, is of any benefit. We have isolated numerous species of anaerobes from genital warts, syphilitic and other ulcers and penile tumours. Heavy colonization of such lesions can lead to contamination of urine samples during collection.

Balanoposthitis

This condition, perhaps more within the remit of the genitourinary physician than the urologist, nevertheless warrants a brief mention here. Although often attributed to *Candida* spp., *Herpes simplex*, *Trichomonas vaginalis* or streptococci rather than to anaerobes, it is usually caused by anaerobes. It results from poor genital hygiene, a tight foreskin and minor trauma. In anaerobic balanoposthitis, the patient's initial complaints are of soreness and itching, but if neglected, the condition may become erosive with purulent offensive discharge and erosions of the prepuce. Erosive and gangrenous balanitis was described nearly a century ago and dubbed a fourth venereal disease,[4] but is seldom seen today. The predominant anaerobes involved are *Bacteroides ureolyticus* and *Porphyromonas* (previously *Bacteroides*) *asaccharolytica* and peptostreptococci. Although cleaning the infected area remains the most important aspect of treatment, metronidazole has also been used with success.

Cowperitis

It would not be surprising to find that cowperitis was caused by anaerobes, but specimens from such cases are rarely subjected to detailed bacteriology; four different anaerobes were isolated from a single case investigated at St Thomas's.

Urethritis

Although some 50% of cases of urethritis are caused by *Chlamydia* and *Neisseria gonorrhoeae*, in at least as many cases no pathogen is defined. Although it has been suggested that anaerobes may be responsible for these cases, proof of this hypothesis is lacking. Interpretation of the microbiology is made difficult by the presence of anaerobes within the urethra as normal flora.

Prostatic infection

Acute prostatitis/prostatic abscess

Acute prostatic abscess and its sequel, prostatic abscess, are rarely seen today. In a review of cases reported over 40 years, Weinberger et al found that cultures had been performed on specimens from 109 of 269 prostatic abscesses, and bacteria isolated in 99 cases.[5] Whilst, overall, coliforms (predominantly *Escherichia coli*) were the commonest pathogens, various anaerobes were isolated from 8 abscesses; in 6 of these 8 cases, aerobes (mostly coliforms) were also isolated. Unless anaerobes are specifically sought in such cases, they will be missed. The culture details for these cases were minimal, and it is likely that in many cases anaerobic cultures were not set up. My own experience is limited to a single case of prostatic abscess from which we recovered *B. fragilis* and *Klebsiella* spp.

Chronic bacterial prostatitis

Genuine chronic bacterial prostatitis is uncommon. It is characterized by relapsing recurrent urinary infection (usually with coliforms) and pus cells are found in prostatic secretions. Provided the urine is sterile at the time, it is possible to localize these infections to the prostate by the Stamey technique of lower tract localization (LTL).[6] Anaerobes have not been reported as pathogens in this infection.

Abacterial (or non-bacterial) prostatitis

Infinitely more common than bacterial prostatitis is this syndrome in which there are symptoms of prostatitis and pus cells found in the prostatic secretions, but there are no documented urinary infections and no defined bacterial cause. We have cultured many hundreds of LTLs from such patients and recovered anaerobic bacteria (always in small numbers) from a few; whether these organisms contribute to the condition or merely represent the urethral commensals is unknown. Some patients with abacterial prostatitis seem to respond to antibiotics at least some of the time, but most do not. A single impressive case report in 1981 attributed the cure of 20 years of prostatitis to metronidazole, initially given to the patient for amoebic dysentery.[7] Anaerobes were not recovered from prostatic samples.

Prostatosis/prostatodynia

Probably as common as abacterial prostatitis is a syndrome characterized by symptoms of prostatitis but without documented urinary infections or pus cells in prostatic secretions. A therapeutically frustrating condition for patient and doctor alike, it has nothing to do with bacteria.

Scrotal abscess

Scrotal abscesses can arise spontaneously, after scrotal surgery, or as a sequel to acute epididymo-orchitis. Those that follow acute epididymo-orchitis are nearly always caused by *Escherichia coli* that can often be cultured from the urine. In all other scrotal abscesses, whether arising spontaneously or after surgery, anaerobes are the predominant pathogens. In the St Thomas's series of 41 scrotal abscesses that were not secondary to epididymo-orchitis, anaerobes alone were isolated from 14, anaerobes with aerobes from 25 and aerobes alone from 2. The commonest anaerobes isolated were the peptostreptococci, *Prevotella* spp. (previously the *Bacteroides melanogenicus–oralis* group) and *Porphyromonas* (previously *Bacteroides*) *asaccharolytica*. *B. fragilis* and related organisms were uncommon (Table 3.2).

Spontaneous scrotal abscesses are often recurrent; one of our patients had suffered from recurrent abscesses for 9 years. They are more common in blacks than whites— an interesting finding since apocrine glands are three times as common in the skin of blacks as in that of whites. Although factors such as obesity, poor hygiene and diabetes may be relevant, it seems likely that the basic defect in anaerobic scrotal abscess, as in anaerobic abscesses involving the breast or axilla, is apocrine blockage, and that the resultant infection is secondary to this. Sometimes patients with recurrent scrotal abscesses have, or have had, anaerobic infections at other sites that are rich in apocrine glands; one of our patients had coincidental hidradenitis suppurativa of the axillae and the same anaerobic species were isolated from axillae and scrotum.

Table 3.2 Bacteria isolated from 41 scrotal abscesses not related to epididymo-orchitis

Anaerobes (39 cases)		Aerobes +/− anaerobes (25 cases)	
Prevotella intermedia	6	**Gram-negative bacilli**	
Prevotella oralis	4	*Escherichia coli*	5
Prevotella bivia	8	*Proteus mirabilis*	3
Prevotella disiens	2	*Citrobacter koseri*	1
Porphyromonas asaccharolytica	23	*Pseudomonas aeruginosa*	2
Bacteroides ureolyticus	21	Coliform (unidentified)	1
Bacteroides fragilis	2	**Gram-positive bacteria**	
Bacteroides ovatus	1	*Staphylococcus aureus*	1
Bacteroides spp.	14	Coagulase-negative staphylococcus	8
Fusobacterium necrophorum	4	*Streptococcus milleri*	6
Fusobacterium spp.	2	Non-haemolytic streptococcus	1
Eubacterium spp.	2	*Enterococcus faecalis*	3
Clostridium sp.	1	Group B streptococcus	3
Peptostreptococcus spp.	69	Group C streptococcus	1
Veillonella spp.	3	*Corynebacterium* spp.	2

Scrotal abscesses after surgery for, for example, hydrocele, scrotal reduction and hypospadias, probably result from infected haematoma. These postoperative infections can be severe; in one of our cases, a scrotal abscess that followed the excision of epididymal cysts resulted in infarction of the testis. Whether prophylactic antibiotics are justified for scrotal surgery is a matter for debate but it seems reasonable to give them.

Conduit-associated infection

Anaerobes occasionally cause infection in association with ileal conduits. Figure 3.1 shows anaerobic cellulitis that developed within 24 hours of a conduitogram performed for a non-functioning conduit. Mixed anaerobes including *B. fragilis* were isolated and there was a prompt response to metronidazole. Such cellulitis is often mistaken for a streptococcal infection, but infections with *Streptococcus pyogenes* produce much greater systemic disturbance than is usual with anaerobes.

Pyonephrosis, renal and perirenal abscesses

These conditions, which are all uncommon, may be associated with anaerobes, particularly *B. fragilis*. In some cases there is a connection with the gut, but even if there is not, the anaerobes that are isolated originate in the gut. Pyonephrosis is sometimes associated with necrotic renal tumours, and

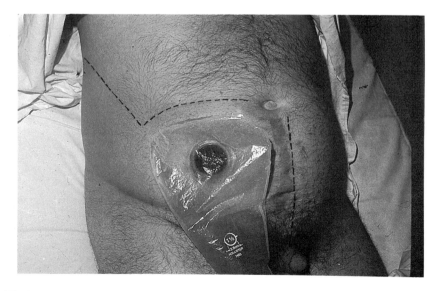

Fig. 3.1 Anaerobic cellulitis that developed within 24 hours of a conduitogram performed for a non-functioning conduit.

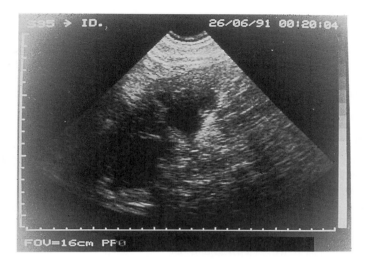

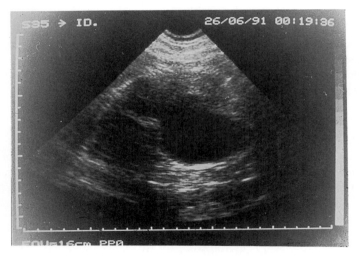

Fig. 3.2   Ultrasound of necrotic renal tumours and associated pyelonephrosis, from which *Bacteroides fragilis* was isolated.

Figure 3.2 shows an ultrasound of a such a case from which *B. fragilis* was isolated.

Wound infection after renal transplantation

Wound infection and abscesses after renal transplantation are often anaerobic. *B. fragilis* was the single most common organism isolated from blood and abscesses in 75 children after renal transplantation,[8] and Ingham et al[9] reported an adult patient with an infarcted transplanted kidney from whom *B. fragilis* was isolated from blood and nephrectomy wound. Our own experience confirms that the commonest organism is *B. fragilis* and suggests that these infections are likely to occur in patients who have developed complications such as urinary leaks.

Necrotizing fasciitis of the male genitalia (Fournier's gangrene)

This uncommon but frighteningly severe condition is eponymously linked with the name of the French dermatologist Fournier, and his original descriptions of the infection (*Gangrène foudroyante de la verge*), published over 100 years ago,[10,11] warrant attention not only for their graphic description of the clinical findings (see below) but also because they show that the disease that he described differs in certain respects from many of those subsequently described as Fournier's gangrene. Fournier described 5 previously healthy men aged 25–30 years with no antecedent local cause or lesion who developed sudden penile pain, swelling and redness that progressed rapidly to penoscrotal gangrene.

La maladie a toujours débuté par une sensation de cuisson, de brûlure, de chatouillement de la verge, douleur d'abord légère, mais qui ne tarde pas a s'exaspérer. . . Tout d'abord, la verge, devenue assez douloureuse, se tuméfie dans son ensemble, elle devient oedémateuse et sa coloration change: elle se transforme en une sorte de gros boudin rose' puis rouge, puis livide. . . .[11]

Remarkably, the testes were spared ('testicules dénudés'). All his patients survived. Fournier attributed the disease to infection and cultures were set up from his cases but there is no record of the results of these. It is of interest that despite such detailed observations of the cases, there is no mention of the smell of the gangrenous tissues and this has been a prominent feature of later reports.

Fournier's papers were followed by various reports of gangrene of the genitalia mostly in the French and German literature, and the condition was variously attributed to many different organisms including anaerobes. Nearly 40 years after Fournier's work was published, the American urologist Randall described 16 cases of 'idiopathic gangrene of the scrotum'.[12] His patients, like those described by Fournier, were previously healthy, but they were older ('past middle life'), and 5 died. Six patients had penoscrotal gangrene, and in the other 10 the scrotum alone was involved. Six of Randell's 16 cases had local lesions including phimosis, chancroidal infection and urethritis that may have acted as portals of entry for the infection. He commented on the 'repulsive fetid odor' of the tissue and predicted that anaerobes were responsible for the infection, although bacteriological studies were 'unproductive' in his cases. Randall's description of the condition cannot be bettered:

About three days from the time that the line of demarcation shows the limits of the gangrenous process, a massive, stinking, slough separates. Where the scrotum is involved the skin, subcutaneous tissues, fascia, dartos, and all the structures of its wall, come away in a stringy, fetid mass. The testes, bared to their tunica vaginales, hang suspended by their cords, shamefully exposed, though remarkably free of gangrene, inured and oblivious to their new surroundings (or possibly I should say lack of surroundings), and can be handled freely without causing the slightest discomfort.[12]

Ten years later, Gibson, another American urologist, reviewed 206 reported cases (including one of his own) of idiopathic gangrene of the scrotum.[13] Whilst most cases were aged 20–50 years, the patients' ages ranged from 5 weeks to 80 years. The mortality rate was 27%. In over half the cases, the gangrenous process involved both penis and scrotum, in a third the scrotum alone and in about a tenth the penis alone. A portal of entry was detected in 40% of cases. Like Randall, Gibson commented on the 'nauseating gangrenous odor' and wondered whether 'all cases of genital gangrene may not be on an anaerobic basis'.

Now, some 60 years later, cases of genital gangrene continue to occur, but infrequently, thus no single clinician can hope to have extensive experience in its management. It is now clear from two recent published series,[14,15] and our own data from the cases seen at St Thomas's (Table 3.3) that these infections are caused by a (presumably synergistic) combination of anaerobes and aerobes; several species of each type of microbe are the norm. They may have a cutaneous, genitourinary or anorectal source and seem to be more likely to occur in diabetics or alcoholics.

Although the condition can apparently occur at virtually any age, it has a predilection for the middle-aged or elderly. The disease that Fournier so

Table 3.3 Clinical characteristics and bacteria isolated in necrotizing fasciitis of the male genitalia (Fournier's gangrene)

	Nickel & Morales[13] (8 cases)	St Thomas's (9 cases)	Clayton et al[14] (57 cases)
Age range (years)	25–82	44–74	5–89
Mean age (years)	58	63	55
Survivors	8/8	6/9	47/57
Diabetic	2	2	18
Alcoholic	1	1	29
Source of infection			
Genitourinary	2		26
Anorectal	1	6	19
Cutaneous	5	3	12
Bacteria isolated			
Anaerobes + aerobes	6	9	35*
Anaerobes only			
Aerobes only	2		9*

*In only 44 cases were specimens cultured anaerobically.

graphically described at the end of the last century seems to occur in a different population today, but his name tends to be given to necrotizing fasciitis of the male genitalia, however it arises.

The predominant anaerobe isolated is *B. fragilis*, but many other species are also usually present. Considerable laboratory expertise is required to determine the true microbial nature of these infections. It is of interest that the excised tissue from one of our cases, who was extremely obese and hairy, but had no definable urinary tract or anorectal predisposing cause, yielded five different anaerobic species on culture, but no gut-specific *Bacteroides*; aerobic cultures grew *Streptococcus milleri* only. These culture results are similar to those obtained from perianal abscesses without a fistula and from scrotal abscesses.

Whatever the underlying cause and whatever bacteria are responsible for necrotizing fasciitis of the genitalia, the mainstay of the treatment of this condition has not altered since before the antibiotic era—immediate (and often repeated) debridement of all necrotic and non-viable tissue. This is the key to a successful outcome. Antibiotics (against aerobes and anaerobes) are always given, but their role is entirely secondary to appropriate surgery, and there is no good evidence that they contribute to the patient's recovery.

Anaerobic bacteraemia in urological patients

Although anaerobic infections are very common, anaerobic bacteraemia is unusual. Anaerobes (most commonly *B. fragilis*) accounted for only 4% of some 4000 documented episodes of bacteraemia at St Thomas' Hospital between 1970 and 1991. During this period there were only 22 episodes of anaerobic bacteraemia in urological patients. Most of these bacteraemias occured in association with infections that have already been considered in this chapter, for example conduit infections, wound infections after renal transplantation and necrotizing fasciitis of the genitalia (Fournier's gangrene). Two infections warrant specific mention here: those associated with lithotripsy and those that follow transrectal biopsy of the prostate.

Infections associated with lithotripsy

A wide variety of bacterial infections are encountered complicating lithotripsy and we have occasionally isolated anaerobes (always *B. fragilis*) from abscesses that have occurred in such cases.

Bacteraemia after transrectal biopsy of the prostate

Although transrectal biopsy of the prostate is generally considered to be a safe procedure, it entails a high risk of subsequent urinary tract infection and febrile reactions.[16] Anaerobic infection was first reported as a complication by Breslin et al who described 2 cases, one with *B. fragilis* bacteraemia and a pelvic abscess from which *B. fragilis* was isolated, and the other who developed clostridal gas gangrene and died.[17] It is not surprising that anaerobic bacteraemia should occur after this procedure considering that the colonic flora consists largely of anaerobes; what is surprising is that it does not occur more often. Even if appropriate prophylactic antibiotics are given, these may not prevent bacteraemia occurring. One of our cases was caused by *B. fragilis*, the other by *B. thetaiotaomicron*.

TREATMENT OF ANAEROBIC INFECTIONS

Most anaerobic infections encountered in urological practice will require drainage or some other surgical procedure, and any antibiotic prescribed is of secondary importance to this. When such a procedure is carried out and concomitant antibiotics given to the patient, it is difficult—often impossible— to define what benefit has accrued from the antibiotic. Occasionally, antibiotics are indicated on clinical grounds. What is appropriate? Without any doubt, the most active agent against anaerobes is metronidazole. This drug (together with other nitroimidazoles such as tinidazole) is, uniquely, only active against anaerobes: it has no activity against aerobic bacteria. Anaerobes other than the *fragilis* group of *Bacteroides* are often sensitive to a wide range of antibiotics including penicillins and cephalosporins; although resistance to the beta-lactams is increasing amongst *Porphyromonas* (previously *Bacteroides*) *asaccharolytica* and *Prevotella* spp. (previously the *Bacteroides melaninogenicus–oralis* group). The *fragilis* group of *Bacteroides* are resistant to most beta-lactam antibiotics, but are usually sensitive to co-trimoxazole, co-amoxiclav, erythromycin, lincomycin, clindamycin, tetracycline and chloramphenicol; these antibiotics are rarely used now to treat anaerobic infection in the UK. Anaerobes are resistant to aminoglycosides and quinolones.

PREVENTION OF ANAEROBIC INFECTIONS

Whilst metronidazole prophylaxis has made a dramatic impact on postoperative anaerobic wound infection in gastrointestinal and gynaecological surgery, such infection seldom follows urological surgery. However when such surgery involves incision or manipulation of the bowel or of the urethra, the commensal anaerobes will contaminate the operative site and prophylaxis seems reasonable if of unproven efficacy. Prophylactic antibiotics should be given (preferably intravenously) at the start of the operative procedure and for not more than 24 hours.

KEY POINTS FOR CLINICAL PRACTICE

- Anaerobes comprise the main part of the commensal flora of all mucous membranes including the genitourinary tract, and anaerobic infections arise from this normal flora.

- Anaerobes are important pathogens in balanoposthitis, scrotal abscess and necrotizing fasciitis (Fournier's gangrene). They are also found as pathogens associated with conduits, causing wound infections after renal transplantation and occasionally causing bacteraemia.
- In common with anaerobic infections at other sites, most anaerobic infections encountered in urological practice will require drainage or other surgical procedure. Antibiotics are secondary, and often unnecessary.
- The preferred and most active antibiotic for anaerobes is metronidazole, but many other agents have useful activity against these organisms.

REFERENCES

1 Finegold SM. Anaerobic bacteria in human disease. New York: Academic Press. 1977
2 Headington JT, Beyerlein B. Anaerobic bacteria in routine urine culture. J Clin Pathol 1966; 19: 573–576
3 Segura JW, Kelalis PP, Martin WJ, Smith LH. Anaerobic bacteria in the urinary tract. Mayo Clin Proc 1972; 47: 30–33
4 Corbus BC, Harris FG. Erosive and gangrenous balanitis. The fourth venereal disease. JAMA 1909; LII: 1474–1477
5 Weinberger M, Cytron S, Servadio C, Block C, Rosenfield JB, Pitlik SD. Prostatic abscess in the antibiotic era. Rev Infect Dis 1988; 10: 239–249
6 Meares EM, Stamey TA. Bacteriologic localization patterns in bacterial prostatitis and urethritis. Invest Urol 1968; 5: 492–518
7 Lockie ACK. Symptomatic cure of prostatitis with metronidazole. Lancet 1981; ii: 475
8 Heseltine PNR, Appleman MD. Retroperitoneal infections. In: Finegold SM, George WL, eds. Anaerobic infections in humans. San Diego: Academic Press, 1989: p 396
9 Ingham HR, Rich GE, Selkon JB et al. Treatment with metronidazole of three patients with serious infections due to *Bacteroides fragilis*. J Antimicrob Chemother 1975; 1: 235–242
10 Fournier AJ. Gangrène foudroyante de la verge. Sem Med 1883; 3: 345–347
11 Fournier AJ. Etude clinique de la gangrène foudroyante de la verge. Sem Med 1884; 4: 69–70
12 Randall A. Idiopathic gangrene of the scrotum. J Urol 1920; 4: 219–235
13 Gibson TE. Idiopathic gangrene of the scrotum. With report of a case and review of the literature. J Urol 1930; 23: 125–153
14 Nickel JC, Morales A. Necrotizing fasciitis of the male genitalia (Fournier's gangrene). Can Med Assoc J 1983; 129: 445–448
15 Clayton MD, Fowler JE, Sharifi R, Pearl RK. Causes, presentation and survival of 57 patients with necrotizing fasciitis of the male genitalia. Surg Gynecol Obstet 1990; 170: 49–55
16 Davison P, Malament M. Urinary contamination as a result of transrectal biopsy of the prostate. J Urol 1971; 105: 545–546
17 Breslin JA, Turner BI, Faber RB, Rhamy RK. Anaerobic infection as a consequence of transrectal prostatic biopsy. J Urol 1978; 120: 502–503

4

Laparoscopic urology

J. E. A. Wickham

The technique of endoscopy has been the main diagnostic and therapeutic tool of the Urologist for over 100 years and of all subspecialties we have more experience in the utilization of these instruments than any other surgical group.

We have pioneered and perfected many intraluminal endoscopic manoeuvres but strangely have not exploited the possibilities of direct inspection and intervention within the peritoneal cavity until very recently.

The history of laparoscopic surgery originates in the original paper by Kelling in 1901;[1] Kelling described the introduction of a cystoscope into the peritoneal cavity of a dog for inspection of the contained viscera. He extended his technique to humans in 1923,[2] although Jacobeus inspected the human peritoneal and pleural cavities in 1910.[4]

In the following years sporadic reports of the use of laparoscopy, usually for diagnostic purposes, appeared and a useful review of this period is given by Gunning.[4] In the decades from 1960 to 1980 increasing use was made of the laparoscope, particularly by gynaecologists and usually for inspection of the pelvic adnexae. More active interventional gynaecological techniques were undoubtedly pioneered by Semm who was one of the first to perform tubal ligation, excision of tubal pregnancies and other adnexal operations.[5] Inspection of the retroperitoneal space for the laparoscopic removal of ureteric calculi was performed by Wickham in 1979[6] but the introduction of intraluminal methods of treating urinary calculi in late 1979 diverted interest away from this approach.

Attempts were made to extend the success of endoscopic nephrolithotomy to the clearance of gall bladder stones[7] but it was the work of Mouret from Lyon in 1988 that initiated the first endoscopic total removal of the gall bladder plus the contained stones. This in turn lit the fuse of the general surgical explosion of interest in the laparoscopic possibilities of intra-abdominal general surgery. The Mouret technique[8] was rapidly exploited by Dubois et al[9] in France and later by Reddick and Olsen[10] in the USA. The beneficial effects of this minimally interventional technique became rapidly apparent and within a 3-year period gave rise to a cataclysmic revival of the fortunes of the almost extinct specialty of general abdominal surgery.

45

Alongside the clinical benefits derived from the adoption of the laparoscopic technique for the treatment of gall bladder disease and disease of other abdominal viscera, a vast commercial enterprise has been set in motion by the manufacturers of endoscopes and more particularly by the companies concerned with the production of disposable ancillary instrumentation. One company is reported as having an annual gross sales return of over two billion dollars in 1991.

So where does this explosion of general surgical interest leave the laparoscopic technique as applied to urology?

What is the justification for the use of such methods over already established techniques of urological surgery? The answer is similar to what has already been overwhelmingly demonstrated in many areas of interventional therapy—reducing the trauma of access for any procedure produces immense benefit in diminution of morbidity and even mortality in most situations. Laparoscopic urology is but a further extension of the 'patient priority concept'.[11]

So what of the technique of laparoscopy as applied to urology?

THE BASIC TECHNOLOGY OF LAPAROSCOPY

To achieve laparoscopy the peritoneal cavity must be initially distended with carbon dioxide gas, which is considered to be the safest medium due to its rapid solubility in the blood and other body fluids. About 200 ml of the gas is absorbed per minute from the peritoneum, but this is rapidly excreted in the expired air. Over prolonged periods of insufflation a considerable acidosis may develop but to some extent this may be corrected by mechanically increasing the tidal respiratory volume during anaesthesia. Carbon dioxide administered over a long period may also cause peritoneal irritation. For shorter periods of operating nitrous oxide may be used as this irritation is avoided, but the danger of gas embolus formation is thought to be slightly higher than when carbon dioxide is used. The risk of any form of gas embolus is however extremely small unless a direct insufflation of gas is inadvertently made into the venous circulation.

Insufflation is carried out by initial peritoneal puncture, usually through the umbilical scar tissue, with a Veress needle, an instrument which possesses a fairly blunt point which retracts automatically on contacting solid tissue within the peritoneal cavity. A fold of abdominal wall is grasped at either side of the umbilicus by the operator and an assistant and the needle is inserted rapidly with a downwards inclination towards the true pelvis. Accurate access to the peritoneal cavity can be tested for by injecting a small volume of saline through a 10.0 ml syringe attached to the needle. If the needle is correctly positioned the saline flows easily into the cavity. Once satisfied that the needle is correctly positioned, a gas line is connected to the luer tap on the needle and the other end is attached to an automatic carbon dioxide insufflator. These machines are now sophisticated and will perfuse gas at a preset volume, rate and pressure. In the average patient about 4.0 l of gas is infused initially at a rate of about 1.0 l/min until the intra-abdominal pressure rises to about 10–12 mmHg. Higher pressures should not be used as compression of the vena cava and other large intra-abdominal veins may occur with occlusion of venous return. Once the pneumoperitoneum is satisfactorily induced the insufflator may be switched to an automatic mode which maintains intra-abdominal pressure at about 10 mmHg, with new gas being infused as necessary to maintain satisfactory distension.

At this point it is usual to insert a wide-bore 10–12 mm cannula or port through the umbilical scar tissue which is partially incised for about 1.0 cm in a small arc below the umbilicus. Modern cannula ports are extremely sophisticated instruments with retractable plastic sheaths. On retraction they expose the triradiate cutting trocar within but resheath the trocar immediately the peritoneum is accessed, thus preventing inadvertent puncture of any subjacent viscus. Once the port is satisfactorily in position the gas lead is transferred from the Veress needle to the luer gas fitting on the port and thereafter gas is fed in from this site.

The next step is to introduce the laparoscopic telescope, usually of 10.0 mm diameter and with either a 0° or 30° angle of view. The peritoneal cavity may then be inspected for pathological processes, such as adhesions or inflammatory responses around organs such as the gall bladder, appendix or ureterine adnexae. It is a good idea to prewarm the telescope to 37°C to prevent fogging of the lens and eye piece due to condensation. Whilst it is possible to place the eye to the endoscope for the initial inspection, it is now more usual to introduce the endoscope with an endoscopic camera pre-mounted and to view the abdominal contents on the television screen.

These cameras can be of two main types, either:

1. Equipped with a beam splitter which allows the operator to view the peritoneal cavity directly whilst still producing a television image

or

2. A directly coupling camera which substitutes or clips on to the eye piece of the endoscope and which provides a television image alone.

These cameras are now very sophisticated devices with integrated control boxes and light sources which may be adjusted to the conditions appertaining for any specific operation. Images produced from the camera are usually displayed on two television monitors, one mounted on each side of the operating table so that both the operator and assistant can have an unobstructed view of the proceedings.

It is usual at this point that the control of the endoscope is passed to the team camera-operator who thereafter becomes responsible for angling and focusing the instrument so that optimum viewing can be maintained for the operator and for the instrumental assistant. Having established a stable view of the peritoneal cavity it is then possible to proceed to a number of the interventional laparoscopic therapeutic operations, which will be considered later.

ANCILLARY INSTRUMENTATION

Whilst laparoscopic visualization of the peritoneal cavity is relatively easy, therapeutic manipulations within the cavity require ancillary instrumentation. Obviously these instruments have to be introduced through other ports of entry and a large range of these are now available for the surgeon.

Ports

Ports usually come in two main classes: non-disposable and disposable. They consist of a primary trocar and cannula which may or may not have a gas insufflation tap attached. These ports obviously have to remain gas-tight when secondary instruments are inserted and removed and the non-disposable ports usually have a simple rubber cap arranged to fit tightly around any secondary instrument and prevent gas leakage. Once the trocar and cannula are inserted the trocar is removed and ancillary instruments may be introduced as necessary.

Disposable ports (Fig. 4.1) are usually made of a combination of metal and plastic, unlike the non-disposable ports which tend to be made of stainless steel, and are rather more sophisticated instruments. They usually have a gas insufflation tap and a small plastic flap valve which prevents extrusion of gas on removal of an ancillary instrument. These ports usually have a protective sheath which is deployed as soon as puncture of the abdominal wall has taken place so that damage does not occur to any subjacent viscera.

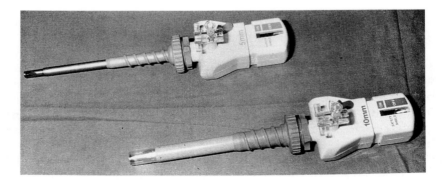

Fig. 4.1   Two sizes of disposable ports — 5 and 10 mm.

Both types of port are supplied in a range of diameters, the usual sizes being 5.0, 10.0 and 12.0 mm. Extra-large sizes are also available for use with the larger stapling devices but the three diameters above are those normally used.

Graspers

A number of endoscopic graspers have been manufactured and again these are disposable or non-disposable. The non-disposable graspers are really endoscopic modifications of grasping forceps and haemostats that are used for open surgery. These instruments are approximately 45 cm long and they may have different types of handle, either non-ratchet or ratcheted, and have different configurations of blades. Most blade configurations however are quite narrow as they must pass easily through the laparoscopic ports. Disposable graspers, again, are a much more sophisticated instrument and quite often also have a rotational movement so that the operator can move the blades of the instrument in a circular motion with one finger without having to disturb the hand grip.

Endoscopic scissors

Endoscopic scissors are again disposable and non-disposable and are miniaturized versions of conventional surgical Mayo or Metzenbaum scissors. Again, the disposables are more sophisticated and usually have a rotational component. Disposable scissors usually have a diathermy attachment, with the added advantage of being able to cut and coagulate tissue at the same time.

The diathermy hook

Small diathermy electrodes with various configurations of hook-type ends are invaluable in the dissection process. These pass simply through the small ports and can transmit a cutting or coagulating current. In the dissection process tissue is hooked up by the hook and then diathermied and transected.

Stapling devices

These instruments, again, can be disposable or non-disposable but are normally of the latter variety. It is here that the epitome of the engineer's art is being rapidly reached. These endoscopic clipping and stapling devices have now reached a high degree of sophistication. It is possible to obtain endoscopic clippers which fire up to 20 clips independently. The clip head reloads automatically from a magazine so that multiple clippings can be achieved without removing the instrument from the laparoscopic port. Such devices not only rotate but also angulate at the tip, making application much easier. Non-disposable stapling devices are usually more cumbersome and only fire and clip one at a time, necessitating removal of the instrument from the port for each manoeuvre, which is time-consuming and disorientating.

Finally, ultrasophisticated disposable stapling devices are now available endoscopically.

Endo-GIA stapler (US Surgical; Fig. 4.2)

Normally this is available with three magazine cartridge heads of different size of staple. These instruments fire parallel rows of six ministaples transversely across the mobilized vessel or duct. An in-built knife then passes between the two rows of staples and transects the vessel or duct in one movement, thus obviating the need for tedious intraperitoneal ligation. Again, these staplers not only rotate but also angulate at the tip to provide ease of application in difficult situations.

Endoscopic ligation

A number of instruments have been developed to enable intra-abdominal endoscopic ligation and knotting of sutures, particularly for the control of large vascular pedicles within the abdominal cavity. These devices are somewhat cumbersome and the knotting process has to be carried out outside the abdominal cavity. The knot is then slid down the endoscope tube with a special knot advancer. Using ligation makes for very long operating procedures. My own feeling is that these ligating and knotting procedures will soon be relegated to the history books as the clipping devices that are already in use

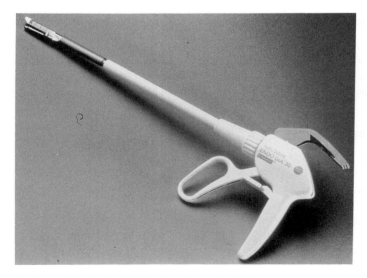

Fig. 4.2   The Endo-GIA stapler (US Surgical, Norwalk, USA).

are becoming sophisticated; I am quite convinced that these will replace any necessity for this type of manoeuvre.

It is thus apparent that the rapid amount of instrumental development and innovation that is being introduced into the application of laparoscopic surgery will inevitably lead to its rapid adoption for specific procedures. The next big leap forward is obviously aimed to be the endoscopic anastomosis of divided bowel and such devices are already being experimentally evaluated. I predict that in the next 5 years the majority of intra-abdominal procedures now being carried out by open surgery will be substituted by endoscopic manipulations of various forms.

LAPAROSCOPIC OPERATIONS IN UROLOGY

These may be grouped into three areas:

1. Established and validated procedures.
2. Procedures already undertaken but still in the stage of development.
3. Procedures projected but at the time of writing not yet carried out in humans.

Established and validated procedures

Varicocele ligation[12]

This is the ideal procedure for gaining familiarity with laparoscopic surgery. Abdominal access is as described above but secondary port placement is required, as shown in Figure 4.3.

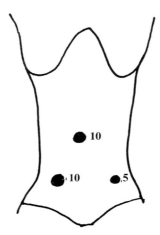

Fig. 4.3 Varicocelectomy. Port sizes in millimetres.

The object of the operation is to clip and divide the dilated testicular vein or veins at the internal inguinal ring. Through the 5.0 mm lateral port, simple grasping forceps are passed and through the midline subumbilical port a pair of endoscissors is inserted (Fig. 4.4). Vessels at the inguinal ring are usually quite visible behind the peritoneal covering which is picked up with forceps and incised with the scissors. The vein or veins are then dissected free from the vas and the testicular artery over a length of about 1.0 cm. Through the lower midline 10 mm port an endoscopic liga-clip applicator is passed and the veins are clipped and divided with the endoscissors.

With experience this operation usually takes about 30 min and patients can usually be treated on a day-case basis.

Pelvic lymph node dissection[13]

The purpose of this operation is at present purely diagnostic and not therapeutic. The aim is to obtain representative biopsies of the draining pelvic lymph nodes in cases of carcinoma of the prostate and bladder to aid in the more accurate staging of the disease processes. In the early stages of both diseases it is necessary to ascertain whether the process is localized to the primary organ or whether the disease is not contained and has spread to draining nodes.

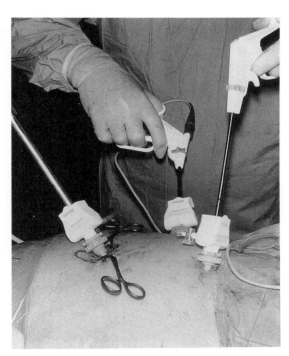

Fig. 4.4   Port placement for varicocele ligation. See text for details.

Previous attempts at accurate staging by lymphography or computed tomography scanning have proved inaccurate but now that direct sampling of nodes for histological evaluation is feasible much unnecessary major surgery may be avoided. During this operative procedure it is usual to obtain node samples from both sides of the pelvis and to retrieve nodes from the obturator, internal iliac and external iliac groups up to the iliac vessel bifurcation.

The operation commences with access being obtained as above. Port placement is indicated in Figure 4.5 and is similar to that used for varicocele ligation, except for the insertion of a second contralateral 5.0 mm port in the iliac fossa (Fig. 4.6). Dissection is commenced by the incision of the posterior parietal peritoneum over the iliac bifurcation on one side. The peritoneum is peeled back to expose the subjacent nodes which are gradually dissected free of the vessels using the diathermy endoscissors or a diathermy hook. The freed nodes are usually removed en bloc through the lower 10.0 mm port and carefully labelled. Dissection is then continued downwards alongside the internal iliac artery and the relevant nodes are removed. Finally, at the limit of the dissection, the obturator nerve is identified crossing the side wall of the pelvis and the related nodes in this area are removed. Some enthusiasts divide the vas at this stage but in my experience it has not been necessary as there is quite easy access to the obturator fossa in most patients. A similar procedure is then carried out on the contralateral side of the pelvis. The pelvic peritoneum is not usually repaired, although it can be roughly approximated and held with a simple clip if desired.

The operating time for this procedure is usually 1½–2 h. It can be carried out as a day-case or a 1-night stay depending on the patient's general condition.

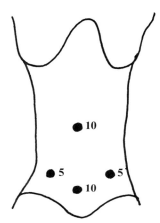

Fig. 4.5   Pelvic lymphadenectomy. Port sizes in millimetres.

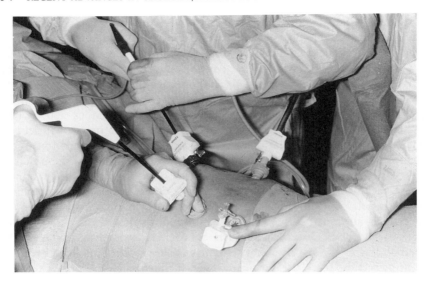

Fig. 4.6   Port placement for pelvic lymph node dissection. A second contralateral 5.0 mm port is inserted in the iliac fossa.

Treatment of cryptorchid testicle

Cortesi et al in 1976[14] appeared to be the first to use the laparoscope for ligation and excision of the intra-abdominal cryptorchid testis. Access is made into the abdominal cavity as usual and the retroperitoneal area and the area of the inguinal ring are inspected. If a reasonable-sized testicle is identified and it is wished to proceed to orchidopexy in due course, Castilho[15] has described the procedure of testicular artery clipping with subsequent staged orchidopexy. If there is a small insignificant testicular remnant, simple dissection and removal may be carried out in a similar way to lymph node dissection.

Procedures already undertaken but still under development

Laparoscopic nephrectomy

This is an operation which was first carried out by Clayman et al in 1991[16] and has since been duplicated at a number of other centres. It must be said that the procedure is a complicated one and should probably not be undertaken by the inexperienced laparoscopist.

The indications for this approach are gradually being defined. It is probably most useful for the removal of the burnt-out glomerulonephritic or pyelonephritic kidney. Shell hydronephroses may also be removed. The burnt-out stone kidney where there has been much perinephric inflammation can be a very difficult problem in dissection. There is current dispute about the value of this procedure for the malignant kidney. Certainly it would not be suitable for large adenocarcinomas but kidneys with small peripheral tumours can be adequately and safely excised using this technique.

The transperitoneal approach (Fig. 4.7). For this procedure the patient is placed on the operating table in the position as for open renal surgery. Endoscopic access is obtained by a 10.0 mm umbilical port or a port placed about 5.0 cm lateral to the midline in the plane of the umbilicus towards the side of the affected kidney. A 5.0 and 12.0 mm port are then placed in the mid clavicular line (Fig. 4.8) and two further 5.0 mm ports are placed in the mid axillary line, all under direct vision. The dissection is commenced, incising the posterior peritoneum along the line of Todt lateral to the colon from the hepatic or splenic flexure, depending on the side, down to the iliac fossa. The colon will then usually be easily displaced immediately and the ureter can be visualized in the retroperitoneum. The ureter is dissected and divided level with the iliac vessels and then traced cranially until the renal pelvis is exposed. Careful dissection of the peripelvic fat will then usually reveal the renal vessels entering the hilum anterior to the pelvis. A 1.0 cm length of each vessel is dissected free and then transected and divided in one movement with the Endo-GIA clamp (US Surgical, Norwalk, USA) passed through the 12.0 mm port. This instrument places two rows of staples across each vessel and divides the vessels automatically between the staples. The convexity of the kidney is then gradually dissected from the surrounding perinephric fat and fascia and ultimately mobilized. Down the 12.0 mm port, a specially made impermeable sac is then introduced into the peritoneal cavity. The margins of the neck of the sac are triangulated open with graspers passed through three of the lateral ports and the kidney is manipulated into the sac. A small

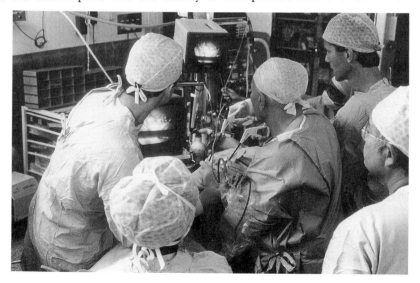

Fig. 4.7 Port placement for the transperitoneal approach to the kidney.

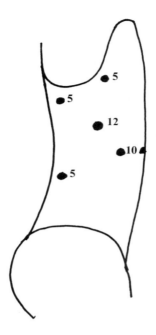

Fig. 4.8 Nephrectomy–nephroureterectomy. Port sizes in millimetres.

drawstring at the neck of the sac is pulled and the neck of the sack withdrawn through either the 10.0 or 12.0 mm port and grasped on the surface by two or three artery forceps. The kidney must then be macerated either with one of the available commercial disintegrators or chopped up with a pair of surgical scissors passed through the neck of the sac. The fragmented kidney is then aspirated and the sac withdrawn from the abdominal cavity. Whilst maceration is being carried out an evaluation of the process can be witnessed laparoscopically.

Finally, all ports are removed with suture of the 10.0 and 12.0 mm ports. The 5.0 mm ports only require simple butterfly dressing.

Retroperitoneal approach (Wickham–Watson).[17] Experience with the exposure of the ureter in the retroperitoneum by laparoscopic means encouraged the author to attempt this approach for endoscopic nephrectomy. The patient is again placed in the lateral position. Access to the retroperitoneum is achieved by primary insufflation with the Veress needle passed through a small puncture in the lumbar fascia below the 12th rib and 2.5 cm lateral to the erectorspinae muscle. About 1–2 l of carbon dioxide is insufflated and a 10.0 mm port is inserted followed by the laparoscope. A second 5.0 mm port is then inserted under direct vision in the mid axillary line. Periureteric and perinephric fat are then dissected to expose the posterior aspect of the kidney, which is elevated and pushed anteriorly to expose the renal artery and vein entering the hilum. Through a 12.0 mm port inserted in the mid axillary line, the Endo-GIA clamp is then passed and the vessels are stapled and transected. The ureter is traced downwards and divided. The kidney is either bagged and macerated or a small 3.0 cm incision is made in the lumbar fascia and the mobilized kidney is removed intact. Often when using the retroperitoneal approach it is very important not to breach the peritoneum itself, for the gas will escape into the peritoneum. If this occurs the peritoneum collapses down on to the cavity in which one is working and obscures the view and one may then have to then revert to a transperitoneal type of operation. More recently the technique has been developed of inserting a balloon into the retroperitoneum; after simple distension of the cavity to a suitable size, the balloon may be removed and a laparoscope passed into the developed space.[18] Mobilization of the kidney is then carried out as described above. The author has had no personal experience of this balloon procedure as yet but intends to try it as soon as possible.

Nephroureterectomy

Nephroureterectomy for transitional cell disease can also be carried out by this method. Preliminary circumcision of the ureteric orifice is carried out in the bladder with cystoscopic diathermy so that the intramural ureter is preliminarily mobilized and sealed. The laparoscopic approach through the retroperitoneum and mobilization are as described above. After kidney mobilization the ureter is traced down into the retroperitoneum, across the iliac vessels and into the pelvis. This is achieved by incising the peritoneum on the side wall of the pelvis. Dissection is usually straightforward and the ureter may be traced down to its insertion into the bladder wall. With simple traction with forceps the ureter is everted from the bladder wall and then cross-stapled with the endostapler. The intramural portion of the ureter is divided and the ureter and kidney removed, as described above, by the bagging manoeuvre. Strict observation of the macerating procedure endoscopically is essential to ensure there is no spillage of malignant material into the peritoneal cavity.

Radical excision for lower ureteric tumour

For the endoscopic treatment of tumour of the lower 5 cm of the ureter, a similar endoscopic technique may be undertaken with the patient supine.[17] The peritoneal cavity is entered as usual (Fig. 4.9) and the lower ureter with contained tumour is mobilized from the retroperitoneal tissues. The ureteric orifice is circumcised to the full depth of the bladder wall and the ureter is completely freed intravesically and retroperitoneally. The mobilized ureter containing the tumour is then drawn down into the bladder with alligator forceps. From the peritoneal aspect the ureteric wall is then stapled to the bladder wall using two or three endostaples. A guidewire is passed into the

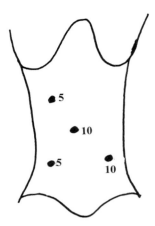

Fig. 4.9   Lower ureteric resection. Port sizes in millimetres.

mobilized ureter in the bladder and the redundant ureter containing tumour is divided and removed from the bladder. Finally a double J stent is passed into the ureter and kidney and the abdominal ports are removed.

Endoscopic colposuspension[19]

Endoscopic colposuspension has been achieved by the retropubic route, closely simulating the conventional procedure.

The retropubic space is entered and insufflated with the Veress needle and a 10.0 mm port is inserted as far superiorly as possible in the midline. A 10.0 mm port is inserted on each side of the abdomen just medial to the inguinal canal (Fig. 4.10). The urethra and bladder neck are freely mobilized using forceps and endoscopic scissors, and then stapled to the back of the pubic ramus and pectineal ligament with an Endo-Hernia stapler (US Surgical, Norwalk, USA) with three or four staples on each side.

Obviously previous retropubic or other types of suspensory surgery will be a contraindication to this approach.

Procedures projected but not yet carried out fully in humans

Much effort is now being expended in trying to extend the frontiers of laparoscopic urological surgery and a number of procedures have undergone animal evaluation.

1. Total cystectomy with urinary diversion.
2. Radical prostatectomy.
3. Ureterolysis for retroperitoneal fibrosis.

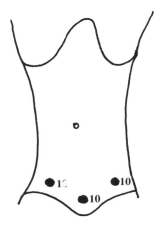

Fig. 4.10   Endocolposuspension. Port sizes in millimetres.

Total cystectomy with urinary diversion

To my knowledge this operation has been performed in the pig both in the USA and in Europe. Mobilization of the bladder provides no great difficulty laparoscopically, although establishment of a satisfactory diversion is obviously more difficult. Implantation of the ureters into the sigmoid endoscopically by ureterosigmoidoscopy and by the simultaneous passage of a colonoscope into the sigmoid to draw the ureters through into the bowel lumen with grasping forceps has been performed and is quite feasible. The ureters are then secured to the bowel wall with endoscopically placed staples. I think that this operation will shortly become utilized in the adult human, particularly in the very elderly person who is unfit for any major conventional abdominal surgery. Once the bladder has been mobilized it will require removal from the abdominal cavity by the bagging technique with subsequent maceration and extraction of the bag contents. Another method has been suggested in females, such that once the bladder is mobilized a small incision is made at the vault of the vagina and the bladder is delivered vaginally. I am aware that this technique is already being carried out by the gynaecologist for laparoscopic-assisted vaginal hysterectomy.

Radical prostatectomy

Kavoussi et al[20] in the USA have attempted radical prostatectomy in humans using a combined laparoscopic and perineal approach. The mobilization and removal of prostate are possibly the easiest part of the procedure. Producing the urethrovesical anastomosis is much more difficult and was achieved by suturing, but I understand there was considerable blood loss during the procedure. I am sure that this technique will be refined, such that the prostate will be removed laparoscopically and the anastomosis will be achieved, possibly by some form of endoscopic or compressive stapling device passed through the urethra. I predict that in the next 3 years this operation will have been satisfactorily achieved.

Ureterolysis for retroperitoneal fibrosis[20]

This operation is perfectly feasible laparoscopically with mobilization of the ureter and dissection of the encased ureter away from the fibrotic area. After mobilization the ureter can easily be displaced laterally away from the involving fibrosis. To my knowledge this operation has not been performed yet in humans but I see no reason why it should not be in the reasonably near future.

The construction of diversionary conduits and pouches

The endoscopic construction of an ileal conduit is now well within the compass of the laparoscopic surgeon. General surgeons are already doing laparoscopic sigmoid bowel resections and small bowel resections using either stapled reanastomosis or an anastomosis produced by compression rings introduced inside and outside of the bowel. These are biodegradable or are passed spontaneously per rectum. If one can endoscopically divide the bowel and reconstitute it, it is a very short step to the performance of an ileal diversionary conduit. The proximal end of the conduit having been divided and sealed by a Endo-GIA stapler, it again would be a fairly easy procedure to pass a flexible endoscope into the distal end of the loop and to draw ureteric implants through into the loop with stapling fixation and then evert the loop on the skin surface. I am sure this technique will evolve very rapidly.

Construction of storage urinary pouches again will possibly come endo-scopically. With the development of even more sophisticated stapling devices it will be quite easy to staple together large lengths of bowel instead of having to close by stitch and also to perform junctional anastomoses between various configurations of bowel. Again, I am sure that endoscopic construction of these type of pouches will come very rapidly in the next 5–10 years.

It must now be obvious to all surgeons, particularly to urologists, that the rapid advances in endoscopic and minimally invasive surgery that have occurred over the last 3–4 years will rapidly impinge upon their practice. There can be little doubt in the minds of those surgeons who have been connected with these minimally invasive techniques that the bonus to the patient in terms of lack of mortality and morbidity is immense.

The safety of these procedures versus an open surgical attack has been questioned and the time taken to complete them in some operations may be considerable. Nevertheless, one has to remember that most of these proce-dures are carried out under very considerable magnification. At open surgery one is working visually about 60 cm from the operative site; with endoscopic surgery one is within millimetres of the target organ or vessel. Difficulties engendered by a little oozing or bleeding in endoscopic surgery make the operator extremely careful to avoid any significant haemorrhage, or vision is rapidly lost. It therefore behoves the surgeon to proceed slowly and meticulously to avoid this haemorrhage, with the obvious secondary fall of the minimization of damage to the target, organ or adjacent structures. Whereas in open surgery one can vigorously retract the abdominal wall and then displace and rearrange the abdominal contents in a somewhat cavalier manner, such an approach would be totally unacceptable endoscopically. Coupled with the fact that if bleeding is encountered at open surgery, it is extremely simple to place a clamp on the involved area and then suck out the haemorrhagic material. Such an event laparoscopically would almost destroy the operation through lack of vision. The laparoscopic surgeon therefore learns very soon to go gently, rapidly and accurately to do the task to the ultimate benefit of him- or herself, but moreover to that of the patient, whose quite often spectacular recovery may even impress the most experienced laparoscopist.

It thus seems that the application of laparoscopy to urology is progressing rapidly and I would encourage my urological colleagues to educate themselves rapidly in this modality. If they do not 'grasp the nettle' then the 'horse and cart' of open surgery will inevitably be overtaken by the minimally invasive horseless carriage speeding by!

REFERENCES

1　Kelling G. Ein in physiologisher Beziehung Beachtens Werther Fall von Magen Resection Nebst Bemerhungen zur Gastro-Enterostomie. Dtsch Z Chir 1901; LX: 155–160
2　Kelling G Colioskopie. Arch Klinchir 1923; 126: 226
4　Gunning JE. History of laparoscopy. In: Phillips JM, Corson SL, eds. Laparoscopy. Baltimore: Williams & Wilkins. 1977: pp 6–16
5　Semm KP. Historical review. From diagnostic laparoscopy to operative pelvioscopy. In: Endoscopic abdominal surgery. Chicago: Year Book. 1987: pp 5–16
6　Wickham JEA. Retroperiotoneal endoscopic ureterolithotomy. Abstracts Int Soc Urol Paris 1979
7　Kellett MJ, Wickham JEA, Russell RCG. Percutaneous cholecystolithotomy. Br Med J 1988; 296: 453–455
8　Mouret P. Personal communication, 1988 (Mouret apparently did not publish, but in France he is credited with the first cholecystectomy)
9　Dubois F, Berthelot G, Levard H. Cholecystectomy par coelioscopy. Nouv Presse Med 1989; 18: 980–982
10　Reddick EJ, Olsen DO. Laparoscopic laser cholecystectomy: a comparison with mini-lap cholecystectomy. Surg Endoscopy 1989; 3: 34–39
11　Wickham JEA. The new surgery. Br Med J 1987; 295: 1581–1582
12　Mehan DJ, Hagod PG, Worischeck JH, Andrus CH, Parro RO. Laparoscopic varicocelectomy: preliminary report of a new technique. J Urol 1991; 145: 242A
13　Schuessler WW, Vancaille TG, Reich H, Griffith DP. Transperitoneal endosurgical lymphadenectomy in patients with localised prostatic cancer. J Urol 1991; 145: 988–991
14　Cortesi N, Ferrari P, Zumbarda E, Maneti A, Baldina A, Pignatti-Morano F. Diagnosis of bilateral abdominal cryptorchidism by laparoscopy. Endoscopy 1976; 8: 33

15 Castilho LN, Ferreira U, Netto N et al. Laparoscopic orchiectomy. J Endourol 1992; 6:
    155–157
16 Clayman RV, Kavoussi LR, Soper NMJ et al. Laparoscopic nephrectomy. N Engl J Med
    1991; 324: 1370
17 Wickham JEA, Watson G. Laparoscopic excision of lower ureteric tumour. Presentation
    to British Association of Urological Surgeons. Annual Meeting Bournemouth 1992
18 Gaur DD. Laparoscopic operative retroperitoneoscopy use of a new device. J Urol 1992;
    148: 1137–1139
19 Vancaille TG. Personal communication, 1992
20 Kavoussi LR, Clayman RV, Brunt LM; Soper NJ. Laparoscopic ureterolysis. J Urol
    1992; 147: 426–429

5

Management of bladder exstrophy

D. S. Peppas   J. P. Gearhart

This chapter will focus on the surgical management of bladder exstrophy and epispadias. The objectives in the genitourinary reconstruction of those patients with exstrophy–epispadias complex are a secure abdominal wall closure; urinary continence with preservation of renal function; and the formation of a functional as well as cosmetically acceptable phallus in the male patient. The most widely accepted surgical approach to achieve these goals is by staged genitourinary reconstruction. In our experience, performance of exstrophy closure, epispadias repair and bladder neck reconstruction as separate, staged procedures insures a higher likelihood for success. This chapter will thus discuss our approach to the management of children with exstrophy–epispadias, to include our results in the staged reconstruction of these patients.

HISTORY

Bladder exstrophy exists as part of a spectrum of anomalies which includes cloacal exstrophy at one extreme and glandular epispadias at the other. The first description of bladder exstrophy appears on an Assyrian tablet from 2000 BC preserved in the British Museum in London. The next written description was in 1597 by Scheuke von Graffenberg, more than 3500 years after its initial description.[1]

In the 1850s, urinary diversion for bladder exstrophy was first employed in its treatment, with little success.[2] Successful diversion via ureterosigmoidostomy began with Coffey;[3] however, because of severe complications (including infection and acidosis) is was not until the contributions by Nesbit in 1949[4] and later by Leadbetter that ureterosigmoidostomy became popular, and remains so in parts of the world.[5]

In 1942 Hugh Hampton Young described the first continent female patient after bladder closure,[6] and in 1948 Michon reported the first success in the male.[7] Despite this initial success, many surgeons preferred treating bladder exstrophy with cystectomy and urinary diversion well into the 1950s.[8,9]

Osteotomy was introduced in 1958 by Schultz.[10] He performed bilateral iliac osteotomies and 2 weeks later bladder closure was performed with symphyseal approximation. A female patient thus treated became continent after removal of her catheter. By approximating the pubic bones into their normal position, it was felt that continence was improved at the level of the urogenital diaphragm.

Despite progressing success with bladder closure in the 1950s and 1960s, success with urinary continence was difficult to achieve. Dees's[11] modification of the Young bladder neck reconstruction, as well as the further improvements made by Leadbetter, resulted in improved dry intervals.[12] This was especially true for the group with epispadias, whereas those with exstrophy tended to do less well in terms of continence.[13,14]

However, over the past three decades, the acceptance of the staged reconstruction in exstrophy management has done much to improve the overall outcome of these children.[15,16] Closure within the first few days of life, with or without osteotomy, epispadias repair to help increase eventual bladder capacity by increasing urethral resistance, and bladder neck reconstruction at a time when bladder capacity has increased have all resulted in increased socialization and participation of these patients.[17,18]

INCIDENCE

Classical bladder exstrophy has an estimated incidence of between 1 in 10 000 and 1 in 50 000 live births.[19–21] The male to female ratio is approximately 2.3 : 1.[22] There appears to be an increased incidence in children of patients with exstrophy or epispadias. In a review by Shapiro et al the risk of extrophy of the bladder in offspring of individuals with exstrophy of the bladder or epispadias was 1 in 70 live births—an almost 500-fold greater incidence than in the general population. There also appears to be an increased risk of having a second family member with this condition. Nine affected siblings were found in 2500 indexed cases, giving a 3.6% overall risk to this group.[23]

Epispadias occurs much less frequently than exstrophy. The incidence is approximately 1 in every 112 000 males and 1 in every 484 000 female births.[24]

EMBRYOLOGY

Normal genitourinary development occurs between the 4th and 12th weeks of gestation.[25] Therefore, interference with the normal developmental processes during this period must be responsible for this spectrum of anomalies.

During the 2nd and 3rd week of gestation, the tail attains a ventral position from its original dorsal location.[26] As this occurs, the common cloaca is formed; this is separated from the amniotic space by the cloacal membrane, which is formed of an inner endodermal layer and an outer ectodermal layer. This cloacal membrane is then bordered laterally by two mesenchymal projections and cranially by the primordia of the genital tubercles. Normally, mesenchymal ingrowth between the layers of the cloacal membrane results in the formation of the lower abdominal muscles and pelvic bones. The division of the common cloaca begins at approximately 5 weeks' gestational age, by the caudal growth of the urorectal septum, and by the lateral infoldings which occur simultaneously. Thus, by the end of the 7th week, the cloaca is divided into a dorsal rectum and a ventral bladder and urogenital sinus.[25,26] The remaining portion of the cloacal membrane, after division of the cloaca into bladder and rectum, will then rupture to become the urethral groove in the male and the vestibule of the vagina in the female.[25] Bladder exstrophy would thus occur if rupture of the cloacal membrane occurred after completion of the urorectal septum, but prior to ingrowth of the mesenchyme forming the abdominal wall. Furthermore, cloacal exstrophy (in which the bladder and hindgut are exposed) would thus occur if membrane rupture occurred before descent of the urorectal septum.[27]

Therefore, the paired genital tubercles and associated mesenchyme would fail to fuse in the midline, resulting in an abnormal communication between the urogenital portion of the cloaca and the amniotic cavity, leading to this malformation.[28,29]

CLINICAL PRESENTATION

Despite the apparent anomaly seen by the parents soon after delivery, the abnormalities seen in bladder exstrophy are relatively confined to the abdomen and perineum, bladder, upper urinary tract, genitalia, spine and bony pelvis. There is foreshortening of the umbilical–anal distance, with the anus being located further anterior than normal. The rectus abdominis muscles are laterally displaced, inserting into the pubic tubercles. As a result of the lateral displacement of the rectus muscles, the internal inguinal canals are widened, placing the internal inguinal ring just beneath the external inguinal ring. Therefore, indirect inguinal hernia is common, occurring in approximately 85% of the population.[30-32]

Imperforate anus is infrequently associated with bladder exstrophy; however, several cases have been reported.[30] In untreated patients and in those with failed initial closures rectal prolapse may be seen. This is associated with poor support by the displaced anal sling mechanism and the Valsalva pressures which occur during crying and grunting.[33] Rectal prolapse is almost never seen after successful bladder closure.

The exposed bladder can vary in size from a very small patch with an estimated capacity of less than 5 ml to one with significant capacity. The epithelium is very sensitive and develops a progressively worsening polypoid appearance as the bladder mucosa remains exposed. Polypoid changes occur as a result of mucosal irritation from salves or clothing. Shortly after birth, microscopic changes in the transitional epithelium can progress to squamous or adenomatous metaplasia which can later lead to squamous cell carcinoma or adenocarcinoma.[34-37] There are some data to suggest that in the unclosed exstrophy patient, the epithelium is at a primitive stage and this may predispose these patients to malignant changes.[38]

The blood supply to the exstrophied bladder is normal. The exstrophied bladder appears to be capable of normal neuromuscular activity, and therefore should demonstrate normal detrusor activity once bladder closure has been successfully accomplished. While a recent study has suggested that there is poor detrusor function in these bladders, muscarinic and cholinergic receptor levels are normal.[39,40]

The ureters course deeply through the bony pelvis and exit into the bladder with markedly shortened submucosal tunnels. As a result, a very large percentage of these patients demonstrate primary vesicoureteral reflux after successful bladder closure.[41] Ureteral activity appears to be normal.[42] The urethra is most commonly completely exposed, but may be covered to the base of the symphysis pubis. In some exstrophy variants, there may be an incomplete epispadias or a normal urethra. Dorsal chordee is the rule.

The male phallus almost always appears shortened. This is due to the widely separate pubic bones, preventing the corpora cavernosa from joining in the midline in their usual position near the base of the pubis. Dorsal chordee is almost always present, and there is often shortening of the urethral groove. In contrast to the normal phallus, the neurovascular bundles which control erectile function in the epispadiac phallus are laterally displaced.[43] Despite the lateral deviation of the neurovascular bundles in exstrophy patients, most patients are capable of satisfactory erections.

The structures derived from the mesonephric (wolffian) duct are normal. Retrograde ejaculation and epididymitis occur in those patients with an open or dysfunctional bladder neck. The reason for this may be the location of the verumontanum and the ejaculatory ducts after successful bladder closure and bladder neck reconstruction. However, there have been reports of exstrophy patients fathering children.[44] Cryptorchidism has been reported to occur with a 10-fold higher incidence compared to the normal population.

In the female there is a hemiclitoris usually present on each side. There may be vaginal duplication, with the orifice or orifices easily seen just inferior to the exposed urethra. Uterine duplication may also be present. The ovaries and fallopian tubes are generally normal.

Virtually all patients with exstrophy or epispadias have pubic diastasis. There is usually outward rotation of the hips. However, few, if any, long-term hip or gait problems result. There has been at least one report of a higher incidence of vertebral malformation in patients with exstrophy.[45]

DIAGNOSIS

With the advent of routine antenatal ultrasound, the diagnosis of exstrophy of the bladder in utero is possible.[46,47] The diagnosis is suspected if on ultrasound the bladder is never seen to fill throughout the study. In addition, the identification of an anterior abdominal mass and/or low-set umbilicus can suggest the diagnosis of bladder exstrophy. Serial ultrasound examinations must be performed, however, because of the low specificity and sensitivity of this diagnosis modality.

Postnatally, the diagnosis of bladder exstrophy is obvious (Fig. 5.1). However, in the spectrum of anomalies thus far discussed, further evaluation may be required prior to treatment. This is especially true with a child with cloacal exstrophy where there is a higher incidence of myelomeningocele, renal anomalies, and where sex of rearing determinations may be necessary.[48]

If the child is to be referred to a specialized center for the treatment of exstrophy, the bladder is to be covered with a square of clear plastic wrap (such as Saran Wrap or cling film) rather than a piece of moist gauze or a diaper. Also to be avoided are salves or petroleum jelly because any of the previous dressings may dry and denude the epithelium.

The bladder is closely inspected. This is especially important in cases of cloacal exstrophy, where portions of hindgut are usually interposed between the hemibladders. Close inspection for the ureteral orifices is also made.

Phallic length in the male needs to be assessed. This is important for the child who may have his sex of rearing altered because of deficient corporal tissue or diminutive size of phallus. In addition the decision as to whether to use paraexstrophy flaps will be based upon the length of the urethral groove and phallic length.

TREATMENT

Ideally, bladder closure should be performed within the first 24–48 hours of birth. If transfer to a medical center familiar with the care of exstrophy

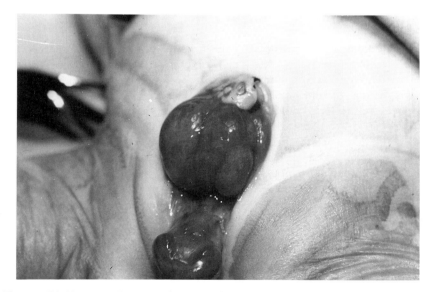

Fig. 5.1   Bladder exstrophy as seen in the newborn.

patients is to occur, then care to provide an adequate dressing for the open bladder is required.

It is of the utmost importance that the parents of the child understand that the treatment of this condition is a staged surgical approach, requiring at a minimum two to three major surgical procedures over a period of several years. They should also understand prior to treatment that, despite the numerous procedures required for the correction of this defect, their child can be expected to lead a normal life.[49]

With close attention to detail and a staged approach to reconstruction, few if any patients need be diverted.[50-53] In 72 children treated exclusively at the Johns Hopkins Hospital for classical bladder exstrophy, only 1 child was diverted initially for what was felt to be inadequate bladder capacity. Children with extremely small bladder capacities have demonstrated good bladder growth following primary closure and epispadias repair.[54]

The initial operative procedure is bladder closure with or without osteotomy. The argument against osteotomy stems from the persistence of maternal relaxin after delivery, lasting up to 72 hours after delivery. Optimally, closure is performed within the first 24–48 hours of life. The argument for osteotomy is that it allows for an unhurried closure, thereby increasing the likelihood of an initial successful closure.

In the male, epispadias repair is performed at approximately 2 years of age. In both males and females, the children are closely observed and regular assessments of bladder capacity under anesthesia are made. At a time when bladder volume exceeds 60 ml bladder neck reconstruction can take place.[16,55] This normally occurs at approximately 3½–5 years of age.

OPERATIVE PROCEDURES

It is important to recognize that at the time of primary bladder closure the goals of the procedure are secure abdominal wall closure; closure of the bladder with displacement to a posterior position deep within the pelvis; approximation of the pubic symphysis; and provision of free urethral drainage. Penile lengthening, if needed, should be performed at the same time.

In some cases, if the child is closed within the first 24–72 hours of life, osteotomy may not be needed (Fig. 5.2). However, if the pubic diastasis is wide or the pelvis is not malleable, either posterior iliac or anterior innominate osteotomy should be performed at the time of initial closure.

In our experience, anterior innominate osteotomy is preferred over posterior (iliac) osteotomy.[56] The advantage of the anterior approach is that there is better pelvic mobilization and both the osteotomy and bladder closure can be completed with the patient in the supine position. In addition, interfragmentary stabilizing pins are placed across the osteotomy to fix the bone fragments; this allows excellent callus formation. The pins are then held in place with an external fixator which is placed at the end of the abdominal

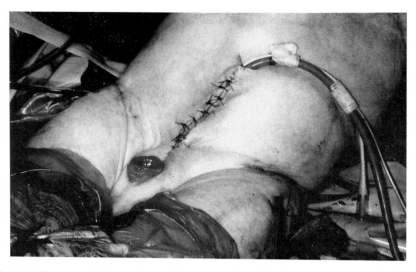

Fig. 5.2   The same child as in Figure 5.1 after functional bladder closure performed without osteotomy. This bladder closure was performed on the second day of life.

closure. In the younger patient, instead of an external fixator, modified Bryant's traction is used.

BLADDER CLOSURE

Prior to performing an incision for bladder closure, any polypoid areas on the bladder mucosa are excised. An incision is then made beginning superior to the umbilicus (following osteotomy, if indicated), using the bladder as a template for the incision. The incision is carried down to the level of the verumontanum in male and to the vaginal orifice in females.[57] Squamous epithelium should not be incorporated into the bladder closure since this may result in squamous metaplasia, which may foster chronic infection. If the phallus in male patients is extremely small, the consideration for genitoplasty and conversion to the female sex of rearing may be entertained. However, this is performed infrequently in classical bladder exstrophy. If the urethral plate is found to be short and there is significant dorsal chordee, then paraexstrophy flaps (the shiny skin adjacent to the area of the bladder neck) may be used to lengthen the urethral plate.[58] If paraexstrophy flaps are used, then the corporal bodies may also be dissected from the body of the pubis. Thus, by bringing the proximal corpora together in the midline, the apparent length of the penis is increased.[58,59]

The bladder is then widely mobilized from the rectus muscles. The peritoneum is bluntly dissected from the posterior wall of the bladder so that the bladder may drop into the pelvis. The dissection is carried laterally to the level of the pubis. At this point, the fibromuscular attachments to the pubis are dissected away from the bone, separating the prostatic and membranous urethra from the pubis. In this manner the urethra will achieve a more posterior position after symphyseal approximation.

In the female, paraexstrophy flaps may also be used to allow further lengthening of the urethra. As opposed to the male, the entire female urethra can be reconstructed at the time of bladder closure. By de-epithelializing the medial aspects of the clitoral halves, the clitoris can be brought together and approximated, leading to a more normal appearance.

Feeding tubes are used to cannulate the ureters bilaterally. The bladder is then closed in two layers with absorbable sutures. Prior to completion of the bladder closure, a suprapubic catheter is placed through a separate stab incision. As one proceeds towards the bladder neck area, it is closed over a sound or catheter (14F) large enough to provide an outlet for urine drainage but small enough to allow some resistance for bladder growth and to prevent bladder prolapse. Urethral catheters should not be used postoperatively. These have been shown to cause necrosis, erosion of the pubic suture and, most importantly, failure of initial closure.[60]

Prior to skin closure, the symphysis pubis is reapproximated. A horizontal mattress suture using number 2 nylon is our suture of choice. The rectus abdominis muscles are brought together in the midline and the abdominal wall closure is completed.

If osteotomy had been performed prior to bladder closure, then the type of immobilization would be dependent upon the type of osteotomy. If anterior innominate osteotomy was performed, an external fixator is placed, insuring against separation of the pubis.[56] If posterior iliac osteotomy has been performed, then a modified Bryant's traction is placed. Bryant's traction is also used in those children who have not undergone osteotomy prior to bladder closure, and in younger patients who have undergone anterior innominate osteotomy, due to the lack of sufficient ossification of the pelvic bones as a site for pin fixation prior to 6 months of age.

Incontinent interval

Follow-up is essential after bladder closure, and begins with calibration of the bladder outlet prior to discharge. Assessment of upper tract drainage by either excretory urography or ultrasound may be performed to rule out hydronephrosis. Since the majority of these children have vesicoureteral reflux, the development of hydronephrosis may indicate stenosis of the bladder neck area.[61] Routine urine cultures are performed at 2-month intervals to rule out any urinary tract infections. If urinary infection occurs, then an evaluation to include cystoscopy is undertaken to look for stones, squamous metaplasia or, more commonly, suture erosion into the posterior urethra.

Most males will undergo an epispadias repair prior to an operation for continence. In our experience the bladder volume must be at least 60 ml for bladder neck reconstruction to be performed. Studies performed at the Johns

Hopkins Hospital have demonstrated that after epispadias repair, bladder volume is further increased in anticipation of bladder neck reconstruction.[54,62] This appears to be true, even for those children who at the time of initial closure may have had a small-capacity bladder, and thus were considered for early diversion.

EPISPADIAS REPAIR

The goals of epispadias repair are to lengthen and straighten the penis. In addition, it should provide an adequate urethra for normal voiding. Along with the creation of a neourethra, the persistent dorsal chordee needs also to be addressed. Preoperatively, testosterone is given intramuscularly to help increase corporal length and availability of penile skin.[63] Usually, testosterone enanthate in oil, 2–3 mg/kg, is given intramuscularly 5 and 2 weeks before epispadias repair. Many different procedures for creation of a neourethra have been proposed.[64] In our experience, the Ransley[65] modification of the Cantwell[66] procedure is the repair of choice (Fig. 5.3 and 5.4).

The procedure is begun by placing a glans-holding suture. A strip along the urethral plate (approximately 1.5 cm in width) is then marked from the glans to the base of the penis. An Ipgam procedure may be performed at this point. The urethral plate is then incised along the axis of the markings. The ventral phallus is degloved in a manner similar to a hypospadias repair. However, care must be taken not to interrupt the leash of vessels which enter the urethral plate ventrally between the corpora. The corporal bodies and the urethral

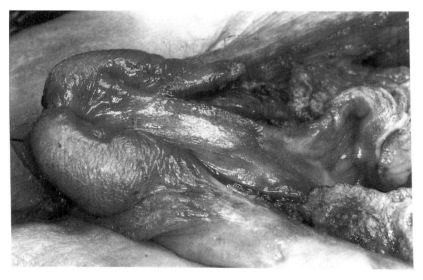

Fig. 5.3 Cantwell–Ransley epispadias repair. The urethral plate has been incised prior to dissection of the corporal bodies.

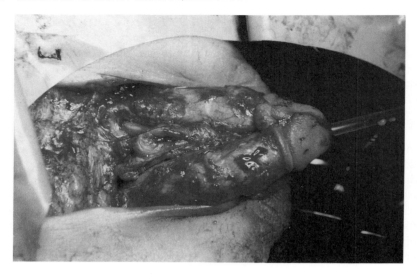

Fig. 5.4 After dissection of the corporal bodies from the urethral plate, the urethra is closed. Following completion of the urethral reconstruction, the corporal bodies will be rotated medially to recreate the normal penile anatomy.

plate are widely mobilized. The urethra is then closed over a soft catheter with a running absorbable suture. After formation of glandular wings, the neourethra is completed. The soft catheter is then sutured to the glans. By rotating the corporal bodies medially, the urethra assumes a more normal position in the penis and dorsal chordee is corrected.[67] The fistula rate is also reduced with this procedure.[68]

BLADDER NECK RECONSTRUCTION

The goal of bladder neck reconstruction is to allow for voluntary voiding with continence. The prerequisites for bladder neck reconstruction include the ability of the child to communicate and a bladder capacity of at least 60 ml. Patience on the part of both the parents and the physician is imperative during this period as the child learns to recognize the sensation of a full bladder and learns to empty the bladder adequately when full. Initial or repeat osteotomy may need to be performed at this time if there is a persistently wide pubic diastasis or a soft interpubic bar is present. Continence appears to be improved if osteotomy is used.[69,70]

The skin is opened through a Pfannenstiel incision, and the bladder is opened vertically. Since the majority of these children have vesicoureteral reflux, ureteroneocystostomy is performed.[71] A cephalotrigonal reimplantation is usually performed, allowing a larger portion of the trigone to be incorporated into the bladder neck reconstruction.[72]

A Young–Dees–Leadbetter bladder neck reconstruction is then performed.[63,73,74] Optimally a 30 mm long × 15 mm wide strip is outlined.

This strip is marked beginning at the penile urethra and proceeding in a cranial direction. The epithelium lateral to the strip is excised (Fig. 5.5). The strip is then rolled over an 8 F catheter into a tube (Fig. 5.6). In a vest-over-pants fashion, the de-epithelialized detrusor muscle is then closed over the tube. The final layer of sutures is left long in order to perform a bladder neck suspension. By suspending the bladder neck, increased urethral pressure can be achieved.[75] A suprapubic catheter and ureteral catheters are brought through separate stab incisions out of the bladder. The bladder is then closed in two layers. A Penrose drain is also placed. Again, as in initial bladder closure, no urethral stents or catheters are left in postoperatively.

RESULTS

Bladder closure

In the years 1975 to 1992, 315 patients with exstrophy were seen. Of these, 72 children with classical bladder exstrophy were referred to the Johns Hopkins for initial treatment. Of the 72 patients, 1 child underwent a diversion because of what was felt to be a small bladder at the time of initial consultation. In retrospect, that child would have been a candidate for initial closure. Of the 72 children closed initially at the Johns Hopkins Hospital, 53 children underwent either bilateral iliac osteotomy or anterior innominate

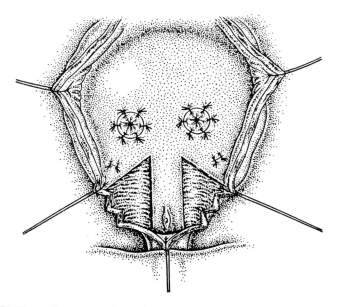

Fig. 5.5 Bladder neck reconstruction. After bilateral ureteral reimplants have been performed, the mucosal strip has been outlined and the lateral areas have been de-epithelialized. Reproduced with permission from Gearhart.[97]

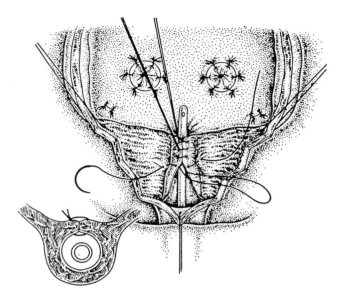

Fig. 5.6 After placement of an 8F catheter, the mucosal strip is rolled into a tube (inset: a cross-sectional view of this stage of the reconstruction). Following the completion of this stage, the detrusor will be brought across in a vest-over-pants fashion to complete the bladder neck reconstruction. Reproduced with permission from Gearhart.[97]

osteotomy at the time of their closure. Only 2 of the remaining 26 children had bladder prolapse postoperatively, requiring reclosure. Three children developed calculi, and 2 patients developed upper tract hydronephrosis requiring augmentation cystoplasty.

Epispadias repair

Prior to the routine use of the Cantwell–Ransley repair, urethrocutaneous fistulae occurred in approximately 30% of our patient population. However, since the advent of the Cantwell–Ransley repair, only 3 fistulae out of 38 patients were noted, and 2 of these closed spontaneously without any further surgery.

Bladder neck reconstruction

Of the 71 patients treated exclusively at the Johns Hopkins Hospital, 45 have undergone bladder neck reconstruction. Stratifying children between the ages of 5–10 and 10 and older, continence rates approaching 90% are seen in the older group.[49] The reason for this is unclear. It is doubtful that the increase in size of the prostate at the time of puberty contributes any increased resistance to urine outflow.[76] It is postulated that these children over the age of 10 mature to the point where they learn to use their continence.[49]

FAILED STAGED REPAIR

Failed initial closure

Children who have experienced dehiscence of the bladder or bladder prolapse have had a failed initial closure. Dehiscence can occur because of infection or, more commonly, as a result of pubic separation. Bladder prolapse can result from either partial wound separation or failure to create a tight-enough bladder neck outlet.[77]

If bladder size is adequate, then a second closure of the bladder 4–6 months after initial attempt can be performed. Repeat closure should be performed with osteotomy or repeat osteotomy. Since 1980, 38 patients with failed initial bladder closure were seen at the Johns Hopkins Hospital. All of these children underwent reclosure with osteotomy. To date, there have been no complications from the repeat closure. However, despite the sucess of repeat closure, the continence rate is less than those with successful initial closures.[77,78]

Failure to gain capacity

A few patients, despite successful initial closure and epispadias repair, fail to gain bladder capacity suitable for bladder neck reconstruction. The development of hydronephrosis and recurrent urinary tract infections may preclude the development of adequate bladder volume. Bladder augmentation with bladder neck reconstruction or augmentation cystoplasty with bladder neck transection and a continent abdominal stoma may be good options in these children.[77]

Failed bladder neck reconstruction

If a continent interval does not develop within 2 years of bladder neck reconstruction continence is rare to occur.[78,79] Repeat bladder neck plasty can be performed in these patients if the capacity seems adequate. In addition to repeat bladder neck reconstruction, bladder augmentation or placement of an artificial urinary sphincter can be performed. Alternatively, bladder neck transection and creation of a continent abdominal stoma with augmentation cystoplasty can also be performed.[80–89]

LONG-TERM OUTCOME

Quality of life

Many patients who have undergone treatment for bladder exstrophy have been followed into adulthood. Many have successful lives as business people, scholars, athletes, physicians, and happily married parents.[90] Survival rates of the patients today far exceed the 40% and 70% expected survival rates in 1925[91,92] and 1947.[93]

Malignancy

The vast majority of tumors in these patients are adenocarcinoma. Adenocarcinoma occurs approximately 400 times more commonly in the exstrophy population than in the normal population. This information is derived from a review of those patients with untreated exstrophy.[94–96] Chronic irritation with transformation of the urothelium to cystitis glandularis and later to malignant degeneration has been postulated.[96] To date, no reports of adenocarcinoma in those patients undergoing closure at birth have been reported. Other tumors can also occur in the bladder exstrophy populations.[96] These include squamous cell carcinoma, rhabdomyosarcoma, and undifferentiated urothelial carcinoma. The long-term results in those patients undergoing successful staged closure is yet to be determined.

Genital function and fertility

Many patients who have undergone staged reconstruction can be expected to have satisfactory sexual relations. Erections adequate enough for sexual function were reported in at least 70% of patients in one series.[52] As a population, males with bladder exstrophy are less fertile than the normal population.[90] Retrograde ejaculation as well as epididymitis can be a problem in these patients.

As a rule, fertility is not a problem in the female patient. In a review of over 2500 exstrophy paitents, only 28 males fathered children, whereas 131 females gave birth to 156 offspring.[23]

KEY POINTS FOR CLINICAL PRACTICE

- As one of the more severe congenital anomalies that urologists face, the genitourinary reconstruction of the child with bladder exstrophy is one of our greatest challenges. Unlike some of our other surgical undertakings, the care of the exstrophy patient require a long-term commitment by the health care provider. A clear understanding of the anatomy and the surgical techniques for correction of this anomaly is paramount.
- In anticipation of bladder closure, the newborn child should have a clear plastic dressing placed over the bladder. This prevents desiccation and irritation of the bladder mucosa.
- Prior to bladder closure a detailed examination is performed and a surgical plan must be prepared. The availability of pediatric orthopedic support in performing either anterior or posterior osteotomy helps avoid a hastily closed bladder. A decision regarding the use of paraexstrophy flaps for

penile lengthening needs to be made, and even the consideration for sex of rearing change needs to be entertained in some cases.

- Once functional bladder closure has been accomplished, the patient must be closely followed to insure maintenance of normal upper tracts, prevention of infection and assessments of bladder volume. At about 2 years of age, the male patient will undergo repair of his epispadias. Our use of the Ransley modification of the Cantwell procedure has reduced our complication rate. Once again, close follow-up is necessary, as previously outlined.

- At 4–5 years of age and when the bladder volume is felt to be appropriate (60 ml at our institution), bladder neck reconstruction is performed. What is most important is that the child should be able to communicate and recognize the new sensation of bladder fullness. The performance of a continence procedure in a child who is uninterested in dryness or who is not mature enough can be an invitation for failure.

- It is at this stage that we as clinicians must be the most patient and persistent in our follow-up. Full continence may take several years to develop and therefore the threshold to perform a repeat bladder neck reconstruction or even urinary diversion needs to be high. With dedication, persistence, and patience, the care of the exstrophy patient is one of the most rewarding endeavors that we can undertake.

REFERENCES

1 Hall EG, McCandles AD, Rickham PP. Vesicointestinal fissure with diphallus. Br J Urol 1953; 25: 219
2 Syme J. Ectopia vesicae. Lancet 1852; 2: 568
3 Coffey RC. Physiological implantation of the severed ureter as common bioduct into intestine. JAMA 1911; 56: 397
4 Nesbit RM. Ureterosigmoid anastomosis by direct elliptical connection: a preliminary report. J Urol 1949: 61: 728
5 Leadbetter WF. Consideration of problems incident to performance of ureteroenterostomy: report of a technique. J Urol 1955; 73: 67
6 Young HH. Exstrophy of the bladder: the first case in which a normal bladder and urinary control have been obtained by plastic operation. Surg Gynecol Ostet 1942; 74: 729
7 Michon L. Conservative operations for exstrophy of the bladder, with particular references to urinary incontinence. Br J Urol 1948; 20: 167
8 Gross RE, Cressen SL. Exstrophy of the bladder; observations from 80 cases. JAMA 1952; 149: 1640
9 Higgins CC. Exstrophy of the bladder: report of 158 cases. Am J Surg 1962; 28: 99
10 Shultz WG. Plastic repair of exstrophy of bladder combined with bilateral osteotomy of ilia. J Urol 1958; 79: 453
11 Dees JE. Epispadias with incontinence in the male. Surgery 1942; 12: 621
12 Leadbetter GW Jr. Surgical correction of total urinary incontinence. J Urol 1964; 91: 261
13 Megalli M, Lattimer JK. Review of the management of 140 cases of exstrophy of the bladder. J Urol 1973; 109: 246
14 Williams DI, Keeton JE. Further progress with reconstruction of the exstrophied bladder. Br J Surg 1973; 60: 203
15 Jeffs RD. Exstrophy and cloacal exstrophy. Urol Clin North Am 1978; 5: 127

16 Jeffs RD, Guice SL, Oesch I. The factors in successful exstrophy closure. J Urol 1982; 127: 974
17 Lattimer JK, Beck L, Yeaw S et al. Long term follow up after exstrophy closure—late improvement and good quality of life. J Urol 1978; 119: 664
18 Woodhouse CRJ, Ransley TC, Williams DI. The exstrophy patient in adult life. Br J Urol 1983; 55: 632
19 Rickham PP. Vesicointestinal fissure. Arch Dis Child 1960; 35: 97
20 Rickham PP. The incidence and treatment of ectopia vesicae. Proc R Soc Med 1961; 54: 389
21 Lattimer JK, Smith MJK. Exstrophy closure: a follow up on 70 cases. J Urol 1966; 95: 356
22 Jeffs RD. Exstrophy of the urinary bladder. In: Welch KJ, Randolph JG, Ravitch MM, O'Neill JA, Rowe MI, eds. Pediatric surgery. Chicago: Yearbook Medical, 1986: p 1217
23 Shapiro E, Lepor H, Jeffs RD. The inheritance of classical bladder exstrophy. J Urol 1984; 132: 308
24 Gearhart JP, Jeffs RD. Exstrophy of the bladder and other bladder anomalies. In: Walsh PC et al, eds. Campbell's urology. 6th edn. Saunders WB, Philadelphia: 1992: p 1772
25 Moore KL. The developing human: clinically oriented embryology. Philadelphia: WB Saunders, 1988: pp 255–297
26 Ambrose SS. The anterior body wall. In: Gray SW, Skandalakis JE, eds. Embryology for surgeons. Philadelphia: WB Saunders, 1972: pp 387–441
27 Patten JF, Barry A. The genesis of exstrophy of the bladder and epispadias. Am J Anat 1952; 90: 35–57
28 Muecke EC. The role of the cloacal membrane in exstrophy: the first successful experimental study. J Urol 1964; 92: 659
29 Marshall VF, Muecke EC. Variations in exstrophy of the bladder. J Urol 1962; 889: 766
30 Gross RE, Cressen SL. Exstrophy of the bladder: observations from 80 cases. JAMA 1952; 149: 1640
31 Husmann DA, McLorie GA, Churchill BM, Ein SH. Inguinal pathology and its association with classical bladder exstrophy. J Pediatr Surg 1990; 24: 332
32 Connolly J, Peppas DS, Gearhart JP, Jeffs RD. The incidence of inguinal hernia in the exstrophy population. J Urol 1993; (in press)
33 Pearl RH, Ein SH, Churchill B. Posterior sagittal anorectoplasty for pediatric recurrent rectal prolapse. J Pediatr Surg 1989; 24: 1100
34 Goyanna R, Emmett JL, McDonald JR. Exstrophy of the bladder complicated by adenocarcinoma. J Urol 1951; 65: 391
35 Culp DA. The histology of the exstrophied bladder. J Urol 1964; 91: 538
36 Gunge RG. Adophlin in treatment of human adenocarcinoma of the bladder. J Urol 1952; 68: 475
37 Engel RM, Wilkinson HA. Bladder exstrophy. J Urol 1970; 104: 699
38 Clark MA, O'Connell KJ. Scanning and transmission of electron microscopic studies of an exstrophic human bladder. J Urol 1983; 110: 481
39 Shapiro E, Jeffs RD, Gearhart JP, Lepor H. Muscarinic cholinergic receptors in bladder exstrophy: insights into surgical management. J Urol 1985; 134: 308
40 Hollowell JG, Hill PD, Duffy PG, Ransley PG. Bladder function and dysfunction in exstrophy and epispadias. Lancet 1991; 338: 926
41 Nisonson I, Lattimer JK. How well can the exstrophied bladder work? J Urol 1972; 107: 664
42 Maloney PK Jr, Gleason DM, Lattimer JK. Ureteral physiology and exstrophy of the bladder. J Urol 1965; 93: 588
43 Woodhouse CRJ, Kellett MJ. Anatomy of the penis and its deformities in exstrophy and epispadias. J Urol 1984; 132: 1122
44 Woodhouse CRJ, Ransley PG, Williams DI. The patient with exstrophy in adult life. Br J Urol 1983; 55: 632
45 Loder RP, Dayioglu MM. Association of congenital vertebral malformations with bladder and cloacal exstrophy. J Pediatr Ortho Pediatr 1990; 10: 389
46 Mirk P, Calisti A, Fileni A. Prenatal sonographic diagnosis of bladder exstrophy. J Ultrasound Med 1986; 5: 291
47 Jaffe R, Schoenfeld A, Ovadia J. Sonographic findings in the prenatal diagnosis of

bladder exstrophy. Am J Obstet Gynecol 1990; 162: 675

48 Howell C, Caldamone A, Synder H et al. Optimal management of cloacal exstrophy. J Pediatr Surg 1983; 18: 365

49 Peppas DS, Gearhart JP, Jeffs RD. Genitourinary reconstruction in classic bladder exstrophy: results of a seventeen year experience in a single institution. J Urol 1993; (in press)

50 Canning DA, Oesterling JE, Gearhart JP, Jeffs RD. A computerized review of exstrophy patients managed during the past 13 years. J Urol 1989; 141: 224A

51 Connor JP, Hensle TW, Lattimer JK, Burbige KA. Long term follow up of 207 patients with bladder exstrophy: an evolution in treatment. J Urol 1989; 142: 793

52 Mesrobian HJ, Kelalis PP, Kramer SA. Long term follow up of 103 patients with bladder exstrophy. J Urol 1988; 139: 719

53 Merguerian PA, McLorie GA, McMullin ND, Khoury AE, Husmann DA, Churchill BM. Continence in bladder exstrophy: determinants of success. J Urol 1991; 145: 350

54 Gearhart JP, Jeffs RD. Bladder exstrophy: increase in capacity following epispadias repair. J Urol 1989; 142: 525

55 Jeffs RD. Exstrophy and cloacal exstrophy. Urol Clin North Am 1978; 5: 127

56 Sponseller PD, Gearhart JP, Jeffs RD. Anterior innominate osteotomies for failure or late closure of bladder exstrophy. J Urol 1991; 146: 137

57 Lepor H, Shapiro E, Jeffs RD. Urethral reconstruction in boys with classical bladder exstrophy. J Urol 1984; 131: 512

58 Duckett JW. Use of paraexstrophy skin pedicle graphs for correction of exstrophy and epispadias repair. Birth Defects 1977; 13: 175

59 Johnston JH. The genital aspects of exstrophy. J Urol 1975; 113: 701

60 Husmann DA, McLorie GA, Churchill BM. Closure of the exstrophic bladder: an evaluation of the factors leading to its success and its importance on urinary continence. J Urol 1989; 142: 522

61 Gearhart JP, Peppas DS, Jeffs RD. The management of the failed initial exstrophy closure. J Urol 1993; (in press)

62 Peters CA, Gearhart JP, Jeffs RD. Epispadias and incontinence: the challenge of the small bladder. J Urol 1988; 140: 1199

63 Gearhart JP, Jeffs RD. The use of parenteral testosterone therapy in genital reconstructive surgery. J Urol 1987; 138: 1077

64 Young HH. An operation for the cure of incontinence associated with epispadias. J Urol 1922; 7: 1

65 Ransley PG, Duffy PG, Wollin M. Bladder exstrophy closure and epispadias repair. In: Spitz L, Nixon HH, eds. Operative surgery (paediatric surgery). London: Butterworths, 1988: pp 620–632

66 Cantwell FV. Operative treatment of epispadias by transplantation of the urethra. Ann Surg 1895; 22: 689

67 Koff SA, Eakins M. The treatment of penile chordee using corporeal rotation. J Urol 1984; 131: 931

68 Gearhart JP, Leonard MP, Burgers JK, Jeffs RD. Epispadias repair using the Cantwell–Ransley technique. J Urol 1992; 148: 851

69 Lepor H, Jeffs RD. Primary bladder closure and bladder neck reconstruction in classical bladder exstrophy. J Urol 1983; 130: 1142

70 Gearhart JP, Jeffs RD. State of the art reconstructive surgery for bladder exstrophy at the Johns Hopkins Hospital. Am J Dis Child 1989; 143: 1475

71 Cohen SJ. Ureterozystoneostomie eine neue antirefluxtechnik. Aktuel Urol 1975; 6: 1

72 Canning DA, Gearhart JP, Peppas DS, Jeffs RD. The cephalo-trigonal reimplant in bladder neck reconstruction for patients with exstrophy or epispadias. J Urol 1993; (in press)

73 Dees JE. Epispadias with incontinence in the male. Surgery 1942; 12: 621

74 Leadbetter GW Jr. Surgical correction of total urinary incontinence. J Urol 1964; 91: 261

75 Gearhart JP, Williams KA, Jeffs RD. Urethral pressure profilometry as an adjunct to bladder neck reconstruction. J Urol 1986; 136: 1055

76 Gearhart JP, Yang A, Jeffs RD, Zerhouni EA. Prostate size and configuration of adult men with classic bladder exstrophy. J Urol 1993; (in press)

77   Gearhart JP, Peppas DS, Jeffs RD. The failed exstrophy closure: strategy for management. Br J Urol 1993; (in press)

78   Oesterling JE, Jeffs RD. The importance of a successful initial bladder closure in the surgical management of classical bladder exstrophy: analysis of 144 patients treated at the Johns Hopkins Hospital between 1975 and 1985. J Urol 1987; 137: 258

79   Arap A, Girln AM, Goes GM. Initial results of the complete reconstruction of bladder exstrophy. Urol Clin North Am 1980; 7: 477

80   Gearhart JP, Jeffs RD. Augmentation cystoplasty in the failed exstrophy reconstruction. J Urol 1988; 139: 790

81   Kramer SA. Augmentation cystoplasty in patients with exstrophy-epispadias. J Pediatr Surg 1989; 24: 1293

82   Hanna MK. Artificial urinary sphincter for incontinent children. Urology 1981; 18: 370

83   Light JK, Scott FB. Treatment of the epispadias–exstrophy complex with the AS792 artificial urinary sphincter. J Urol 1983; 129: 738

84   Dector RM, Roth DR, Fishmen IJ et al. Use of the AS800 device in exstrophy and epispadias. J Urol 1988; 140: 1202

85   Quinlan DM, Leonard MP, Brendler CB, Gearhart JP, Jeffs RD. Use of the Benchekroun hydraulic valve as a catheterizable continence mechanism. J Urol 1991; 145: 1151

86   Aliabadi H, Gonzalez R. Success of the artificial urinary sphincter after failed surgery for incontinence. J Urol 1990; 143: 987

87   Mitchell ME, Piser JA. Intestinocystoplasty and total bladder replacement in children and young adults: followup in 129 cases. J Urol 1987; 138: 579

88   Gonzalez R, Nguyen DH, Koleilat N, Sidi AA. Compatibility of enterocystoplasty and the artificial urinary sphincter. J Urol 1989; 142: 502

89   Leonard MP, Gearhart JP, Jeffs RD. Continent urinary reservoirs in pediatric urological practice. J Urol 1990; 144: 330

90   Lattimer JK, Beck L, Yeaw S et al. Long-term follow up after exstrophy closure: late improvement and good quality of life. J Urol 1978; 119: 664

91   Gross D. Diseases and injuries of the urinary bladder. In: Gross D. System of surgery: pathological, diagnostic, therapeutic, and operative. Philadelphia: Blanchard and Lea, 1862: pp 270–272

92   Mayo CH, Hendricks WA. Exstrophy of the bladder. Surg Gynecol Obstet 1926; 43: 129

93   Harvard BM, Thompson GJ. Congenital extrophy of the bladder: late results of treatment by the Coffey–Mayo method or ureterointestinal anastomosis. J Urol 1951; 65: 223

94   Mostofi FK. Potentialities of bladder epithelium. J Urol 1954; 71: 705

95   Kandzari SJ, Majid A, Orteza AM, Milam DF. Exstrophy of urinary bladder complicated by adenocarcinoma. Urology 1974; 3: 496

96   Krishmansetty RM, Rao NK, Hines CR et al. Adenocarcinoma in exstrophy and dysfunctional ureteral sigmoidostomy. Kentucky Med Assoc 1988; 86: 409

97   Gearhart JP. Bladder neck reconstruction in the incontinent child. In: Frank JD, Johnston JH, eds. Operative paediatric urology. Edinburgh: Churchill Livingstone, 1990; pp 192, 193

6

Advances in management of renal cell carcinoma

M. E. Gore

There are over 3500 cases of kidney cancer per year in the UK and over 2500 deaths. This represents 1.6% of all malignant neoplasms and of all deaths related to malignant neoplasia. The disease is commoner in males than females (1.6 : 1), and has a peak incidence between the ages of 50 and 70 years.[1,2] The commonest symptoms are haematuria, pain and the presence of an abdominal mass, which occur in 56, 38 and 36% of patients respectively, but the classic triad of all three occurs in only 9% of patients; other symptoms that are common include weight loss and anaemia (20–30%). Occasionally, in less than 10% of patients, symptoms are those of metastatic disease, and include pyrexia, erythrocytosis, hypercalcaemia, acute varicocele; or the neoplasm may be found incidentally.[3,4] Paraneoplastic syndromes are common with renal cell carcinoma and when patients present with one of these syndromes there may be a delay in the diagnosis. These syndromes occur through the overproduction of proteins and hormones that are either normally produced by the kidney, e.g. renin, erythropoietin, prostaglandins, or not normally derived from renal tissue, such as parathyroid hormone, insulin, glucagon, enteroglucogon, chorionic gonadotrophin and ferritin.[5] Paraneoplastic syndromes include hypertension, non-metastatic rises in liver function tests associated with fever and focal hepatic necrosis (Stauffer's syndrome[6]), Cushing's syndrome, galactorrhoea, erythrocytosis and disorders of iron metabolism and transport. Common features of renal cell carcinoma such as fever, which occurs in about 20% of patients and hypercalcaemia, which has been reported in 3–13% of patients, may have multiple aetiologies, including the secretion of ectopic humoral factors.[5]

AETIOLOGY

The aetiology of renal cell carcinoma remains uncertain, although a number of factors have been associated with an increased risk of developing renal cell carcinoma, including cigarette smoking, obesity and phenacetin abuse. A number of occupations have been implicated, such as leather tanners, shoe workers, workers exposed to cadmium, particularly if they smoke, and possibly those exposed to the contrast medium thorotrast. There has also been a suggestion that those exposed to petroleum products may be at increased risk. Patients with acquired cystic disease of the kidney have a 5.8% incidence of renal cell carcinoma and the development of cysts is, in turn associated with long-term dialysis, a situation where 35–47% of patients acquire cystic disease.[7]

Animal studies have identified a number of chemical carcinogens: dimethyl nitrosamine, diethylnigrosoamine, nitrosoureas, fluoro-biphenyl acetamide, cycasin and the food additive potassium bomate. Classic data from the late 1940s and early 1950's showed that chronic administration of oestrogen to males in animal models induced renal cell carcinoma.[8]

Familial renal cell carcinoma is rare, but in the well-known autosomal dominant von Hippel–Lindau syndrome (cerebelloretinal haemangioblastomatosis) there is a high risk of developing the disease, which frequently occurs at an earlier age than usual and is often bilateral. Occasional familial cases that are not part of this syndrome have been described and they also tend to be bilateral and occur at an earlier age.[9,10] A number of studies have now looked at the molecular genetics of familial renal cell carcinoma and, although no single chromosomal change has been found, it appears that where an abnormal karyotype is found it tends to be located on chromosome 3. The main abnormalities involve a 3;11 or 3;8 translocation[11,12] or deletions of the short arm of chromosome 3.[13,14]

Most of the chromosomal abnormalities described in spontaneous renal cell carcinoma involve deletions in the short arm of chromosome 3[14-16] and include loss of 3p 12-14, 3p 14.ter and 3p 21-3. Interestingly, this latter site is part of the region that contains two loci genetically linked to von Hippel–Lindau disease[17,18] and these data suggest that one locus is responsible for this disease, with loss of a tumour suppressor gene being part of the mechanism for the development of both hereditary and sporadic renal cell carcinoma. However, it has also been proposed that different loci may be responsible for different histological types of renal cell carcinoma.[16] Allele loss has been described in other chromosomes (13 and 11p) but most notably it has been demonstrated that the allelic loss on 17p found in 60% of the renal cell carcinomas examined involved the locus of the tumour suppressor gene, p53.[19]

A number of additional molecular abnormalities have also been associated with renal cell carcinoma, e.g. the overexpression c-fms[20] the presence of mutated *ras*[21,22] and alterations in c-*myc* expression.[23] This c-*myc* abnormality is of particular interest as the c-*myc* sequence is sited on chromosome 3. *Ras* mutations are found in <2% of renal cell carcinomas, although these tumours can be induced by infection of normal proximal tubule cells with *ras*.[22,24] Nanus et al have also induced renal cell carcinoma and its commonly associated chromosomal abnormalities by infecting proximal tubule cells with V-*sarc*,[25] suggesting a role for tyrosine kinase in the genesis of this tumour type.

Finally, growth factors may be involved in the aetiology of renal cell carcinoma. Several investigators have found an overexpression of transforming growth factor beta and the messenger RNA for epidermal growth factor receptor in specimens of renal cell carcinoma and correlations have been made with levels of these and stage of cancer.[26,27]

TREATMENT OF THE PRIMARY LESION

The definitive treatment for primary renal cell carcinoma is radical nephrectomy. The place of adjuvant lymph node dissection remains controversial, as does the place of adjuvant radiotherapy combined with nephrectomy. The earliest study of the role of postoperative radiotherapy[28] suggested an improvement in 5-year survival from 37 to 56%, but subsequent studies have not confirmed this.[29,30] In both these latter studies the 5-year survival in the radiotherapy group was lower (38 and 47% against 62 and 63%, respectively), with a high complication rate due to the radiotherapy, which was mainly gastrointestinal and in some cases fatal.

Spontaneous remission has been reported in 5 out of 1447 cases (0.35%), whereas remission following nephrectomy occurred in 4 out of 663 cases (0.6%) in one retrospective analysis.[31] Although remission after nephrectomy appears to be almost twice as common as spontaneous remission, because it occurs in less than 1% of patients this would mean that 199 patients with metastatic disease are being nephrectomized for 1 patient to respond. In addition, the reported incidence of remission after nephrectomy is almost certainly an overestimate in view of the fact that these figures are inevitably based on cumulative data and retrospective analyses. Thus, nephrectomy in the face of metastatic disease is not indicated if the sole aim is to induce a response in the metastatic lesions.

The indications for nephrectomy in the face of metastatic disease are as follows:

1. Large primary tumour (asymptomatic) associated with very small-volume metastatic disease and if it is likely that the patient will develop local problems before any symptoms associated with the metastases occur.

2. Large primary tumour (symptomatic) associated with small- to moderate-volume metastatic disease. Local symptoms, including pain, haematuria and recurrent infection, are well-palliated by nephrectomy, which may in addition be less morbid than radiotherapy or embolization. Similarly, in patients with systemic constitutional symptoms from their cancer, such as fever, malaise and anorexia, nephrectomy may improve or even completely reverse these symptoms by substantially reducing the tumour burden.

3. Certain experimental protocols, particularly those involving immunotherapy, require patients to be nephrectomized prior to entry into the study. Nephrectomy is justified in these circumstances but not in patients who are undergoing immunotherapy outside clinical trials as the relationship between nephrectomy and response to immunotherapy remains unproven.

CHEMOTHERAPY

Response to all treatment modalities including chemotheraphy is defined according to WHO criteria[32] as follows: complete response is the disappearance of all detectable lesions for at least 1 month and partial response is the decrease in the sum of the products of two bidimensionally measured lesions by 50% or more for at least 1 month, without progression in any other lesion or reappearance of new tumours. The overall response rate is the sum of the complete and partial responses.

In 1983 Harris[33] reviewed the literature on the use of single-agent chemotherapy in renal cell carcinoma. He reported 38 agents which had been given to 1011 patients with an overall response rate of 9%. Some drugs in this series gave response rates of 10–20% (nitrogen mustard, chlorambucil, CCNU, thiotepa, ifosfamide, bleomycin, hydroxyurea, 6-mercaptopurine) and three drugs resulted in response rates of 20–25% (cyclophosphamide, vinblastine, dibromodulcitol). Among the drugs with a less than 10% response rate are agents which form the mainstay of chemotherapy regimens in other tumour types, namely, cyclophosphamide, Mitomycin-C, Adriamycin, 5-fluorouracil, methotrexate, DTIC, cisplatin.

Most attention has been focused on vinblastine. In Harris's review there were 135 patients who had received this drug and the overall response rate was 24%. It has been suggested that there is a steep dose–response curve for vinblastine, with doses of 0.2–0.3 mg/kg per week resulting in a response rate of 31% (12 out of 39 patients), whereas below this dose only 15% of patients responded (14 out of 96 patients[34]). Vinblastine has also been administered by continuous intravenous infusion but results have been disappointing, with response rates below 10%.[35,36]

Since Harris's review, ifosfamide has been the subject of two further phase II studies but only one partial response out of 25 patients treated has been reported.[37,38] Other agents that have been examined since that report include a new nitrosourea (PCNU), streptozocin, deoxydoxorubicin, fludarabine, diaziquone, bisantrene, doxycytidine, carboplatin, elliptinium and echinomycin;[39–49] there were only 8 responses out of 340 patients treated in these studies (2%), with only 1 patient achieving a complete remission (on elliptinium). Recently, there has been considerable interest in the use of fluorodeoxyuridine (FUDR). Hrushesky and colleagues[34a,b] showed that FUDR infused according to the circadian rhythm with the peak dose occurring around 6 p.m. resulted in a response rate of 24%. However, this finding has not been confirmed by other workers and there have only been 5 responses reported out of 38 patients (13%) treated since then in three studies.[50–52]

A number of groups have attempted to modulate the cytotoxicity of single-agent chemotherapy by biochemical means and/or by reversing mechanisms of drug resistance in order to improve response rates. Quinidine has been added to vinblastine,[53] misonidazole has been added to cyclophosphamide,[54] metronidazole has been added to Mitomycin-C,[55] dipyridamole has been added to vinblastine[56] and leucovorin and interferon have been added to FUDR;[57] these manoeuvres have resulted in response rates of <5%.

Attempts to improve response rates by combining cytotoxic agents have also been unsuccessful. Harris[33] reviewed 22 combination regimens which had been used to treat 406 patients with a cumulative response rate of 17% but very few patients achieved complete remission. Five combinations resulted in response rates of 10–20%: vincristine + Adriamycin + methyl CCNU, 37 patients; bleomycin + CCNU + methylprednisolone + Adriamycin, 30 patients; vinblastine + hydroxyurea + cyclophosphamide + medroxyprogesterone acetate (MPA) + prednisolone, 42 patients; Adriamycin + bleomycin + vincristine + cyclophosphamide + BCG, 13 patients; vinblastine + bleomycin, 15 patients. Three studies gave response rates of 32–35%: CCNU + mega ace + BCG transfer factor, 14 patients; vinblastine + methotrexate + bleomycin + tamoxifen, 28 patients: vincristine + Adriamycin, MPA, BCG, 31 patients. More recently, a study has confirmed the activity of vinblastine + bleomycin + high-dose methotrexate to be 30%[58] but a complicated regimen including Adriamycin, vindesine, cyclophosphamide, cisplatin and DTIC produced only 1 response out of 14 patients, albeit it was a complete remission.[478] Vinblastine has been combined with CCNU in four studies in which 127 patients have been treated, with a response rate of 14% with three complete remissions.[59–62]

The duration of remissions to chemotheraphy is short and measured in months. This observation that renal cell carcinoma is an inherently chemoresistant disease is supported by the finding that renal tubular epithelium, from which this tumour derives, expresses the multidrug-resistant gene, MDR 1[63] This gene encodes for a 170 kDa glycoprotein known as p-glycoprotein, which is present in the cell membrane and is responsible for actively transporting cytotoxic drugs out of cells. Goldstein and colleagues[64] have found that the MDR 1 gene was over-expressed in 38 out of 46 human renal cell carcinomas specimens analysed. There are no randomized prospective studies on the use of adjuvant chemotheraphy in this condition but it would be very unlikely that a therapeutic modality with such a low response rate in advanced disease would have any impact in this setting.

HORMONE THERAPY

MPA has been the standard systemic treatment for advanced renal cell carcinoma since Bloom[65] reported a 16% 'significant objective response' to this drug, given at a dose of 300 mg/day. Since then Harris[33] reviewed the literature and found that the cumulative response rate to MPA in 173 patients treated in 10 trials was 10%. Two recent studies[66,67] reported 4 partial responses in a total of 41 patients treated (10%) with high doses of MPA, 500/day. Interestingly, 2 out of Bloom's original 11 responders had been treated with other hormones (testosterone in 1 case and testosterone plus hydroxyprogesterone caproate in another). Thus if the original data are recalculated to exclude these 2 patients as well as 2 further patients who had stabilization of their disease rather than an objective response, then the overall response rate in this important study falls to 11% (9 out of 79 patients), almost exactly the efficacy that has been found in subsequent studies. The duration of remission for the 9 patients that we reanalysed from Bloom's report[65] ranges from 2 to 24 months, with a median of 3 months.

Progesterones other than MPA seem to be less active, with 3 responses being reported out of 47 patients (6%) in four studies, and a similar response rate is found for testosterone.[33] Tamoxifen at low dose appears to be virtually inactive–response rate 2% in 103 patients–but 2 out of 15 patients responded to tamoxifen given at high doses, 80 mg/day.[33] Combinations of hormones or hormones with chemotherapy do not seem to add anything to response rates and newer agents such as lonidamine have not shown significant activity.[68] Hormonal agents, particularly MPA, are frequently used despite their very low activity because of the symptomatic improvement they can afford. The majority of patients feel well on MPA, increase their appetite and gain weight. Fluid retention is sometimes seen with these agents but is rarely a major problem. MPA is relatively expensive and it still remains open to question whether simpler palliative measures such as low-dose prednisolone may be more cost-effective for this patient population.

INTERFERONS

The interferons are a group of proteins classified as alpha, beta or gamma. Interferon-alpha is encoded by more than 20 genes, producing a small family of proteins, whereas beta and gamma interferon are encoded by a single gene, producing a single protein each. Interferons have a wide variety of biological actions but they all seem to have antiviral and immunoregulatory activity as well as the ability to enhance the cytotoxicity of a variety of leukocytes. Interferon-alpha and -beta have additional antiproliferative effects on normal and malignant cells and interferon-gamma enhances T- and B-cell responses as well as activating macrophages.

Horoszewicz and Murphy[69] reviewed 56 published studies in which 1684 patients were treated with interferons. They analysed 1112 patients treated with interferon-alpha and found that the overall response rate was 15%, with 20 patients (2%) obtaining a complete remission. The overall response rates for interferon-beta and gamma were 10 and 9% respectively, although the number of patients studied was very much less (31 and 112 respectively). Combination therapy with different types of interferon has been reported in 15 studies with an overall response rate of 19% (420 patients treated), but again the complete remission rate is low, 3%.

The duration of remission to interferon-alpha can vary widely from patient to patient, e.g. Buzaid and colleagues[70] have reported a range of 1–17 + months and there are patients who have even maintained a partial response for 25 + and 31 + months.[71] The median durations of remission reported in the literature range from 5 to 16 months[70–74] and they do not appear to be significantly different for interferon-beta or gamma.

Unlike chemotherapy, where response occurs within weeks and sometimes days, the time taken to respond to interferons may be very prolonged and varies widely–1–11 months.[75] However, most patients who respond have done so by 3–4 months and it would be very unusual for patients who progress on interferon to respond subsequently. It can be argued that patients with stable disease after this length of time should remain on interferon indefinitely, as stabilization of the disease may be a consequence of treatment with interferon. For patients who have achieved a partial remission there is a similar dilemma with regard to the duration of treatment and there are no data addressing this problem. It is probably reasonable to stop treatment after 1 year but in practice, this author continues treatment indefinitely for those patients with stable disease or in partial remission, provided they are able to tolerate the side-effects. However, treatment is stopped as soon as progressive disease occurs.

Muss[76] has addressed the issue of the dose–response relationship for interferon-alpha in renal cell carcinoma. Analysing the results of 17 studies involving 593 patients he showed that the response rate to daily doses <5 Mu/day was 11%, whereas for doses of 5–10 or >10Mu/day, response rates were 20 and 15% respectively. Daily dosing is no longer commonly used and usually interferon-alpha is given three times a week (Mondays, Wednesdays, Fridays). Patients should be started on a low dose so that they can get used to the side-effects and the aim is to reach 10–18 Mu per dose (i.e. 4–8 Mu/day equivalent) within 1–2 increments. The final dose used can be adjusted to take vial size into account for the sake of economy. There is little value in using high doses of interferon-alpha and indeed there is evidence that higher doses are associated with lower response rates. The subcutaneous as opposed to the intramuscular or intravenous route is recommended because of ease of administration and it is associated with fewer side-effects. Muss and colleagues[71] have clearly shown in a randomized study that response rates are equivalent (7 and 10% respectively) whether the drug is given subcutaneously or intravenously but patients treated via the latter route have a much higher incidence of toxicities such as flu-like symptoms, somnolence, nausea, anorexia and other gastrointestinal disturbances. However, a criticism of this study is that the dose and scheduling of interferon-alpha differed between the two arms of the study (subcutaneous: 2 Mu/m^2 × 3 per week; intravenous: 30 Mu/m^2 daily × 5 q. 21 days) and this could account for the differences seen, but data from non-randomized studies support this observation.

A number of patient characteristics have been proposed as predictors of response to interferons. An analysis of cumulative data suggested that prior nephrectomy was a feature in 83% of responders, whereas only 79% of all patients in the studies analysed had been nephrectomized prior to interferon therapy.[75] A similar analysis suggested that patients with pulmonary metastases were more likely to respond than those with disease at other sites: 83% of responders had pulmonary metastases whereas only 66% of the study population had disease at this site. Nephrectomy is not a prerequisite for treatment with interferons but other authors have noted that pulmonary metastases are a favoured site for response.[72] Other characteristics that have been suggested as predictors of response include performance status, no prior systemic treatment, white blood cell count, disease-free interval, age and sex but none of these data are reliable as the numbers involved in the analyses are small and neither the presence nor absence of any of these features should be used to withhold interferon treatment from a patient. The single exception to this is performance status, but this is a general consideration when any systemic treatment is proposed for incurable metastatic cancer and does not apply specifically to this tumour type or to this modality of treatment.

The development of anti-interferon antibodies has been reported in 5–40% of patients.[71,77–79] The relationship however between the development of antibodies, response and severity of side-effects remains uncertain. Their development has been associated with loss of response in other tumour types such as hairy cell leukaemia, lymphoma, chronic granulocytic leukaemia, carcinoid as well as occasionally renal cell carcinoma.[72,78] Theoretically, there are considerable worries about the development of neutralizing antibodies being associated with a reduction in efficacy but the routine measurement of interferon antibodies is not indicated in general clinical practice.

There has been one randomized study of adjuvant interferon-alpha after nephrectomy. There was a no-treatment control arm and with 270 patients in the study no difference in survival has been noted.[80] Interferon-alpha is therefore never indicated after removal of the primary in the absence of residual or metastatic disease.

A number of trials have combined interferon-alpha with chemotherapy, steroids, hormonal agents and immunemodulators, including other interferons. The combination of interferon-alpha with cimetidine or MPA does not appear to increase its efficacy.[81,82] Of particular interest is the work of Fossa et al[83] who combined prednisone with interferon without a reduction in efficacy while increasing tolerability. This is a particularly interesting observation in view of the theoretical interaction between steroids and interferon-alpha, that should reduce the latter's efficacy because of the down-regulation of the cellular enzyme 2,5-oligosynthetase, which forms part of the intracellular signalling pathway following interferon-alpha's binding to its cell surface receptor.

There has been much attention paid to the combination of interferon-alpha with vinblastine, and Bergerat and colleagues[84] have reported a 41% response rate for patients treated with this combination in 58 evaluable patients.

Cumulative data from 10 other phase 2 studies where 320 patients have been treated suggest that the response rate is only 17% (complete remission rate 3%) and the median duration of remission similar to that seen for patients who respond to interferon alone.[85-94] Bergerat's study[84] involved 30 Mu/m^2 of interferon-alpha per week and, although most of the other studies employed lower doses of interferon, most patients in these reports were receiving a daily dose equivalent of 5-10 Mu. Dose differences may account for the discrepancy between the response rate found in Bergerat's study but it may also be accounted for by the characteristics of the patients treated: there was a high percentage of patients with pulmonary lesions (51%), nearly all patients had been nephrectomized, a good performance status was mandatory before study entry and there was a high male to female ratio, which some have reported as a prognostic factor for response. There have, however, been two randomized studies including 165 and 145 patients[95,96] and neither of these studies have shown a survival benefit for the combination and the response rates in both arms of Smalley's study[95] were in fact only of the order of 10%. The combination of vinblastine and interferon-alpha can therefore not be recommended outside the context of a clinical trial.

Other chemotherapy–interferon combinations have been studied in renal cell carcinoma, including BCNU[97] and cyclophosphamide[98] but they are not active. Dexeus and colleagues[99] combined cisplatin, 5-Fluorouracil, doxorubicin and Mitomycin-C and randomized 36 patients to receive interferon with this regimen or not: only 2 responses were seen in each arm. More recently, the combination of FUDR and interferon has shown activity with a 40% response rate in a very small study.[100] Other combinations have included interferon with MPA[82] with a very low response rate (5%) but, more interestingly, aspirin has been combined with interferon-alpha in 29 patients, giving an overall response rate of 34%, and 1 patient achieved a complete remission.[101]

Interferons have also been combined with each other, in particular interferon-alpha and -gamma, in view of the in vitro synergism that has been seen in respect of their antiviral and antiproliferative properties. A randomized study failed to show any advantage for the combination[102] but this group has since looked at escalating doses within this combination and overall response rates of 24–28% were seen in two studies involving 29 and 25 patients respectively. In these two studies a total of 6 complete remissions were seen, some of which were durable, and these new combinations of interferon-alpha and -gamma at different doses are now being studied in a randomized setting under the auspices of the EORTC Genitourinary Tract Cancer Group.[102] Tumour necrosis factor given as a single agent is not active in any human cancer but in one report when combined with interferon-gamma in a small study of 22 patients, 3 obtained a complete remission and 1 patient had a partial remission.[103] Of particular interest is the combination of tumour necrosis factor and interferon-alpha;[104] these authors have reported a small study of 19 patients with 2 complete remissions and an overall response rate of 47%. These remarkable results are now the subject of a confirmatory phase 2 study being carried out at the Royal Marsden Hospital, London.

Recently, two randomized studies of MPA versus interferon have been started, one in Scandinavia from which there has been a preliminary report; the other mounted by the Medical Research Council in the UK. The interim analysis of the Scandinavian study has reported 1 out of 30 responders in the MPA arm and 2 out of 30 in the interferon arm.[105] These are important trials as interferon treatment is invasive, relatively expensive and associated with side-effects but is probably associated with more objective responses which are of longer duration.

Most patients receiving interferons find these flu-like symptoms often abate after the first few weeks of treatment. Tolerance to these side-effects can also be increased by administering interferon at night together with paracetamol. Occasionally the fatigue continues and does not improve, in which case it may be severe enough to become dose-limiting. Gastrointestinal side-effects also occur, although in less than 50% of patients, and these can include a reduction in taste, nausea and vomiting, anorexia and weight loss. Myelosuppression is sometimes seen and elevated serum transaminases but not clinical hepatitis have also been reported. Occasionally, central nervous system side-effects such as paraesthesia, somnolence, depression, memory impairment, confusion and personality change occur. The side-effects of interferons tend to be dose-related and are rapidly reversible on cessation of treatment.[106]

INTERLEUKIN-2

Interleukin-2 is a cytokine that was first identified as a T-cell growth factor but has since been shown to have a variety of effects, including stimulation of macrophage cytotoxicity, stimulation of B-cell growth and differentiation, and the production of other cytokines. Animal studies in the mid 1980s showed that interleukin-2 could lead to the in vitro generation of lymphocyte-derived killer cells and the mediation of tumour regression in established tumours in animals. These observations led to a large number of studies on the effects of interleukin-2 in human cancers, especially renal cell carcinoma, as this tumour appears to be particularly responsive to this form of therapy.

Initial clinical studies performed by Rosenberg et al[107] suggested that bolus doses of interleukin-2 resulted in an overall response rate of 22% and some remissions were shown to be durable, continuing over 3 years. However, when interleukin-2 was combined with adoptive immunotherapy, that is, the transfer of immunologically active cells with antitumour activity, a much higher response rate was found (35%) and over 10% of patients achieved a complete remission. Rosenberg and colleagues used in vitro interleukin-2-stimulated T cells (lymphokine-activated killer cells, LAK) for their adoptive immunotherapy combined with intravenous interleukin-2.[7] Table 6.1 shows the published results of interleukin-2 given either by continuous infusion or

Table 6.1   Non-randomized studies of interleukin-2 (IL-2) given by bolus intravenous injection or continuous intravenous infusion (CI) with and without lymphokine-activated killer (LAK) cells

	n	Complete response	Partial response
Bolus IL-2–LAK			
Rosenberg et al (1989)[107]	54	4	8
Abrams et al (1990)[108]	16	0	0
Bukowski et al (1990)[109]	41	1	4
Poo et al (1991)[110]	15	0	4
Escudier et al (1992)[111]	88	0	16
Total	214	5(2%)	32(15%)
CI IL-2-LAK			
Negrier et al (1989)[112]	32	2	4
Galligioni et al (1990)[113]	18	3	3
von der Masse et al (1991)[114]	51	2	6
Total	101	7(7%)	13(13%)
Bolus + LAK			
Rosenberg et al (1989)[107]	72	8	17
Fisher et al (1988)[115]	32	2	3
Total	104	10(10%)	20(19%)
CI IL-2 + LAK			
Negrier et al (1989)[112]	51	5	11
West (1989)[116]	20	2	4
Gaynor et al (1990)[117]	25	2	2
Parkinson et al (1990)[118]	47	2	2
Thompson et al (1992)[119]	42	4	10
Total	185	15(8%)	29(16%)

bolus intravenous injection with or without LAK cells. The overall response rates are: bolus interleukin-2 without LAK cells, 17%; continuous infusion interleukin-2 without LAK cells, 20%; bolus interleukin-2 with LAK cells, 29%; continuous infusion interleukin-2 with LAK cells, 24%. A randomized study of interleukin-2 with and without LAK cells has been performed by Rosenberg and colleagues and with 88 patients evaluated, the overall response rate for those receiving LAK cells was 33%, with 7 patients obtaining a complete remission and for those treated by bolus interleukin-2 alone, 24%, with 3 patients achieving complete remission.[7] Bolus interleukin-2 administered with and without LAK cells has also been compared in a randomized study by McCabe and colleagues;[120] response rates were 8% in the 37 patients treated with interleukin-2 alone and 13% in the arm treated with interleukin-2 plus LAK cells (32 patients). A randomized study of interleukin-2 given as a continuous infusion or by bolus injection with both arms of the study receiving LAK cells has been reported. Sixty-one patients were randomized into the study and the response rate in both arms was 22%. Interestingly, toxicities were similar for both schedules, although more pulmonary toxicity was observed with the bolus schedule.[121]

These treatments can be associated with considerable toxicity but this is very dose- and schedule-dependent. Common side-effects include nausea and vomiting, diarrhoea, hypotension, fevers and weight gain due to the retention of fluid within tissues consequent on endothelial leakage. Moderate rises in serum creatinine and liver function tests are also seen commonly and occasionally these may be very marked. Other uncommon side-effects include respiratory distress due to pulmonary oedema, cardiac dysrhythmias and hypothyroidism due to the induction of autoimmune T-cell-mediated thyroid disease. Myocardial infarction and severe encephalopathy occur in less than 5% of patients and the overall mortality of interleukin-2 treatment is approximately 1%.[122] Interleukin-2 has a very short half-life and toxicities are rapidly reversible within days and sometimes hours once the treatment has been discontinued. Interleukin-2 given as a bolus is more toxic than when it is given by continuous infusion and very much more toxic when LAK cells are also administered. Therefore one of the major issues surrounding the use of interleukin-2 in renal cell carcinoma is whether, by using the less toxic schedule of continuous infusion interleukin-2 without LAK cells, efficacy is compromised. It must also be remembered that LAK cell therapy is not only more toxic but also very much more labour-intensive and expensive as it involves considerable resources to culture and generate these cell in vitro. Most workers in the field feel that the small increase in response rate seen with LAK cells (26% from 18%; see Table 6.1) is not worthwhile and indeed, dose intensity, not the administration of LAK cells appears to correlate with response when the results from a large number of trials are pooled.[123] Attempts have been made to reduce further the toxicity of interleukin-2 therapy by lowering the intravenous dose but response rates have been very disappointing.[124,125] However, interleukin-2 can be given subcutaneously and thus can be delivered as outpatient treatment. Sleijfer and colleagues[126] treated 21 patients with a subcutaneous outpatient schedule and observed 2 complete remissions and 4 partial responses, but not all studies have shown activity for this mode of administration.

Criticisms of the above studies have included the fact that many have been performed in specialist centres and that the treatment may not be applicable to more general hospitals. A recently analysed multicentre study in Europe in which 109 evaluable patients were treated with interleukin-2 alone by the continuous infusion schedule has shown that the overall response rate is 14%, with 4 patients achieving complete remission in a relatively unselected group of patients.[127]

Three studies have attempted to improve the response rates to interleukin-2 and adoptive immunotherapy by either using tumour-infiltrating lymphocytes taken at operation[128] or by using peripheral blood lymphocytes stimulated by means other than interleukin-2.[129,130] There were no responses seen to interleukin-2 given together with tumour-infiltrating lymphocytes but encouraging results have been seen with mitogen-activated lymphocytes given together with interleukin-2: Wang and colleagues[129] observed 6 responses in

30 patients and Bernstein and coworkers[130]observed 6 responses in 17 patients.

A number of groups have attempted to combine interferon-alpha with interleukin-2 given either subcutaneously, intravenously, or as a combination of the two. Table 6.2 shows the results of these studies: the cumulative data suggest that 28% of patients respond to this combination, with an 8% complete remission rate. However, there has been a randomized study of interleukin-2 versus interleukin-2 plus interferon-alpha where both treatments were given by bolus intravenous injection. Three out of 28 patients treated on the combination regimen responded compared to 8 out of 30 patients who received single-agent interleukin-2.[138] The authors are unclear as to the reason for this discrepancy but have closed accrual into the combination arm. A number of other agents have been used in combination with interleukin-2 and these are shown in Table 6.3. The data in this Table largely consist of small studies and results clearly require confirmation.

Table 6.2 Non-randomized studies of interleukin-2 combined with interferon-alpha

	n	Complete response	Partial response
Rosenberg et al (1989)[131]	46	4	11
Hirsh et al (1990)[132]	12	3	3
Bergmann et al (1991)[132]	29	2	5
Pichert et al (1991)[134]	6	0	0
Atzpodien et al (1991)[135]	34	4	6
Demchak et al (1991)[136]	29	0	5
Figlin et al (1991)[137]	30	0	9
Total	186	13(7%)	39(21%)

Table 6.3 Non-randomized studies of interleukin-2 (IL-2) combined with other cytokines and/or other immunomodulators and/or chemotherapy

	Agent(s) in combination with IL-2	Complete response n	Overall response rate
Rosenberg et al (1989)[107]	Tumour necrosis factor	10	30%
	Cyclophosphamide	3	0%
Lindeman et al (1989)[139]	Cyclophosphamide	14	0%
Krigel et al (1990)[140]	interferon-beta	22	27%
Wershall et al (1991)[141]	Cyclophosphamide + Interferon-alpha	16	19%
Escudier et al (1991)[142]	Interferon-gamma	31	23%
Bramwell et al (1991)[143]	Indomethacin + ranitidine	25	9%
Pinto et al (1991)[144]	Vinblastine	15	0%
Markowitz et al (1991)[145]	Interferon-alpha + cyclophosphamide	10	30%
Fink et al (1992)[146]	Vinblastine	33	15%
Sosman et al (1992)[124]	Anti-CD 3	34	9%

MISCELLANEOUS TREATMENTS

A variety of immunomodulatory treatments have recently been applied to renal cell carcinoma. In 1987 Marshall and colleagues[147] reported 3 complete remissions and 11 partial remissions out of 42 patients treated with a combination of cimetidine (300 mg q.d.s.) and coumarin (100 mg q.d.s.). This study has been repeated but only 3 out of 50 patients responded[148] and when the dose of coumarin was dropped to 100 mg/day, no responders at all were seen.[149] Cimetidine given as a single agent is inactive[150] but has antisuppressor cell activity. It was used as the control arm in a randomized study of autolymphocyte therapy. Ninety patients were randomized to receive autologous lymphocytes that had been activated in the presence of the mitogenic monoclonal antibody OKT3 which is directed against the CD3 portion of the T-cell receptor. The response rate to autologous lymphocyte treatment was 21% against 5% for cimetidine and early survival data suggested that the group treated with autologous lymphocytes had a 2.5 times longer survival than the cimetidine group,[151] with the survival advantage being particularly marked in the male patients.

Experimental immunotherapy with cancer vaccines against renal cell carcinoma using autologous tumour, allogeneic tumour or subcellular units has been used for some time. Recently, augmentation of the immune response to vaccination has been possible using exogenous cytokines such as interleukin-2[152] or gene therapy by inserting cytokine genes into the inoculum (tumour cells or lymphocytes). Scharfe and colleagues[153] reported 10 objective responses in 89 patients using an autologous tumour vaccine and Ross and colleagues[154] used autologous lymphocytes sensitized in vitro to autologous tumour to treated patients while on oral cimetidine. Unfortunately, the response rate to this latter approach was very low (5.5%), but there was a suggestion that patients may have prolonged survival compared to historical controls.

CONCLUSIONS

Metastatic renal cell carcinoma is an incurable condition but 10–20% of patients with metastatic disease are alive at 2–4 years. A number of prognostic factors determine the survival of patients who present with metastatic disease and survival data from non-randomized studies must therefore be interpreted with considerable caution as patients are often highly selected before entering these trials, particularly where they involve intensive treatments. Study entry criteria are often precisely those that predict for response and good survival, e.g. good performance status, nephrectomy, etc. Results may therefore not be applicable to the metastatic renal cell carcinoma patient population as a whole.

Radical nephrectomy is the treatment of choice for primary lesions and there is no evidence that postoperative radiotherapy improves survival.

Nephrectomy may be indicated in patients with metastatic disease but only for specific reasons, usually concerning local palliation. Standard systemic treatment lies between MPA, interferon and interleukin-2. The increased response rates seen with interferon-alpha compared to MPA need to be confirmed in randomized trials and any benefit considered against financial cost, mode of administration and side-effects. The place of interleukin-2 remains controversial as cumulative data do not suggest an improvement in response rate over interferon-alpha. However, there may be subgroups of patients who will benefit from interleukin-2 therapy but whether there is a survival advantage over interferon-alpha remains to be demonstrated. Current experimental studies are concentrating on three main areas:

1. Combination cytokine therapy, e.g. combinations of interferons, tumour necrosis factor + interferon, interleukin-2 + interferons.
2. Tumour vaccination with or without immunemodulation using cytokines such as interleukin-2 delivered exogenously or as gene therapy.
3. Adoptive transfer techniques using subsets of autologous peripheral blood lymphocytes or tumour-infiltrating lymphocytes stimulated in vitro by a variety of methods.

REFERENCES

1 Facts on Cancer, Factsheet 3.2 and 3.3. Cancer Research Campaign 1989.
2 Facts on Cancer, Factsheet 1.2 and 1.3. Cancer Research Campaign 1990.
3 Skinner DG, Colvin RB, Vermillion CD et al. Diagnosis and management of renal cell carcinoma: a clinical and pathological study of 309 cases. Cancer 1971; 28: 1165–1177
4 Ritchie AWS, Chisholm GD. The natural history of renal cell carcinoma. Semin Oncol 1983: 10: 390–400
5 Stenzl A, de Kernion JB. Pathology, biology and clinical staging of renal cell carcinoma. Semin Oncol 1989; 16 (suppl 1): 3011
6 Boxer RJ, Waisman J, Lieber MM et al. Non metastatic hepatic dysfunction associated with renal cell carcinoma J Urol 1978; 119: 468–471
7 Linehan WM, Shipley WU, Longo DL. Cancer of the kidney and ureter. In: DeVita VT, Hellman S, Rosenberg SA, eds. Cancer: principles and practice of oncology. 3rd edn, JB Lippincott, Philadelphia, 1989: p 994
8 Outzen HC, Maguire HC. The etiology of renal cell carcinoma. Semin Oncol 1983; 10: 378–384
9 Richards RD, Melust WK, Schrinke RN. A prospective study of von Hippel–Lindau Disease. J Urol 1973: 110: 27–30
10 Goldman SM, Gishman EK, Abeshouse G et al. Renal cell carcinoma diagnosed in three generations of a single family. South Med J 1979; 72: 1457–1459
11 Coen AJ, Li FP, Berg S et al. Hereditary renal cell carcinoma associated with a chromosomal translocation. N Engl J Med 1979; 301: 592–595
12 Pathak S, Strong LC, Ferrel RE et al. Familial renal cell carcinoma with 3; 11 chromosome translocation limited to tumour cells. Science 1982; 217: 939–941
13 King CR, Schmike RN, Arthur T et al. Proximal 3p deletion in renal cell carcinoma cells from a patient with von Hippel–Lindau disease. Cancer Genet Cytogenet 1987; 27: 345–348
14 Zbar B, Branch H, Talmadge C, Linehan M. Loss of alleles of loci on the short arm of chromosome 3 in renal cell carcinoma. Nature 1987; 327: 721–724
15 Kovacs G, Szucs S, De Rise W, Baumgartl H. Specific chromosome aberration in human

renal cell carcinoma. Int J Cancer 1987; 40: 171–178

16   Ogawa O, Kakehi Y, Ogawa K, Koshiba M, Sugiyama T, Yoshida O. Allelic loss at
     chromosome 3p characterizes clear cell phenotype of renal cell carcinoma. Cancer Res
     1991; 51: 949–953

17   Seizinger BR, Rouleau GS, Ozelius LJ et al. Von Hippel–Lindau disease maps to the
     region of chromosome 3 associated renal cell carcinoma. Nature 1988; 332: 268–269

18   Hosoe S, Branch H, Latif F et al. Localisation of the von Hippel-Lindau disease gene to
     a small region of chromosome 3. Genomics 1990; 8: 634–640

19   Yoshida O. Oncogenes in renal cell carcinoma. In: Proceedings of second international
     symposium on immunobiology of renal cell carcinoma, Cleveland, USA. Saunders,
     Philadelphia, 1991: p 9

20   Slamon DJ, de Kernion JB, Verma IM et al. Expression of cellular oncogenes in human
     malignancies. Science 1984; 224: 256–262

21   Karthaus HF, Bussemakers MJ, Schalken JA et al. Expression of proto-oncogenes in
     xenografts of human renal cell carcinomas. Urol Res 1987; 15: 349–353

22   Nanus DM, Ebrahim SAD, Bander NH et al. Transformation of human kidney proximal
     tubule cells by ras containing retroviruses: implications for tumour progression. J Exp
     Med 1989; 169: 953–973

23   Drabkin HA, Bradley C, Hart I et al. Translocation of c-myc in the hereditary renal cell
     carcinoma associated with a t(3;8) (p14.2; 924.13) chromosomal location. Proc Natl Acad
     Sci USA 1985; 82: 6980–6984

24   Nanus DM, Mentle IR, Motzer RJ, Bandes NH, Albino AP. Infrequent point mutations
     of ras oncogenes in renal cell carcinoma. J Urol 1990; 143: 175–178

25   Nanus DM, Lynch SA, Rao PH, Anderson SM, Jhanwar SC, Albino AP. Transformation
     of human kidney proximal tubule cells by src-containing retroviruses. Oncogene 1991; 6:
     2105–2111

26   Weidner U, Peter S, Strohmyer T, Hussnatter R, Ackermann R, Sies H. Inverse
     relationship of epidermal growth factor receptor and HER2 new gene in renal cell
     carcinoma. Cancer Res 1990: 50: 4504–4509

27   Mydlo JH, Michaeli J, Cordon-Cardo C, Giddenberg AS, Heston WDW, Fair WR.
     Expression of transforming growth factor of and epidermal growth factor receptor
     messenger RNA in neoplastic and non-neoplastic human kidney tissue. Cancer Res
     1989; 49: 3407–3411

28   Rafla S. Renal cell carcinoma: natural history and results of treatment. Cancer 1970; 25:
     26–40

29   Juusela H, Malmio K, Alfthan D et al. Preoperative irradiation in the treatment of renal
     adenocarcinoma. Scand J Urol Nephrol 1977; 11: 277–281

30   Kjaer M, Frederiksen PL Engelholm SA. Postoperative radiotherapy in stage II and III
     renal adenocarcinoma. A randomized trial by the Copenhagen Renal Cancer Study
     Group. Int J Radiat Oncol Biol Phys 1987; 13: 665–772

31   Possinger K, Wagner H, Beck R et al. Renal cell carcinoma. Contrib Oncol 1988; 30:
     195–207

32   World Health Organization. Handbook for reporting results of cancer treatment. Offset
     publication 48. WHO, Geneva, 1978

33   Harris DT. Hormonal therapy and chemotherapy of renal cell carcinoma. Semin Oncol
     1983; 10: 422–430

34a Hrushesky WJ, Murphy GP. Current status of the therapy of advanced renal carcinoma. J
     Clin Oncol 1977; 9: 277

34b Hrushesky WJM, von Roemeling R, Lanning M, Rabatin JT. Circadian-shaped infusions
     of floxuridine for progressive metastatic renal cell carcinoma. J Clin Oncol 1990; 8:
     1504–1513

35   Crivellari D, Tumulo S, Frusaci S et al. Phase II study of five-day continuous infusion of
     vinblastine in patients with metastatic renal cell carcinoma. Am J Clin Oncol 1987: 10:
     321

36   Elson PF, Kvols LK, Vogl SE et al. Phase II trials of 5-day vinblastine infusion (NSC
     49842), L-alanosine (NSC 153353), acivicin (NSC 163501), and aminothiadiazole (NSC
     4728) in patients with recurrent or metastatic renal cell carcinoma. Invest New Drugs
     1988; 6: 97

37   de Forges A, Droz JP, Ghosn M, Theodore C. Phase II trial of ifosfamide/mesna in

metastatic adult renal carcinoma. Cancer Treat Rep 1987; 71; 1103

38   Bodrogi I, Baki M, Sinkovics I, Eckhardt S. Ifosfamide chemotherapy of metastatic renal cell cancer. Semin Surg Oncol 1988; 4: 95

39   Licht JD, Garnick MB. Phase II trial of strepotozocin in the treatment of advanced renal cell carcinoma. Cancer Treat Rep 1986; 71: 97

40   Braich IA, Salmon SE, Robertone A et al. Phase II trial of esorubicin in cancers of the breast, colon, kidney, lung and melanoma. Invest New Drugs 1986; 4: 269

41   Stephens RL, Kirby R, Crawford ED, Bukowski R, Rivkin SE, O'Bryan RM. High dose AZQ in renal cancer. Invest New Drugs 1986; 4: 57–59

42   van Oosterom AT, Bono AV, Kaye SB et al. 4-Deoxydoxorubicin in advanced renal cancer. Eur J Cancer Clin Oncol 1987; 22: 1531

43   Elson PJ, Earhart RH, Kvols LK et al. Phase II studies of PCNU and bisantrene in advanced renal cell carcinoma. Cancer Treat Rep 1987; 71: 331

44   Shevrin DH, Lad TE, Kilton LJ et al. Phase II trial of fludarabine phosphate in advanced renal cell carcinoma: an Illinois Cancer Council study. Invest New Drugs 1989; 7: 251

45   Balducci L, Blumenstein B, Von Hoff DD et al. Evaluation of fludarabine phosphate in renal cell carcinoma: a Southwest Oncology Group study. Cancer Treat Rep 1987; 71: 543

46   Abele R, Clavel M, Dodion P et al. The EORTC early clinical trials cooperative group experience with 5-Aza-2'-deoxycytidine (NSC 127716) in patients with colo-rectal, head and neck, renal carcinomas and malignant melanomas. Eur J Cancer Clin Oncol 1987; 23: 1921

47   Tait N, Abrams J, Egorin MJ, Cohen AE, Eisenberger M, Van Echo DA. Phase II carboplatin (CBDCA) for metastatic renal cell cancer with a standard dose (SD) and a calculated dose (CD) according to renal function. Proc Am Soc Clin Oncol 1988; 7: 125

48   Droz JP, Theodore C, Ghosn M et al. Twelve-year experience with chemotherapy in adult metastatic renal cell carcinoma at the Institute Gustave-Roussy. Semin Surg Oncol 1988; 4: 97

49   Marshall ME, Taylor S, Wolf M, Flanigan R, Blumenstein B, Crawford ED. Phase II trial of echinomycin in advanced renal cell carcinoma: a Southwest Oncology Group Study. Proc Am Soc Clin Oncol 1992; 11; 637

50   Geoffrois L, Conroy T, Jubert J, Krakowski F, Guillemin F, Volff D. Circadian modified FUDR infusion in patients with metastatic renal cell cancer: a confirmatory phase II study. Proc Am Soc Clin Oncol 1991; 10: 595

51   Marsh R de W, Agaliotis D. Treatment of metastatic renal cell carcinoma with 5 FUDR circadian shaped infusion. Proc Am Soc Clin Oncol 1992; 11: 644

52   Clark JW, Cummings F, Muray C, Browne M, Beitz J, Weitberg A. Circadian varied intravenous infusional floxuridine for renal cell cancer. Proc Am Soc Clin Oncol 1992; 11: 686

53   Szumowski J, Ernstoff MS, Bahnson MS et al. Chemotherapy (vinblastine, V) and inhibitor (quinidine sulfate, Q) multi-drug resistance (MDR) in the treatment of metastatic renal cell carcinoma (RCC). Proc Am Soc Clin Oncol 1989; 8: 145

54   Glover D, Trump D, Kvols L, Elson P, Vogl S. Phase II trial of misonidazole (MISO) and cyclophosphamide (CYC) in metastatic renal cell carcinoma. Int J Radiat Oncol Biol Phys 1986; 12: 1405

55   Stewart DJ, Futter N, Irvine A, Danjoux C, Moors D. Mitomycin-C and metronidazole in the treatment of advanced renal-cell carcinoma. Am J Clin Oncol 1987; 10: 520

56   Murphy B, Rynard S, Pennington K, Grosh W, Loehrer PJ. A phase II trial of vinblastine (VLB) plus dipyridamole (DP) in advanced renal cell carcinoma (RCC): a Hoosier Oncology Group Study. Proc Am Soc Clin Oncol 1991: 10: 569

57   Stadler W, Charette J, Whitman G, Vogelzang NJ. A phase II study of 5 day continous infusion FUDR, leucovorin (LV) and high dose interferon-alpha 2b (IFN) in metastatic renal carcinoma (RC). Proc Am Soc Clin Oncol 1992; 11: 698

58   Bell DR, Aroney RS, Fisher RJ et al. High-dose methotrexate with leucovorin resue, vinblastine and bleomycin with or without tamoxifen in metastatic renal cell carcinoma. Cancer Treat Rep 1984; 68: 587

59   Merrin C, Mittleman A, Fanous A et al. Chemotherapy of advanced renal cell carcinoma with vinblastine and CCNU. J Urol 1975; 113: 21

60   Davis, TE, Manalo FB. Combination chemotherapy of advanced renal cell cancer with CCNU and vinblastine. Proc Am Soc Clin Oncol 1978; 19: 316
61   Hahn RG, Begg CB, Davis R. Phase II study of vinblastine-CCNU, triazinate, and dactinomycin in advanced renal cell cancer. Cancer Treat Rep 1981; 65: 711
62   Kuhbock J, Potzi P, Madaras T. Palliative and adjuvant chemotherapy of metastatic renal cancer. Semin Surg Oncol 1988; 4: 116
63   Fojo A, Shen DW, Mickley LA, Pastan J, Gottesman MM. Intrinsic drug resistance in human kidney cancer is associated with expression of a human multidrug-resistance gene. J Clin Oncol 1987; 5: 1922
64   Goldstein L, Galski H, Fojo A, et al. Expression of multi-drug resistance gene in human tumors. Proc Am Assoc Cancer Res 1988; 29: 298
65   Bloom HJG. Medroxyprogesterone acetate (Provera) in treatment of metastatic renal cancer. Br J Cancer 1971; 25: 250–265
66   Kjar M, Frederiksen PL. High-dose medroxyprogesterone acetate in patients with renal adenocarcinoma and measurable lung metastases: a phase II study. Cancer Treat Rep 1986; 70: 431–432
67   Ljungberg B, Tomic R, Roos G. Deoxyribonucleic acid content and medroxyprogesterone acetate treatment in metastatic renal cell carcinoma. J Urol 1989; 141: 1308
68   Weinerman BH, Eisenhauer EA, Besner JG, Coppin CM, Stewart D, Band PR. Phase II study of lonidamine in patients with metastatic renal cell carcinoma: a National Cancer Institute of Canada Clinical Trials Group study. Cancer Treat Rep 1986; 70: 751
69   Horoszewicz JS Murphy GP. An assessment of the current use of human interferons in therapy of urological cancers. J Urol 1989; 142: 1173–1180
70   Buzaid AC, Robertone A, Kisala C, Salmon SE. Phase II study of interferon alpha 2a, recombinant (Roferon A) in metastatic renal cell carcinoma. J Clin Oncol 1987; 5: 1083
71   Muss HB, Costanzi JJ, Leavitt R et al. Recombinant alfa interferon in renal cell carcinoma: a randomized trial of two routes of administration. J Clin Oncol 1987; 5: 1083
72   Figlin RA. Biotheraphy with Interferon—1988. Semin Oncol 1988; 15: 3–9
73   Torrecillas L, Erazo A, Cervantes G, Fuentes H, Rosales F. Metastatic renal cell carcinoma (RCC) treatment with interferon alfa 2b (IFN). Proc Am Soc clin Oncol 1991; 10: 549
74   Fujita T, Inagaki J, Asano H et al. Effects of low-dose interferon-alpha following nephrectomy in metastatic renal cell carcinoma. Proc Am Soc Clin Oncol 1992; 11: 685
75   Muss HB. Interferon therapy for renal cell carcinoma. Semin Oncol 1987; 14: 36–42
76   Muss HB. The role of biological response modifiers in metastatic renal cell carcinoma. Semin Oncol 1988; 15 (suppl 5): 30–34
77   Krown SE, Einzig AI, Abramson JA et al. Treatment of advanced renal cell cancer with recombinant leukocyte A interferon. Proc Am Soc Clin Oncol 1983; 2: 58
78   Quesada JR, Rios A, Swanson D et al. Antitumour activity of recombinant-derived interferon alpha in metastatic renal cell carcinoma. J Clin Oncol 1985; 3: 1522–1528
79   Umeda T, Niijima T. Phase II study of alpha interferon on renal cell carcinoma: summary of three collaborative trials. Cancer 1986; 58: 1231–1235
80   Porzolt F on behalf of the Delta-P Study Group. Adjuvant therapy of renal cell cancer (RCC) with interferon alfa-2A. Proc Am Soc Clin Oncol 1992; 11: 622
81   Porzolt F, Messerer D, Hautmann R et al. Treatment of advanced renal cell cancer with recombinant interferon alpha as a single agent and in combination with medroxyprogesterone acetate. J Cancer Res Clin Oncol 1988; 114: 95
82   Kinouchi T, Saiki S, Kuroda M et al. The treatment of metastatic renal cell carcinoma with human lymphoblastoid alpha interferon. J Jpn Soc Cancer Ther 1986; 21: 767
83   Fossa SD, Gunderson R, Moe B. Recombinant interferon-alpha combined with prednisolone in metastatic renal cell carcinoma. Reduced toxicity without reduction of the response rate—a phase II study. Cancer 1990; 65: 2451–2454
84   Bergerat JP, Ford J, Herbrecht R et al. Recombinant alpha-interferon plus vinblastine in metastatic renal-cell cancer: Analysis of response and survival in 58 evaluable patients. In: Bollack CG, Jacquim D, eds. EORTC Genitourinary Group monograph 9: basic research and treatment of renal cell carcinoma metastasis. Wiley-Liss, New York, 1990: pp 137–150

85   Ravdin P, Tuttle R, Davis TE, Trump DL. Phase I/II trial of human lymphoblastoid interferon (L-IFN), Wellferon and continuous infusion vinblastine (VBL-c i) in advanced renal cell cancer. Proc Am Soc Clin Oncol 1985: 4: 101
86   Fossa SD, de Garis ST, Heier MS et al. Recombinant inteferon alfa-2a with or without vinablastine in metastatic renal cell cancer. Cancer 1986; 57: 1700
87   Jacquim D, Bergerat JP, Dufour P et al. Metastatic renal cell carcinoma. Interferon alpha 2 and vinblastine combined therapy. Results of a series of 21 patients. J Urol 1987: 133: 329A
88   Sarna G, Figlin R, de Kernion J. Interferon in renal cell carcinoma. The UCLA experience. Cancer 1987; 59: 610
89   Neidhart J, Harris J, Tuttle R. A randomized study of Wellferon (WFN) with or without vinblastine (VBL) in advanced renal cancer. Proc Am Soc Clin Oncol 1987; 3: 153
90   Fossa SD, De Garis ST. Further experience with recombinant interferon alfa-2a with vinblastine in metastatic renal cell carcinoma: a progress report. Int J Cancer 1987; (suppl 1): 36
91   Rizzo M, Bartoletti R, Selli C, Sicignano A, Criscuolo D. Interferon alpha-2a and vinblastine in the treatment of metastatic renal cell carcinoma. Eur Urol 1989; 16: 271
92   Otto U, Bauer JW, Jager N, Wander J, Schneider E. Alpha-2 recombinant interferon treatment of metastatic renal cell cancer. Semin Surg Oncol 1988; 4: 184
93   Schornagel JH, Verweij J, ten Bokkel Huinink WW et al. Phase II study of recombinant interferon alpha-2A and vinblastine in advanced renal carcinoma. J Urol 1989; 142: 253
94   Cetto GL, Franceschi T, Turrina G et al. Recombinant alpha-inteferon and vinblastine in metastatic renal cell carcinoma: efficacy of low doses. Semin Surg Oncol 1988; 4: 184–190
95   Smalley R, Neidhart J, Harris J et al. Pulmonary metastases from renal cell carcinoma responsive to alpha interferon. Proc Am Soc Clin Oncol 1989; 8: 131
96   Fossa SD, Martinelli G, Otto U et al. Recombinant interferon alfa-2a with or without vinblastine in metastatic renal cell carcinoma: results of a European multicenter phase III study. Ann Oncol 1992: 3: 301–305
97   Creagan ET, Kovach JS, Long HJ et al. Phase I study of recombinant leukocyte A human interferon combined with BCNU in selected patients with advanced cancer. J Clin Oncol 1986; 4: 408
98   Wadler S, Einzig AI, Dutcher JP et al. Phase II trial of recombinant alpha-2b interferon and low-dose cyclophosphamide in advanced melanoma and renal cell carcinoma. Am J Clin Oncol 1988; 11: 55–59
99   Dexeus F, Logothetis C, Chong C, Sella A, Finn L. Phase III study in metastatic renal cell carcinoma (RCC) comparing combination chemotherapy (CT) versus interferon (IFN) alternating with combination chemotherapy. Proc Am Soc Clin Oncol 1988; 15: 396
100   Falcone A, Cianci C, Pfanner E, Lencioni M, Conte PF. Alfa-2b interferon (IFN) + floxuridine (FUDR): a feasible and active combination in metastatic renal carcinoma (MRC). Proc Am Soc Clin Oncol 1992; 11: 642
101   Creagan ET. Buckner JC, Hahn RG et al. An evaluation of recombinant leukocyte A interferon with aspirin in patients with metastatic renal cell cancer. Cancer 1988; 61: 1787–1791
102   de Mulder PHM, Debruyne FMJ, Beniers AJMC. Interferons in renal cell carcinoma: status and prospects. In: Bollack CG, Jacquim D eds, EORTC Genitourinary Group monograph 9: Basic research and treatment of renal cell carcinoma metastasis. Wiley-Liss, New York 1990; pp 49–59
103   Sohn M, Markos-Pusztai S, Kempeni J, Jakse G, von Broen G. Tumor necrosis factor alpha and interferon gamma or alpha: multicenter trials in metastatic renal cell carcinoma. Proc Am Soc Clin Oncol 1992; 11: 639
104   Otto U, Conrad S, Schneider AW. Combined therapy with TNF-alpha and IFN-alpha-2A in metastatic renal cell carcinoma—promising preclinical and clinical results. In: Proceedings of second international symposium on immunobiology of renal cell carcinoma, Cleveland. Saunders, Philadelphia 1991; 99
105   Steineck G, Strander H, Carbin BE et al. Recombinant leukocyte interferon alpha-2a

and medroxyprogesterone in advanced renal cell carcinoma. Acta Oncol 1990; 29: 155–162

106   Goldstein D, Laszlo J. Interferon therapy in cancer: from imaginon to interferon. Cancer Res 1986; 46: 4315–4329

107   Rosenberg SA, Lotze MT, Yang JC et al. Experience with the use of high-dose interleukin-2 in the treatment of 652 cancer patients. Ann Surg 1989; 210: 474–485

108   Abrams JS, Raynor AA, Wiernik PH et al. High-dose recombinant interleukin-2 alone: a regimen with limited activity in the treatment of advanced renal cell carcinoma. J Natl Cancer Inst 1990; 82: 1202–1206

109   Bukowski RM, Goodman P, Crawford ED, Serji JS, Redman BG, Whitehead RP. Phase II trial of high-dose intermittent interleukin-2 in metastatic renal cell carcinoma: a Southwest Oncology Group study. J Natl Cancer 1990; 82: 143–146

110   Poo WI, Fynan T, Davis C, Flynn S, Durivage H, Todd M. High-dose recombinant interleukin-2 alone in patients with metastatic renal cell carcinoma. Proc Am Soc Clin Oncol 1991; 10: 557

111   Escudier B, Rossi JF, Ravaud A et al. French experience of high dose IL-2 on a two-days a week schedule in metastatic renal cell carcinoma: a multicentric study. Proc Am Soc Clin Oncol 1992; 11: 651

112   Negrier S, Philip T, Stoter G et al. Interleukin-2 with or without LAK cells in metastatic renal cell carcinoma: a report of a European multicentre study. Eur J Cancer Clin Oncol 1989; 25 (suppl 3): S21–S28

113   Galligioni E, Sorio R, Quala M et al. Clinical aspects of treatment with recombinant interleukin-2 in metastatic renal cell cancer: experience of the comprehensive cancer center, Aviano, Italy. Insights Immunother 1990; 1: 37–40

114   von der Masse H, Geertsen P, Thatcher N et al. Recombinant Interleukin-2 in metastatic renal cell carcinoma—a European multicentre phase II study. Eur J Cancer 1991; 27: 1503–1509

115   Fisher RI, Coltman CA, Doroshow JH et al. Metastatic renal cancer treated with interleukin-2 and lymfokine-activated killer cells. A phase II clinical trial. Ann Intern Med 1988; 108: 518

116   West WH. Continuous infusion recombinant interleukin-2 in adoptive cellular therapy of renal carcinoma and other malignancies. Cancer Treat Rev 1989; 16 (suppl A): 83–89

117   Gaynor ER Weiss GR, Margolin KA et al. Phase I study of high dose continuous-infusion recombinant interleukin-2 and autologous lymphokine-activated killer cells in patients with metastatic or unresectable malignant melanoma and renal cell carcinoma. J Natl Cancer 1990: 82: 1397–1402

118   Parkinson DR, Fisher RI, Rayner AA et al. Therapy of renal cell carcinoma with interleukin-2 and lymphokine-activated killer cells: phase II experience with a hybrid bolus and continuous infusion interleukin-2 regimen. J Clin Oncol 1990; 8(10): 1630–1636

119   Thompson A, Shulman K, Benyunes M et al. Prolonged continuous intravenous infusion interleukin-2 and lymphokine-activated killer cell therapy for metastatic renal cell carcinoma. Proc Am Soc Clin Oncol 1992; 11: 824

120   McCabe MS, Stablein D, Hawkins MH. The modified group C experience—phase III randomized trials of IL-2 vs IL-2/LAK in advanced renal cell carcinoma and advanced melanoma. Proc Am Soc Clin Oncol 1991: 10: 714

121   Weiss GR, Margolin K, Aronson FR et al. A randomized phase II trial of continuous infusion (CI) interleukin-2 (IL-2) or bolus injection (BI) IL-2 plus lymphokine-activated killer cells (LAK) for advanced renal cell carcinoma. Proc Am Soc Clin Oncol 1989; 8: 509

122   Margolin KA, Rayner AA, Hawkins MJ et al. Interleukin-2 and lymphokine-activated killer cell therapy of solid tumors: analysis of toxicity and management guidelines. J Clin Oncol 1989; 7: 486–498

123   Bradley EC, Louie AC, Paradise CM et al. Antitumor response in patients with metastatic renal cell carcinoma is dependent upon regimen intensity. Proc Am Soc Clin Oncol 1989; 8: 519

124   Sosman J, Fisher RI, Weiss G et al. Phase 1A/1B trial of anti-CD3 monoclonal antibody with high dose IL-2 in renal cell and melanoma. Proc Am Soc Clin Oncol

1992; 11: 826

125 Marshall ME, Butler K, Dickson L, Phillips B, McConnell W, Macdonald JS. Treatment of metastatic renal cell carcinoma with "low dose" interleukin-2 and lymphokine-activated killer cells. Proc Am Soc Clin Oncol 1989; 8: 525

126 Sleijfer D, Janssen R, Willemse P et al. Subcutaneous (s.c.) interleukin-2 (il-2) (Cetus) in patients (pts) with metastatic renal cell cancer (RCC). Proc Am Soc Clin Oncol 1991; 10: 517

127 Gore ME, Galligioni E, Keen CW et al. The treatment of metastatic renal cell carcinoma by cutaneous infusion of recombinant interleukin 2. 1993 submitted

128 Hanson J, Petit R, Walker M et al. Tumor infiltrating lymphocyte (TIL) therapy for metastatic renal cancer (RC) using interleukin-2 (IL-2). Proc Am Soc Clin Oncol 1992: 11: 682

129 Wang JCL, Walle A, Novogrodsky A et al. A Phase II clinical trial of adoptive immunotherapy for advanced renal cell carcinoma using mitogen-activated autologous leukocytes and continuous infusion interleukin-2. J Clin Oncol 1989; 7: 1885–1891

130 Bernstein ZP, Walther PJ, Vaickus L et al. Treatment of renal cell carcinoma with interleukin-2 (IL-2) and pheylalanine methyl ester (PME) pretreated lymphokine activated killer cells (LAK). Proc Am Soc Clin Oncol 1991; 10: 587

131 Rosenberg SA, Lotze MT, Yang JC et al. Combination therapy with interleukin-2 and alpha-interferon for the treatment of patients with advanced cancer. J Clin Oncol 1989; 7: 1863–1874

132 Hirsh M, Lipton A, Harvey H et al. Phase I study of interleukin-2 and interferon alpha-2 as outpatient therapy for patients with advanced malignancy. J Clin Oncol 1990; 8: 1657–1663

133 Bergmann L, Frenchel K, Enzinger HM Weidmann E, Jahn B, Mitrou PS. Daily alternating schedule with interferon-alpha and interleukin-2 in advanced renal cell cancer—clinical results and biological effects. Eur J Cancer 1991; (suppl 2); 584

134 Pichert G, Jost LM, Fierz W, Stahel RA. Clinical and immune modulatory effects of alternative weekly interleukin-2 and interferon alpha-2a in patients with advanced renal cell carcinoma and melanoma. Br J Cancer 1991; 63: 287–292

135 Atzpodien J, Korfer A, Menzel T, Poliwoda H, Kirchner H. Home therapy using recombinant human IL-2 and IFN-alpha2b in patients with metastatic renal cell carcinoma. Proc Am Soc Clin Oncol 1991; 10: 571

136 Demchak P, Atkins M, Sell K, Givant E, Lipton A. Phase II study of interleukin 2 (IL-2) and interferon-2α (IFNα) outpatient therapy for metastatic renal cell cancer (RCC). Proc Am Soc Clin Oncol 1991; 10: 565

137 Figlin RA, Belldegrun A, deKernion J. Recombinant interleukin-2 and interferon alpha: an active outpatient regimen in metastatic renal cell carcinoma. Proceedings of 2nd International Symposium on Immunobiology of renal cell carcinoma, Cleveland, Saunders, Philadelphia, 1991; 81.

138 Atkins M, Sell K, Givant E, Lipton A. Phase II study of interleukin-2 and interferon alpha-2a outpatient therapy for metastatic renal cancer. Proc Am Soc Clin Oncol 1991; 10: 565

139 Lindemann A, Hoeffken K, Schmidt RE et al. A multicenter trial of interleukin-2 and low-dose cyclophosphamide in highly chemotherapy-resistant malignancies. Cancer Treat 1989; 16 (suppl A): 53–57

140 Krigel RL, Padavic-Shaller KA, Rudolph AR, Konrad M, Bradley EC. Renal cell carcinoma: treatment with recombinant interleukin-2 plus beta-interferon. J Clin Oncol 1990: 8: 460–467

141 Wersall JP, Masucci G, Froden JE, Mellstedt H. Low dose cyclophosphamide, alpha-interferon and continuous infusions of r-IL-2 in kidney cancer. A phase II clinical study. ECCO-6. Eur J Cancer 1991; (suppl 2): 581

142 Escudier B, Farace F, Droz JP et al. Lymphokine activated natural killer cells may induce shift from partial into complete response in metastatic renal cell carcinoma: an hypothesis. Proc Am Soc Clin Oncol 1991; 10: 527

143 Bramwell VHC, Mertens WC, Lala PK. Continuous oral indomethacin and ranitidine and continuous venous infusion interleukin-2 in advanced renal carcinoma. Proc Am Soc Clin Oncol 1991; 10: 546

144 Pinto HA, Yahanda A, Reese J et al. Chemoimmunotherapy with recombinant

interleukin-2 and vinblastine in metastatic renal cell carcinoma. Proc Am Soc Clin Oncol 1991; 10: 579

145   Markowitz A, Parkinson D, Itoh K et al. Phase 1B study of tumour infiltrating lymphocytes combined with recominant interferon alpha2A and cyclophospamide in patients with advanced renal cell carcinoma (RCC) and malignant melanoma. Proc Am Soc Clin Oncol 1991; 10: 726

146   Fink KI, Valone FH, Myers FJ, Zukiwski AA, Louie AC, Aronson FR. Interleukin-2 and vinblastine for advanced renal cell carcinoma: a phase I-II study. Proc Am Soc Clin Oncol 1992; 11: 664

147   Marshall ME, Mendelsohn L, Butler K et al. Treatment of metastatic renal cell carcinoma with coumarin (1, 2-bendzopyrone) and cimetidine: a pilot study. J Clin Oncol 1987; 5: 862

148   Dexeus FH, Logothetis CJ, Sella A et al. Phase II study of coumarin and cimetidine in patients with metastatic renal cell carcinoma. J Clin Oncol 1990; 8: 325–330

149   Hermann R, Egri T, Manegold C, Matthiesen W. Coumarin and cimetidine in the treatment of metastatic renal cell carcinoma. Proc Am Soc Clin Oncol 1988; 7: 131

150   Inhorn L, Pennington K, Miller M et al. Phase II study of high dose cimetidine in renal cell carcinoma: a trial of the Hoosier Oncology Gorup (HOG). Proc Am Soc Clin Oncol 1989; 8: 148

151   Osband ME, Lavin PT, Babayan RK et al. Effect of autolymphocyte therapy on survival and quality of life in patients with metastatic renal-cell carcinoma. Lancet 1990; 335: 994–998

152   McCune CS. Cytokines as possible adjuvants to vaccines in active specific immunotherapy for renal cell carcinoma. In: Staehler G, Pomer S, eds Basic and clinical research on renal cell carcinoma. Springer-Verlag, Berlin, 1992: pp 189–199

153   Scharfe T, Muller S, Riedmiller H, Jacobi GH, Hohenfellner R. Immunotherapy of metastasizing renal cell carcinoma: results of multicentered trial. Urol Int 1989: 44: 1

154   Ross S, Osband M, Kane R, Laun P. Prolonged survival in patients with metastatic renal cell carcinoma (RCC) treated with autolymphocyte therapy (ALT): a low toxicity, outpatient approach to adoptive immunotherapy without interleukin-2. Proc Am Soc Clin Oncol 1989; 8: 142

7

Orthotopic bladder substitutes

M. A. Ghoneim

Attempts to create a sphincter-controlled bladder substitute began at the turn of this century. One of the earliest trials was by Tizzoni & Foggi in 1888.[1] Operating on a dog, a loop of intestine was isolated. One month later, the ureters were transplanted into this blind loop which in turn was sutured to the neck of the bladder. The history of these early experiments was recently reviewed by Studer et al.[2]

With a better understanding of intestinal physiology, the implications of incorporation of segments of intestine in the urinary tract and increasing knowledge of the anatomical and urodynamic aspects of urinary continence, there has been a revived interest on behalf of urologists to re-explore, modify and optimize the surgical techniques employed for orthotopic bladder substitution.

BACKGROUND

A wide range of procedures involving almost all segments of the gastrointestinal tract in different configurations has been utilized. A critical review of these techniques is necessary to find our way through this maze and establish some principles based on physiological and urodynamic principles for proper selection of the bowel segment, its length and configuration.

The stomach

The use of a gastric segment to augment or replace the bladder was first described by Leong & Ong.[3] These authors used the pyloric antrum based on the left gastroepiploic artery. Later, Adams et al[4] utilized a gastric wedge based on the right gastroepiploic vessels. The isolated wedge is cross-folded and anastomosed to the urethra. The ureters were implanted by a submucous tunnel.

The advantages advocated for the use of a gastric segment include a minimal production of mucous and a reduced incidence of infection[5] The stomach segment seems to be quite satisfactory in terms of providing a compliant low-pressure system.[4] In addition, gastric tissue has an excellent

103

muscle backing which allows a submucous tunnelled implantation of the ureter.

The ileum

The ileum was the earliest and currently is the most frequently employed segment for construction of an orthotopic bladder substitute. Couvelaire,[6] in 1951, reported the first clinical attempt for creation of a functional bladder from a segment of ileum and demonstrated its clinical feasibility. The same surgical principle was tried later by several investigators.[7-11] Credit however remains for Camey, who worked for 25 years with patience and perseverance to modify and refine the original technique.[12] His method (currently known as Camey I procedure) entails isolation of a 40 cm long segment of ileum. The ends of the loop are closed and the mid-point of the antimesenteric border anastomosed to the urethral stump. The ureters are implanted by an antireflux technique originally proposed by Le-Duc et al.[13] Deklerk and coworkers[14] modified the procedure by incision of the antimesenteric border of the isolated segment and suturing the medial margins together to form a U-shaped reservoir (currently known as Camey II). A common feature of all of these procedures was nocturnal enuresis in the majority of cases. The explanation was later provided by Roehrborn et al,[15] who noted that tubular-shaped ileal reservoirs maintained their physiological contraction waves which can reach an amplitude of greater than 50 cm water and overcome the urethral resistance at night, causing enuresis.

Parallel with these developments, and following extensive laboratory experiments and clinical trials, Kock and associates[16] presented a new form of urinary diversion with a continent cutaneous stoma. By splitting the intestine at its antimesenteric border and folding the intestinal plate twice, a low-pressure highly compliant reservoir was formed. Two intussusception valves were fashioned to provide an antireflux mechanism and a continent stoma. The recognition of these principles had overcome many of the functional problems which were previously encountered and set the stage for the birth of the many surgical procedures which are currently in vogue.[17-21]

The ileocaecal region and the ascending colon

The ileocaecal region was first utilized for urine diversion by Verhoogen in 1908.[22] It was not until 1965 that Gil-Vernet reported its use as a bladder substitute.[23] In a series of 130 patients, Khafagy and coworkers[24] in 1987 reported that day and night continence could only be achieved among 7% of their patients. A study of the dynamic characteristics of this segment could explain the cause of this problem. Spontaneous bowel contractions with a mean maximum pressure of 90 cm water and lasting for a mean of 60 s were recorded by Light.[25] Similar observations were also noted by other investigators.[26,27] To overcome this functional problem, the procedure has been modified by patching the caecum with a segment of ileum.[28-30]

Alternatively, Goldwasser & Benson[31] in 1986 utilized the caecum and ascending colon. The segment was longitudinally incised, folded and sutured horizontally. The reconfigurated segment was then anastomosed to the urethral stump.

The sigmoid colon

The sigmoid colon as well was used for bladder substitution by Gil-Vernet,[32] Deleveliotis & Macris[33] and Kuss and coworkers.[34] Reddy et al[35] reported their experience in 10 patients in whom this procedure was utilized. All the 7 patients who were free from disease were incontinent at night. In a recent publication, the same authors modified their procedure by detubularization and folding of the isolated sigmoid to improve its compliance.[36]

The rectum

Lemoine[37] in 1913 was the first to describe the utilization of an isolated rectal pouch joined to the posterior urethra for bladder substitution. Farah & Rifaat[38] in 1977 isolated a segment of rectum and re-established the continuity of the intestinal tract by the technique of low anterior resection. The isolated rectum was anastomosed to the urethra through a perineal urethrostomy. This approach did not gain popularity apparently due to its technical complexity.

THE CHOICE

The multiplicity of the available procedures renders the choice of an ideal or nearly ideal operation difficult. Each group of investigators advocate certain advantages for the procedure of their choice. The problem is compounded by the fact that many of these techniques were christened with the name of an institute, town or even a state. Objectivity is thus often subdued for reasons of personal or national pride. In order to establish certain selection criteria with some degree of objectivity certain issues have certainly to be addressed:

1. What is the most suitable segment of bowel for utilization as a bladder substitute?
2. What is its optimal length and configuration?
3. Should an antireflux system be provided, and by what means?

Choice of the segment of bowel

Again, for proper selection of a given segment of bowel, an inquiry into the following issues should be made:

1. What are the consequences of its exclusion from the gastrointestinal tract?
2. What are the consequences of its incorporation in the urinary tract?
3. Would it provide a compliant neobladder with an adequate capacity at low pressure?
4. What are the potentials for the future development of tumours?

Resection of parts of the stomach can lead to a dumping syndrome due to jejunal distension. A hypokalaemic, hypochloraemic metabolic alkalosis can occur.[39] Decreased excretion of the intrinsic factor results in a decreased absorption of vitamin B_{12} with consequent development of a megaloblastic anaemia. However, the most potentially serious problem is chemical urethritis and ulcerations in the neobladder or in the residual stomach itself as a result of increased gastrin production. Gastrin is produced in response to the mechanical stretching of the bladder substitute or by local chemical stimulation. Experimental studies have demonstrated increased serum levels of gastrin when portions of the stomach have been used for urinary reconstruction.[40] Patients may require long-term therapy with an H_2-blocker (cimetidine) or a proton blocker (omeprazole).[41] Accordingly, the technique is only suitable for children with acidosis who require a reconstruction or substitution of their bladder. One wonders what would happen if the patient become anuric or oliguric while the stomach patch was continuing to secrete acid in the bladder—an unmitigated disaster.

To our knowledge, the use of a jejunal segment to construct a bladder substitute has not been reported. Resection of jejunal segments should not be associated with malabsorption problems. Nevertheless, the expected severe metabolic consequences resulting from its incorporation in the urinary tract deter attempts at its use. Although they require a much shorter length of bowel, jejunal urinary conduits are infrequently used. The large jejunal surface (tall villi) loses large amounts of sodium chloride, leading to a severe hypochloraemic acidosis, hyponatraemia and hyperkalaemia.[42]

The ileum is the sole site for absorption of bile acids and vitamin B_{12}. In addition it impedes the intestinal transit time to allow greater absorption of water and electrolytes. The potential risks of malabsorption following resection of ileum depend on the length of the resected segment and the integrity of the ileocaecal valve.[43] Evidence has been provided that resection of an ileal segment measuring up to 60 cm is without significant sequelae among patients with a normal terminal ileum and an intact ileocaecal valve. The absorption of bile acids is reduced but compensated for by an increased production by the liver. In addition, there is experimental and clinical evidence that the absorptive power improves with time after resection of ileum as a function of an increase in the number of absorptive cells per unit length.[44] Resection of longer segments of ileum may be associated with diarrhoea due to the increased amount of bile acids reaching the colon. The loss of bile acids exceeds the increased production by the liver, resulting in impaired absorption of lipids and fat-soluble vitamins. A concomitant resection of the ileocaecal valve aggravates the condition due to a short contact time and bacterial overgrowth in the terminal ileum. Clinically, patients develop malabsorption, steatorrhoea and vitamin B_{12} deficiency.[45]

The main function of the colon is to absorb sodium actively with water following passively. The total absorptive capacity of a normal colon is 5–6 l/day. Resection of a considerable length of colon is possible without significant problems as long as the ileocaecal region and the right colon remain intact. The more distal the resected area, the better is the tolerance.

The incorporation of ileum or colon within the urinary tract can lead to metabolic acidosis secondary to active absorption of urinary constituents, particularly chlorides. The active and passive transport systems for reabsorption are similar among the ileum and colon but are much more efficient in the latter.[46] Bony demineralization can complicate the state of metabolic acidosis[47,48]—a problem of special concern in children and women. A strong correlation exists between the length of bowel used for bladder substitution and the incidence of postoperative metabolic acidosis. In a study by Studer and associates,[49] none of their patients in whom a pouch was constructed from a length of ileum of 40 cm or less developed acidosis. Furthermore, following exposure of the ileal mucosa to urine, the height of the villi and absorptive capacity is reduced with time.[50,51] Evidence has also been provided that the rate of reabsorption of chlorides correlates with the process of villous atrophy.[52] These changes are a unique property of the ileum and were not observed when the colon was similarly exposed to the urinary stream.[53] This may provide an explanation for the several studies which demonstrated that when comparable amounts of ileum and colon were used there was a greater risk of metabolic disorders with the colonic segments.[52,54,55]

The precise risk of malignancy in intestinal segments used for urinary reconstruction is not known. The risk of developing colonic tumours following ureterosigmoidostomy ranges between 5 and 40%, with a latent period of approximately 20 years.[56] The pathogenesis for the development of such tumours appears to be multifactorial. The pioneering animal work of Crissey and associates[57] had shed light on some of the involved mechanisms. Shands and coworkers had provided evidence that the presence of a faecal stream is not a prerequisite for tumour formation.[58] Filmer & Spencer reported 14 tumours following cystoplasty and 9 following conduit diversion.[59] Of the cystoplasty cases, 9 were in an ileocystoplasty, 3 in a colocystoplasty and 2 in a caecocystoplasty. Of the conduit cases, 3 were in an ileal and 3 in a colonic conduit. Clinical data regarding ureterosigmoidostomy and urinary augmentations seem to indicate that proliferative instability at the urointestinal anastomotic line is an important factor in tumour initiation. Consequently all forms of continent diversion regardless of the segment of bowel utilized are at risk. However one should consider that the incidence of adenocarcinoma of the ileum is less than 2% that of the colon. Furthermore, the incidence of colorectal cancer in the USA is 6%, and 25% of these develop in the sigmoid.[59] One can contemplate that with ileal segments the probability of tumorgenesis is less than that of the colon, with the sigmoid particularly at high risk.

Compliance is defined as the change in volume as a function of a change in pressure.[60] The bowel wall is viscoelastic. Elasticity allows lengthening in response to stretch. Viscosity delays recovering following stretch. The stronger-walled colon, at least initially, is less compliant than the ileum.[61] In addition, while both ileum and colon exhibit tonal basal activity with superimposed segmental contractions, the latter, especially with stimuli, exhibits the so-called mass contractions seen after substitution with intact colon. The superiority of the urodynamic characteristics of ileum over those of the colon has been observed in several clinical reports. Berglund and associates[62] demonstrated the superiority of ileal versus caecal reservoirs. Lytton & Green[63] reported that ileal reservoirs can accommodate larger volume at a lower pressure when compared to those derived from the right colon. Davidsson et al[64] compared the urodynamic characteristics of the neobladders derived from the ileum and the right colon. Although the volume capacity was the same, the pressure at maximum capacity was much lower with ileal reservoirs.

Considering all the above-mentioned data and outlined issues, I favour the use of an ileal segment for construction of an orthotopic bladder substitute. The sigmoid is a viable second alternative but one should consider the higher probability of tumorigenesis. Furthermore, the sigmoid could be the seat of several pathological disorders—ulcerative colitis, diverticulosis and schistosomiasis—which limit its utilization.

The optimal length and configuration

Choosing a length of ileum is a balance between two factors: it should provide a future reservoir with an adequate capacity, yet its exclusion from the gastrointestinal tract and/or incorporation in the urinary system should not be associated with untoward side-effects. A length of approximately 40 cm of terminal ileum would satisfy both requirements.[49] It can provide a reservoir with an adequate capacity provided it has been fashioned in a proper configuration. Its exclusion from the gastrointestinal system would not be associated with problems of malabsorption provided the rest of the intestine is healthy and the ileocaecal valve is intact. Its incorporation within the urinary system should not be complicated by metabolic acidosis requiring therapy.

The necessity for detubularization and reconfiguration of the isolated segment has been clearly outlined by Hinman[61] on a mathematical basis. The configuration of the neobladder should take advantage of the geometric fact that volume increases by the square radius. Accordingly, spherical or near spherical pouches have a larger capacity. These can accommodate to filling more readily because, as Laplace's law states, the container with the greater radius and thus a greater mural tension will hold larger volumes at lower pressure. The contractile ability is blunted by the failure of segmental contractions to encompass the entire circumference. The more complex the folds of the bowel segment, the more blunted is the pressure increase. These theoretical considerations were supported by experimental data[65,66] as well as by many clinical investigations.[17,49,67,68] The best possible configuration that can meet the above mentioned criteria is by splitting the bowel and double folding (Kock[69]) or by rearrangement of the isolated segment in a W configuration (Hautmann[70]). It was calculated that if a 40 cm loop of ileum is constructed in a Kock's fashion, it would yield a reservoir of 500–700 ml in capacity at a pressure less than 40 cm water.[49,68] Our own experience, as well as that of Skinner, supports these calculations in the clinical setting.[20,71]

The necessity and technique of reflux prevention

The importance of incorporation of an antireflux mechanism with orthotopic bladder substitutes does not need any emphasis. These systems are frequently infected at least initially and regurgitation of their contents could be deleterious to renal function. Furthermore, absence of reflux allows progressive enlargement and maturation of the pouch, otherwise it would remain small in size with a limited capacity.[71] Several operative techniques were utilized for reflux prevention. The creation of an intussuscepted nipple valve was first described by Perl in 1949.[72] To improve the stability of the valve, Kock and associates applied diathermy coagulation to the serosal surface and used non-absorbable sutures.[73] However, eversion and dessusception were frequent complications. Kock and coworkers believed that this was due to traction by the bulk of the mesentery of the intussuscepted ileum. Accordingly, the technique was modified by defattening of the mesentery and by stapling of the nipple rather than using non-absorbable sutures.[16] An additional row of staples was also applied to anchor the nipple to the wall of the pouch, providing enhanced stability. Creation of a window in the mesentery opposite the intussusception would prevent any traction and add further stability to the nipple. This additional refinement was proposed by Skinner and associates[67] on the basis of a method originally described by Hendren.[74]

Several methods were described to create intussuscepted valves without the use of a stapling technique. Melchior and associates[75] utilized an antiperistaltic nipple valve, fixed in place by transmural sutures. The ureters were pulled through the intussusception and anastomosed to the mucosa of the bowel. Human fibrin was used to glue the adventitia of the ureters and the serosa of the intussuscepted bowel. Atta[76] made a full circumferential incision in both nipple layers except for the mesenteric border down to the mucosa of the inner layer. The seromuscular layers on each side of the incision are then closed. The author reported his experience in 6 cases with good outcome. It must be stated, however, that a long follow-up of a large number of cases for these methods has yet to be reported.

Creation of a mucosal sulcus in which the ureter is embedded, as described by Le-Duc and associates,[13] appears an attractive alternative in view of its technical simplicity and the possibility of using a shorter segment of bowel. Furthermore, the use of stapling is not required. Critical evaluation of the published data and our own results indicates that the procedure has a complication rate of the order of 20–30%.[13,19,77–79] Catalona[79] maintains that the incidence of reflux following this technique is much less if a large-capacity low-pressure system is utilized. The unpredictable results following this technique may be attributed to the irregular and often delayed creeping of the intestinal mucosa to cover the bare ureter. Ureteric adventitia exposed to urine may be the seat of inflammatory reaction with subsequent scarring. It is of interest to note that when the intestinal mucosa was sutured in front of the embedded ureter, the complication rate was significantly reduced.[68]

Studer and associates[80] proposed the utilization of a long afferent loop for reflux prevention. On the basis of a controlled study, they maintained that the functional results are comparable to those with an intussuscepted valve. However, it may be argued that the fate of this segment in the long run has yet to be determined. Previous experience with replacement of the ureter by ileum indicates that such a segment may undergo dilatation and become non-propulsive.[81,82]

In summary, an isoperistaltic intussuscepted nipple valve into which the spatulated ureters are implanted by an end-to-side anastomosis appears to yield the best long-term functional results, at least in our hands. This could be achieved with a high degree of reliability if the above-mentioned technical modifications were strictly observed.

INDICATIONS AND LIMITATIONS OF ORTHOTOPIC BLADDER SUBSTITUTES

The main indication for bladder substitution is after cystectomy for cancer. The extent of the operation should remain a radical cystoprostatectomy and should not be compromised in favour of a bladder substitute. It could legitimately be argued that the urethra may be the site of future recurrence or development of a new tumour. The reported risks of urethral recurrence after radical cystectomy vary between 4 and 18% and the time lag averages 3 years (1–11 years).[83] According to Schellhammer & Whitmore,[84] premalignant changes were observed in 5% of urethras removed prophylactically with cystectomy. On the other hand, the retained urethra was the site of malignancy in 7% of 348 patients who underwent cystectomy only. Recently, Hardeman & Soloway[85] reported urethral recurrence in 37% of patients with tumour in the prostate, compared to only 4% in those with all other types of tumour involvement exclusive of disease in the prostate. Accordingly, in transitional cell carcinoma of the bladder, prophylactic urethrectomy should be carried out only in a high-risk subpopulation of patients. These include tumours infiltrating the prostate, carcinoma-in-situ of the prostatic urethra or multifocal tumours involving the upper tract. Assessment of candidates for orthotopic substitution should include mucosal cup biopsies from the prostatic urethra and deep transurethral resection biopsies of the prostate if the primary tumour involves the trigone. With squamous cell carcinoma of the bladder, the risk is minimal. In a study by Khafagy et al[86] the trigone was involved in only 2.3% of their cases. The investigators could not demonstrate carcinoma-in-situ of the prostatic urethra in any of the 86 studied specimens. When these criteria are well-observed, the risk of developing a urethral recurrence should be in the order of 2%.[68,87,88]

Traditionally, radical cystectomy in the female includes a urethrectomy as well. Consequently, orthotopic substitution was considered unsuitable for female patients. Nevertheless, Holmes et al[89] reported the utilization of the procedure in 4 female patients following subtotal cystectomy for carcinoma of the bladder. This development should be of interest since the introduction of neoadjuvant chemotherapy may allow the employment of such procedures in the future more frequently. A different concept for functional bladder replacement in the female after cystectomy was recently tried in an experimental investigation by Hubner et al[90]. This involves the utilization of the caecoappendicular junction as a neobladder neck and the vermiform appendix as a neourethra.

Orthotopic bladder substitutes may also be used for complete functional reconstruction of incontinent epispadias or exstrophy. The initial idea was proposed by Arap and associates.[91] The whole of the bladder remnant is utilized to construct a musculoelastic tube 5–6 cm in length that would act as the future sphincter mechanism. An isolated segment of bowel is then anastomosed to the urethral tube to function as a reservoir. This idea was later modified and optimized by others.[92,93]

Refluxing contracted bladder resulting from interstitial cystitis, tuberculosis and bilharziasis can also be successfully treated by subtotal cystectomy and orthotopic substitution.

AN EXPERIENCE WITH ORTHOTOPIC BLADDER SUBSTITUTE USING A HEMI-KOCK'S POUCH

The patients

We have been using a hemi-Kock's pouch for orthotopic substitution since 1986. So far, 280 such cases have been carried out in our institute. The material included 269 males, 6 females and 5 children. The indications are outlined in Table 7.1.

Table 7.1 Indications for orthotopic bladder substitution

	Number of patients
Bladder cancer	241
Contracted bladder	31
Bladder exstrophy	5
Extensive bladder leukoplakia	2
Complicated vesicovaginal fistula	1
Total	280

The cystectomy

A standard radical cystoprostatectomy is carried out.[94] However, the final stages of the operation have to be carried out carefully with attention to detail in order to avoid damage to the urethra and periurethral musculature. The integrity of these structures plays a central role in the functional success of orthotopic substitution. The reader's attention is directed to anatomical contributions that shed light on the precise anatomy, innervation and components of the distal urethral sphincter.[95,96]

Following the lymphadenectomy and control of the pedicles, the endopelvic fascia on either side of the prostate is opened by the tip of a blunt pair of scissors. A right-angled clamp is used to lift the fascia from the underlying venous plexus and then it is further incised medially until the puboprostatic ligaments are reached. These ligaments are carefully severed at the point of their insertion in the pubic bone. The prostatic venous plexus is controlled by one or two suture ligatures of 3/0 polyglactin acid just distal to the vesicoprostatic junction. A transverse incision is made proximal to these sutures and extended by sharp dissection with scissors towards the apex of the prostate. The catheter is palpated in the urethra, the anterior wall of which is then incised just distal to the prostatic apex. The exposed Foley's catheter is transected, and held for traction. At this point three stay sutures of 4/0 polyglactin acid are placed through the urethra at the 3, 9 and 12 o'clock positions, incorporating the mucosa as well as the periurethral musculature. These prevent retraction of the urethra following its complete transection and can be used later for the urethroileal anastomosis. The posterior urethral wall is then incised to expose the dorsal fibrous raphe formed by the fascia of Denonvillier. This is lifted from the anterior surface of the rectum by a right-angled clamp and divided. The divided fascia is then included in two posterior stay sutures at the 5 and 7 o'clock positions for its later incorporation in the urethrointestinal anastomosis. According to Klein,[97] this step results in early regain of continence postoperatively.

The intestinal pouch

A 45–50 cm long segment is isolated from the distal ileum. The continuity of the bowel is re-established by an end-to-end anastomosis. The proximal

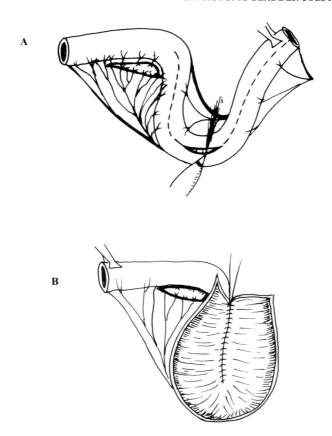

Fig. 7.1 (**A**) A 45 cm long loop of ileum is isolated. The antimesenteric border of the distal two-thirds is incised by diathermy. The proximal one-third will be used for construction of the reflux-preventing valve. (**B**) The opened intestine is folded into a U-shaped configuration. Adjacent sides of the U are joined by continuous 3/0 polyglactin acid.

third of the isolated segment is preserved for construction of the reflux-preventing valve and the inlet of the reservoir. The distal two-thirds are used for the formation of the pouch (Fig. 7.1a). The antimesenteric border of the distal two-thirds of the isolated segment is opened by electrocautery. The opened intestine is folded into a U-shaped configuration with its convexity towards the left side of the patient. The adjacent sides of the U are then united by continuous 3/0 polyglactin acid sutures (Fig. 7.1b). This is followed by construction of the reflux-preventing valve from the intact afferent segment. This is a critical step in the operation and must be done carefully with attention to detail to avoid subsequent deintussusception. An 8–10 cm long window is created in the mesentery of the segment destined for intussusception. The bowel wall is grasped through its opened lumen and is intussus-

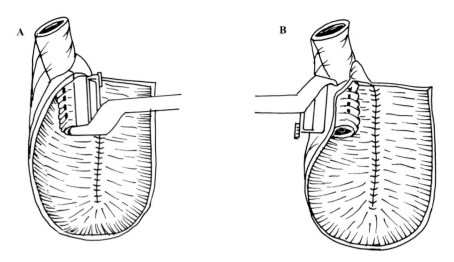

Fig. 7.2 (**A**) A 5 cm nipple valve is constructed from the intact proximal segment. The intussuscepted position is maintained by three rows of staples. (**B**) The position of the stapler is then reversed and an additional row is applied to fix the valve to the wall of the pouch.

cepted to form a 5 cm long nipple valve. The intussuscepted position is maintained by two to three rows of 4.8 mm staples (Fig. 7.2a). As recommended by Skinner and associates,[67] the staples that ordinarily would be placed near the tips of the nipple are removed to reduce the incidence of stone formation.

The position of the stapler is now reversed and an additional row is applied to fix the valve to the wall of the pouch (Fig. 7.2b). The intussuscepted position is further secured by the application of interrupted 3/0 polyglactin acid seromuscular sutures at the base of the valve. The intestinal plate then is folded up and the reservoir is closed with a layer of continuous inverting 3/0 polyglactin acid sutures (Fig. 7.3a). The corners of the pouch are then pushed downwards between the mesenteric leaves so that the posterior aspect of the reservoir is brought anteriorly (Fig. 7.3b). This manoeuvre changes the configuration of the pouch and provides several distinct advantages. It allows the pouch to be positioned in the pelvis with the apex facing the urethral stump. Furthermore, the position of the open end of the inlet becomes cranial, facilitating its anastomosis to the ureters (Fig. 7.4).

The suture line of the most dependent portion of the pouch in close proximity to the urethral stump is reopened for a distance of 2 cm. The security of the suture line is maintained by 2 interrupted sutures at both ends of the aperture. The urethral stump is anastomosed to the thus-created hole, using interrupted 4/0 polyglactin acid sutures. After the posterior row of sutures has been applied, a balloon catheter is inserted through the urethra and into the pouch. The anterior sutures are then applied using the stay

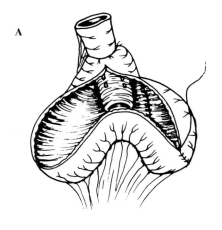

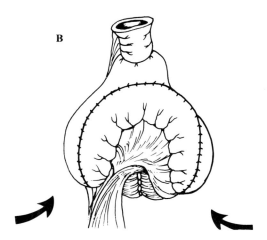

Fig. 7.3 **(A)** The intestinal plate is folded up and the reservoir closed. **(B)** Corners of the pouch are pushed downwards between the mesenteric leaves.

sutures, which were already holding the urethral stump. Finally, a stented end-to-side anastomosis is performed between the spatulated ends of the ureters and the inlet of the pouch. Two tube drains are placed in the pelvic cavity and brought out through separate incisions in the abdominal wall. Gravity drainage only is used. Intravenous alimentation is necessary until normal bowel functions are resumed. Prophylactic antibiotics are routinely administered. The tube drains are removed once fluid drainage has ceased. The urethral catheter is retained for 3 weeks.

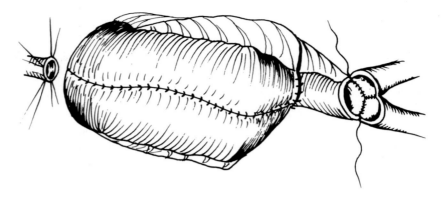

Fig. 7.4 Final configuration of the reservoir, with its apex facing the urethral stump and its inlet facing the ureters.

EVALUATION

Postoperative mortality and morbidity

In spite of the complex nature of the procedure and the length of time required to carry out a one-stage cystectomy and substitution, the postoperative mortality and morbidity were extremely low (Table 7.2). Two patients died postoperatively—a rate of less than 1%. Similar figures have also been reported in other series,[20,68] and all compare very favourably with those for cystectomy and conventional diversion.

All complications were treated conservatively. Eight patients required temporary percutaneous nephrostomy drainage for the treatment of extensive urinary leak from the ureteroileal anastomosis.

The urinary tract

On the basis of follow-up observations that ranged between 6 and 60 months, improvement or stability was demonstrated in the majority of renal units

Table 7.2 Early complications

	Number of patients
Urinary leaks	28*
Pelvic collections	19
Septicaemia	8
Prolonged ileus	6
Deep venous thrombosis	5
Mortality (pulmonary embolism)	2
Total	68

*Eight required temporary percotaneous nephrostomy (PCN).

A

B

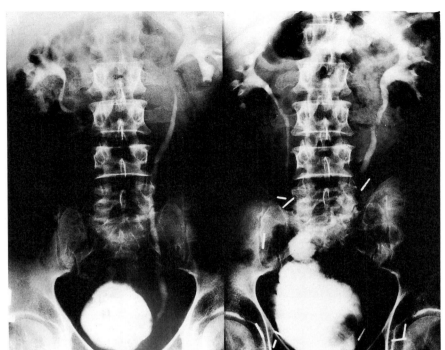

Fig. 7.5 **A** Preoperative intravenous urogram. **B** Intravenous urogram taken 6 months postoperatively. Note the perfect function and configuration of the upper tract.

studied by urography (Fig. 7.5). Back-pressure changes were noted in 34 renal units (8%) due to a failing antireflux valve in 23 or a ureteroileal stricture in 11. Surgical revision was carried out for correction of dessuscepted valves in 17 cases, followed by stability of the upper tract function. Endourological antegrade dilatation was successful in the management of 3 anastomotic strictures;[98] the remainder required open surgical revision.

Ascending and micturition studies were carried out to evaluate the stability of the reflux-preventing valve, test for the presence of residual urine and determine the patency of the urethroileal anastomosis and distal urethra (Fig. 7.6). It was noted that the rate of valve failure was less than 1%, if attention to detail was observed during their construction.[87,88] Using air and contrast, one can clearly demonstrate the length of the valve and its fixity to the wall of the pouch (Fig. 7.7).

Urodynamic characteristics

The capacity of the reservoir to accommodate urine increases gradually with time to reach its maximum after 6 months.[71] Figure 7.8 is a cystometrogram

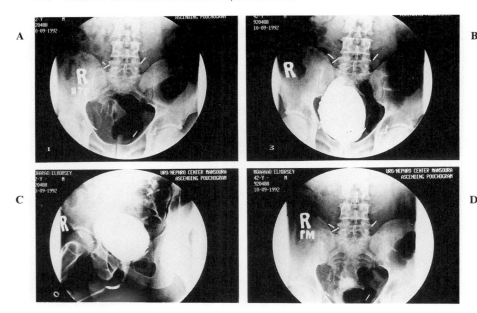

Fig. 7.6 (A–D) Micturition cycle. Note the adequate capacity with no reflux with a patent urethroileal anastomosis. A minimal amount of residual urine is seen in the postvoiding film.

of a fully mature pouch. A maximum capacity of 800 ml could be attained at a pressure of 35 cm water. The amplitude of segmental contractions is extremely blunted. Voiding is achieved by voluntary increase of the intra-abdominal pressure. It is an effective driving force leading to complete evacuation so long as there is no reflux and the urethroileal anastomosis is non-stenotic.

Continence

Continence is a critical parameter in the evaluation of the functional success of an orthotopic substitute. It depends on a balance between the pressure within the reservoir and the urethral closure pressure. A distinct advantage of detubularized ileal reservoirs is that they can accommodate large volumes of fluid at low pressure. The significance of this feature should be emphasized in view of the absence of normal sacral route reflexes after cystoprostatectomy, with lack of response in urethral resistance to bladder filling.[99] A review of the continent status following orthotopic ileal bladder substitutes is given in Table 7.3. While the daytime continence has always been better than 90%, night-time continence ranges between 70 and 80%. A possible explanation for the pathogenesis of nocturnal incontinence was proposed by Jakobsen et al.[103] They reported that the maximal urethral pressure was reduced by a factor of ±20% during sleep. This reduction correlated with the stage of sleep as

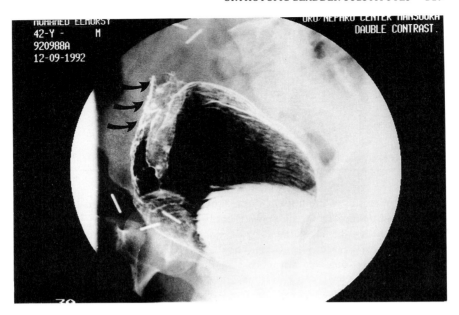

Fig. 7.7 Ascending pouchogram with air and contrast. Note the adequate length of the nipple valve and its fixity to the wall of the valve (arrows).

determined by electroencephalography. Some 40% of our enuretic patients had a remarkable improvement with imipramine hydrochloride. This is presumably since it reduces the depth of sleep and thus prevents the concomitant reduction of the urethral closure pressure. It is always gratifying to try to find a correctable cause for enuresis such as reflux, asymptomatic

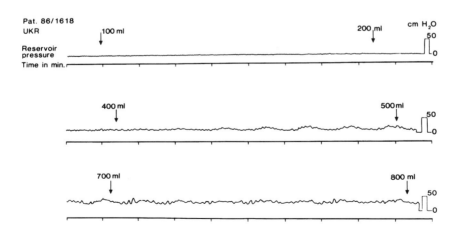

Fig. 7.8 Cytometrogram of a fully mature pouch. Note the large capacity, low pressure and blunting of segmental contractions.

Table 7.3   Continence status after orthotopic ileal bladder substitutes

Authors	Number of patients	Continence		Frequency of voiding		Time of evaluation
		Daytime (%)	Night-time (%)	Day time	Night-time	
Studer et al[49]	80	91	82	6	3	6 months
Wenderoth et al[68]	95	87	82	3–9	0–3	>3 months
Pagano et al[100]	16	87	81	3–5	0–1	>3 months
Skinner et al[101]	121	94	84	3–5	2–3	>9 months
Ghoneim et al[102]	248	93	74	3–5	0–1	>6 months

infection or stones in the pouch. Control of these problems is usually followed by rapid improvement in the state of continence. Furthermore, it was noted by some investigators[49] as well as by us that a nerve-sparing cystectomy would lead to an early regain of continence. There is some evidence that the rhabdosphincter receives autonomic as well as somatic innervation.[104,105] Further studies are however necessary to determine if the improved continence with nerve-sparing cystectomy is due to preservation of the pelvic nerve or because the required dissection avoids iatrogenic damage to the distal sphincter system.

Other observations

Stone formation in the pouch was encountered among 12% of our patients. Invariably the stones formed on the metallic staples used for the construction of the reflux-preventing valve. Most of the stones were tiny, allowing spontaneous passage. Nevertheless, endoscopic retrieval was required for 6%. Skinner and associates[101] reported a much lower incidence (<1%). This may be due to the fact that they used only one half-length of the staple lines. A randomized study is currently underway in our centre, comparing metallic staples with ones made from synthetic absorbable material relative to valve stability and rate of stone formation.

None of our patients had a metabolic acidosis of a degree that warranted alkali therapy. This is because we have always used a segment of bowel less than 50 cm in length. A similar observation was noted by Studer et al[49] and Skinner et al.[88] When segments of ileum longer than 50 cm were used, Wenderoth and associates[68] reported that mild metabolic acidosis was encountered in 50% of their patients and all received routine alkali therapy.

CONCLUSIONS

Orthotopic bladder substitution is feasible. The functional results are remarkable. Contemporary cystectomy should not be associated with a serious functional loss or a need for an external appliance or self-catheterization.

Consequently patients' quality of life and self-image are significantly better than those with conventional methods of urinary diversion.[106] Postoperative mortality, morbidity and long-term complications are not significantly different from those of standard urinary diversion.[107] This does not mean that a Utopia has been reached. There is always room for improvement and refinement. The availability of a new synthetic material for bladder substitution and the feasibility of electronic or hydraulic drive for the sphincters provide promising channels that have also to be pursued.[108]

ACKNOWLEDGEMENT

Our experience with continent diversion has been realized in collaboration with Prof. Nils G. Kock, Emeritus Professor of Surgery, the University of Göteborg, Sweden. His efforts were always stimulating, his thoughts inspiring, and his advice invaluable.

REFERENCES

1   Tizzoni G, Foggi A. Die Wiederherstellung der harnblase. Exp Untersuchungen Zenteralbl Chir 1888: 15: 921–924
2   Studer UE, Casanova GA, Zingg EJ. Historical aspects of continent urinary diversion. In: Rowland RG, Paulson DF eds. Problems in urology, vol 5, no 2 Philadelphia: JB Lippincott, 1991: pp 197–202
3   Leong CH, Ong GB. Gastrocystoplasty. Br J Urol 1975; 47: 236
4   Adams MC, Mitchell ME, Rink RC. Gastrocystoplasty: an alternative solution to the problem of urological reconstruction in the severely compromised patient. J Urol 1988; 140: 1152–1156
5   Nguyen DH, Mitchell ME. Gastric bladder reconstruction. Urol Clin North Am 1991; 18: 649–657
6   Couvelaire R. Le reservoir ileal de substitution apres la cystectomie totale chez l'homme. J Urol Nephrol 1951; 57: 408–417
7   Mellinger GT, Klatte PB. Uretero-ileo-urethral anastomosis. J Urol 1959; 82: 459–461
8   Gandin MM. Uretero-ileo-urethral anastomosis: a case report. J Urol 1960: 83: 279–282
9   Hradec EA. Bladder substitution indications and results in 114 operations. J Urol 1965; 94: 406–417
10 Barry JM, Pitre TM, Hodges CV. Ureteroileourethrostomy: 16-year follow up. J Urol 1976; 115: 29–31
11 Kirkegaard P, Lyndrup J, Walter S, Ejby Poulsen P. Long-term results after uretero-ileo-urethrostomy. Br J Urol 1982; 54: 226–229
12 Camey M, Le-Duc A. L'enterocystoplastie apres cystoprostatectomie totale pour cancer de la vessie. Indications, technique operative, surveillance et resultats sur quatre-vingt-sept cas. Ann Urol 1979; 13: 114–123
13 Le-Duc A, Camey M, Teillac P. An original antireflux uretero-ileal implantation technique: long-term follow-up. J Urol 1987; 137: 1156–1158
14 Deklerk JN, Lambrechts W, Viljoen I. The bowel as substitute for the bladder. J Urol 1979; 121: 22–24
15 Roehrborn CG, Teigland CM, Sagalowsky AI. Functional characteristics of the Camey ileal bladder. J Urol 1987; 138: 739–742
16 Kock NG, Nilson AE, Nilsson LO, Norlen LT, Philipson BM. Urinary diversion via a continent ileal reservoir: clinical results in 12 patients. J Urol 1982; 128: 469–475
17 Ghoneim MA, Kock NG, Lycke G, Shehab El-Din A. An appliance-free, sphincter controlled bladder substitute: the urethral Kock pouch. J Urol 1987; 138: 1150–1154
18 Tscholl R, Leisinger HJ, Hauri D. The ileal S-pouch for bladder replacement after

cystectomy: preliminary report of 7 cases. J Urol 1987; 138: 344–347

19 Hautmann RE, Egghart G, Frohneberg D, Miller K. The ileal neobladder. J Urol 1988; 139: 39–42

20 Skinner DG, Lieskovsky G, Boyd S. Continent urinary diversion. J Urol 1989; 141: 1323–1327

21 Studer UE, Ackermann D, Casanova GA, Zingg EJ. Three years' experience with an ileal low pressure bladder substitute. Br J Urol 1989; 63: 43–52

22 Verhoogen J. Neostomie uretero-cecale. Formation d'une nouvelle poche vesicale et d'un nouvel uretre. Assoc Franc Urol 1908; 12: 352–365

23 Gil-Vernet JM. The ileocolic segment in urologic surgery. J Urol 1965; 94: 418–426

24 Khafagy MM, Kalawy M, Ibrahim A, Safa M, Meguid HA, Bassioni M. Radical cystectomy and ileocaecal bladder reconstruction for carcinoma of the urinary bladder. Br J Urol 1987; 60: 60–63

25 Light JK. Enteroplasty to ablate bowel contractions in the reconstructed bladder: a case report. J Urol 1985; 134: 958–959

26 Sidi AA, Reinberg Y, Gonzalez R. Influence of intestinal segment and configuration on the outcome of augmentaion enterocystoplasty. J Urol 1986; 136: 1201–1204

27 Steven K, Klarskov P, Jakobsen H, Bay-Nielsen H, Rasmussen F. Transpubic cystectomy and ileocecal bladder replacement after preoperative radiotherapy for bladder cancer. J Urol 1986; 135: 470–475

28 Light JK, Engelmann UH. Le bag: total replacement of the bladder using an ileocolonic pouch. J Urol 1986; 136: 27–31

29 Thuroff JW, Alken P, Riedmiller H, Engelmann U, Jacobi GH, Hohenfellner R. The Mainz pouch for bladder augmentation and continent diversion. J Urol 1986; 136: 17–26

30 Marshall FF. Creation of an ileocolic bladder after cystectomy. J Urol 1988; 139: 1264–1268

31 Goldwasser B, Benson RC. Bladder replacement using the detubularized right colon. A preliminary report of a new technique. Mayo Clin Proc 1986; 61: 615–621

32 Gil-Vernet JM. Technique for construction of a functioning artificial bladder. J Urol 1960; 83: 39–50

33 Develeliotis A, Macris SG. Replacement of the bladder with an isolated segment of sigmoid. J Urol 1961; 85: 564–568

34 Kuss R, Bitker M, Camey M, Chatelain C, Lassau JP. Indications and early and late complications of intestino-cystoplasty: a review of 185 cases. J Urol 1970; 103: 53–63

35 Reddy PK, Lange PH, Fraley EE. Bladder replacement after cystoprostatectomy: efforts to achieve total continence. J Urol 1987; 138: 495–499

36 Reddy PK, Lange PH, Fraley EE. Total bladder replacement using detubularized sigmoid colon. Technique and results. J. Urol 1991; 145: 51–55

37 Lemoine G. Creation d'une vessie nouvelle par un procede personnel apres cystectomie totale pour cancer. J Urol 1913; 4: 367–372

38 Farah GR, Rifaat MA. Rectal vesico-urethroplasty updated with ten years evaluation. Br J Urol 1977; 49: 391–400

39 McDougal WS. Metabolic complications of urinary intestinal diversion. J Urol 1992; 147: 1199–1208

40 Tiffany P, Vaughan ED Jr, Marion D, Amberson J. Hypergastrinemia following antral gastrocystoplasty. J Urol 1986; 136: 692–695

41 Mitchell ME. Electrolyte transport in gastric mucosa in contact with urine. Scand J Urol Nephrol 1992; 142 (suppl): 33–35

42 Golimbu M, Morales P. Electrolyte disturbances in jejunal urinary diversion. Urology 1973; 1: 432–438

43 Koivisto P, Miettien TA. Adaptation of cholesterol and bile acid metabolism and vitamin B_{12} absorption in the long-term follow-up after partial ileal bypass. Gastroenterology 1986; 90: 984–990

44 Einarsson K. Metabolic effects caused by exclusion of intestinal segments. Scand J Urol Nephrol 1992; 142 (suppl): 21–26

45 Steiner MS, Morton RA. Nutritional and gastrointestinal complications of the use of bowel segments in the lower urinary tract. Urol Clin North Am 1991; 18: 743–754

46 Mohler JL. Metabolic acidosis after bladder replacement: comparison of severity and reversibility in ileal and colonic reservoirs. J Urol 1988; 139: 628–633

47 McDougal WS, Koch MO, Shands C, Price RR. Bony demineralization following urinary intestinal diversion. J Urol 1988; 140: 853–855

48 Mundy AR, Nurse DE. Calcium balance, growth and skeletal mineralization in patients with cystoplasties. Br J Urol 1992; 69: 257–259

49 Studer UE, Gerber E, Springer J, Zingg EJ. Bladder reconstruction with bowel after radical cystectomy. World J Urol 1992; 10: 11–19

50 Akerlund S, Nilsson LO. Water and electrolyte absorption in ileal segments surgically transposed to the urinary bladder in the cat. Scand J Urol Nephrol 1986; 20: 63–69

51 Akerlund S, Jagenburg R, Kock NG, Philipson BM. Absorption of L-phenyl alanine in human ileal reservoirs exposed to urine. Urol Res 1988; 16: 321–323

52 Nurse DE, Mundy AR. Metabolic complications of cystoplasty. Br J Urol 1989; 63: 165–170

53 Mansson W, Willen R. Mucosal morphology and histochemistry of the continent caecal reservoir for urine. J Urol 1988; 139: 1199–1201

54 Kosko JW, Kursh ED, Resnick MI. Metabolic complications of urologic intestinal substitutes. Urol Clin North Am 1986; 13: 193–200

55 Wagstaff KE, Woodhouse CRJ, Rose GA, Duffy PG, Ransley PG. Blood and urine analysis in patients with intestinal bladders. Br J Urol 1991; 68: 311–316

56 Gittes RF. Carcinogenesis in ureterosigmoidostomy. Urol Clin North Am 1986; 13: 201–205

57 Crissey MM, Steele GD, Gittes RF. Rat model for carcinogenesis in ureterosigmoidostomy. Science 1980; 207: 1079–1080

58 Shands C, McDougal WS, Wright EP. Prevention of cancer at the urethro-ileal enteric anastomotic site. J Urol 1989; 141: 178–181

59 Filmer RB, Spencer JR. Malignancies in bladder augmentations and intestinal conduits. J Urol 1990; 143: 671–678

60 Bates P, Bradley WE, Glen E et al. First report on the standardization of terminology of lower urinary tract function. Br J Urol 1976; 48: 39–42

61 Hinman F Jr. Selection of intestinal segments for bladder substitution: physical and physiological characteristics. J Urol 1988; 139: 519–523

62 Berglund B, Kock NG, Norlen L, Philipson BM. Volume capacity and pressure characteristic of the continent ileal reservoir used for urinary diversion. J Urol 1987; 137: 29–34

63 Lytton B, Green DF. Urodynamic studies in patients undergoing bladder replacement surgery. J Urol 1989; 141: 1394–1397

64 Davidsson T, Poulsen AL, Hedlund H, Steven K, Mansson W. A comparative urodynamic study of the ileal and the colonic neobladder. Scand J Urol Nephrol 1992; 142 (suppl): 143

65 Schmidbauer CP, Chiang H, Raz S. The impact of detubularization on ileal reservoirs, J Urol 1987; 138: 1440–1445

66 Shaaban AA, El-Nono IH, Abdel-Rahman M, Ghoneim MA. The urodynamic characteristics of different ileal reservoirs; an experimental study in dogs. J Urol 1992; 147: 197–200

67 Skinner DG, Lieskovsky G, Boyd SD. Continuing experience with the continent ileal reservoir (Kock pouch) as an alternative to cutaneous urinary diversion: an update after 250 cases. J Urol 1987; 137: 1140–1145

68 Wenderoth UK, Bachor R, Egghart G, Frohneberg D, Miller K, Hautmann RE. The ileal neobladder: experience and results of more than 100 consecutive cases. J Urol 1990; 143: 492–497

69 Shaaban AH, Dawaba MS, Gaballah MA, Ghoneim MA. Urethral controlled bladder substitution: a comparison between parks S pouch and hemi-Kock pouch. J Urol 1991; 146: 973–976

70 Bachor R, Frohneberg D, Miller K, Egghart G, Hautmann R. Continence after total bladder replacement: urodynamic analysis of the ileal neobladder. Br J Urol 1990; 65: 462–466

71 Kock NG, Ghoneim MA, Lycke G, Mahran MR. Replacement of the bladder by the urethral Kock pouch: functional results, urodynamics and radiological features. J Urol 1989; 141: 1111–1116

72 Perl JI. Intussuscepted conical valve formation in jejunostomies. Surgery 1949; 25: 297–299

73 Kock NG, Nilson AE, Norlen L, Sundin T, Trasti H. Urinary diversion via a continent ileum reservoir. Clinical experience. Scand J Urol Nephrol 1978; 49 (suppl): 23–31

74 Hendren WH. Reoperative ureteral reimplantation: management of the difficult case. J Pediatr Surg 1980; 15: 770–786

75 Melchior H, Spehr C, Wagemann IK, Persson MC, Juenemann KP. The continent ileal bladder for urinary tract reconstruction after cystectomy: a survey of 44 patients. J Urol 1988; 139: 714–718

76 Atta A. A new technique for ileal nipple fixation: preliminary report. J Urol 1990; 144: 1192–1193

77 Allen TD, Peters PC, Sagalowsky AI, Roehrborn C. The Camey procedure: preliminary results in 11 patients. World J Urol 1985; 3: 167–171

78 Lockhart JL, Bejany DE. Antireflux uretero-ileal reimplantation: an alternative for urinary diversion. J Urol 1987; 137: 867–870

79 Catalona WJ. Personal communication, 1990

80 Studer UE, Casanova GA, Ackermann DK, Zingg EJ. Ileal bladder substitute: antireflux nipple or afferent tubular segment. J Urol 1990; 143 (suppl): 398A

81 Tanagho EA. A case against incorporation of bowel segments into the closed urinary system. J Urol 1975; 113: 796–802

82 Shokeir AA, Gaballah MA, Ashamallah AA, Ghoneim MA. Optimization of replacement of the ureter by ileum. J Urol 1991; 146: 306–310

83 Alken P. The risk of urethral recurrence after radical cystectomy. Scand J Urol Nephrol 1992; 142 (suppl): 95

84 Schellhammer PF, Whitmore WF Jr. Transitional cell carcinoma of the urethra in men having cystectomy for bladder cancer. J Urol 1976; 115: 56–60

85 Hardeman SW, Soloway MS. Urethral recurrence following radical cystectomy. J Urol 1990; 144: 666–669

86 Khafagy MM, El-Bolkainy MN, Mansoura A. Carcinoma of the bilharzial urinary bladder: a study of the associated mucosal lesions in 86 cases. Cancer 1972; 30–150–159

87 Ghoneim MA, Shaaban AA, Mahran MR, Kock NG. Further experience with the urethral Kock's pouch. J Urol 1991; 147: 361–365

88 Skinner DG, Boyd SD, Lieskovsky G, Bennett C, Hopwood B. Lower urinary tract reconstruction following cystectomy: experience and results in 126 patients using the Kock ileal reservoir with bilateral uretero-ileal urethrostomy. J Urol 1991; 146: 756–760

89 Holmes SAV, Christmas TJ, Kirby RS, Hendry WF. Cystectomy and substitution enterocystoplasty: alternative primary treatment for T2/3 bladder cancer. Br J Urol 1992; 69: 260–264

90 Hubner WA, Trigo-Rocha F, Plas EG, Tanagho EA. Functional bladder replacement in the female after radical cystectomy: experimental investigations on a new concept. Scand J Urol Nephrol 1992; 142 (suppl): 144–145

91 Arap S, Nahas WC, Giron AM, Bruschini H, Mitre AI. Incontinent epispadias: surgical treatment of 38 cases. J Urol 1988; 140: 577–581

92 Fisch M, Wammack R, Sert U, Muller SC, Hohenfellner R. Continent urinary diversion in childhood. World J Urol 1992; 10: 107–114

93 Woodhouse CRJ. Lower urinary tract reconstruction in young patients. Br J Urol 1992; 70: 113–120

94 Ghoneim MA, El-Hammady SM, El-Bolkainy MN, Ashamallah AK, Mansour MA, Soliman EH. Radical cystectomy for carcinoma of bilharzial bladder. Technique and results. Urology 1976; 8: 547–552

95 Oelrich TM. The urethral sphincter muscle in the male. Am J Anat 1980: 158: 229–246

96 Myers RP, Goellner JR, Cahill DR. Prostate shape, external striated urethral sphincter and radical prostatectomy: the apical dissection. J Urol 1987; 138: 543–550

97 Klein EA. Early continence after radical prostatectomy. J Urol 1992; 148: 92–95

98 Mahran MR, El-Diasty T, Ghoneim MA. Endourologic management of urinary leakage and uretero-ileal stricture in patients with orthotopic bladder replacement. Scand J Urol Nephrol 1992; 142 (suppl): 156–157

99 Goldwasser B, Mansson W, Davidsson T, Hedlund H, Brooks M, Roman J.

Cystoureterometric findings in patients with detubularized right colonic segment for bladder replacement. J Urol 1991; 145: 538–541

100 Pagano F, Artibani W, Ligato P, Piazaza R, Garbeglio A, Passerini G. Vesica ileale Padovana: a technique for total bladder replacement. Eur Urol 1990; 17: 149-154

101 Skinner DG, Boyd SD, Lieskovsky G, Bennet C, Hopwood B. Lower urinary tract reconstruction following cystectomy: experience and results in 126 patients using the Kock ileal reservoir with bilateral uretero-ileal urethrostomy. J Urol 1991; 146: 756–760

102 Ghoneim MA, Shaaban AA, Abdallah HA, Mahran MA, Kock NG. Results of orthotopic bladder replacement by Kock pouch. Scand J Urol Nephrol 1992; 142 (suppl): 165

103 Jakobsen H, Steven K, Stigsby B, Klarskov P, Hald T. Pathogenesis of nocturnal urinary incontinence aftter ileocaecal bladder replacement. Br J Urol 1987; 59: 148–152

104 Elbadawi A, Schenk EA. A new theory of the innervation of bladder musculature. Part 4, Innervation of the vesicourethral junction and external urethral sphincter. J Urol 1974; 111: 613–615

105 Kumagai A, Koyanagi T, Tokahashi Y. The innervation of the external urethral sphincter. An ultrastructural study in male human subjects. Urol Res 1987; 15: 39–43

106 Bjerre BD, Johansen C, Steven K. Quality of life after cystectomy for bladder cancer: bladder substitution compared with ileal conduit diversion. A questionnaire survey. Scand J Urol Nephrol 1992; 142 (suppl): 164

107 Benson MC, Slawin KM, Wechsler MH, Olsson CA. Analysis of continent versus standard urinary diversion. Br J Urol 1992; 69: 156–162

108 Griffith DP, Gleason MJ. The prosthetic bladder—perhaps the technology has arrived. Scand J Urol Nephrol 1992; 142 (suppl): 109–122

8

Chemotherapy for invasive bladder cancer

J. Waxman   H. Wasan

Bladder cancer is a common tumour. In the UK, it is the fourth most frequent cancer of men, and the sixth commonest cause of cancer deaths. The most recent Department of Health statistics described 9991 registrations and 4851 deaths. In the USA, there are approximately 40 000 new cases of bladder cancer annually and nearly 11 000 deaths. Bladder cancer is much less frequent in women than in men and this difference is thought to relate to the different exposure of men and women to workplace carcinogens and cigarettes.

Current treatments for locally advanced muscle-invasive bladder cancer by radiotherapy or surgery are relatively ineffective in controlling the disease. Urologists and oncologists recognize the inadequacy of radiation and cystectomy in limiting the progression of bladder cancer and have welcomed the observation that these tumours are chemosensitive. Pragmatically, they have introduced chemotherapy into the management of urothelial cancers both as adjuvant treatments and for metastatic or locally recurrent tumours.

Philosophically, the idea of adjuvant therapies given when tumour bulk is small and the therapeutic ratio increased is attractive. It might be hoped that the advances seen with adjuvant chemotherapy in many other solid tumours such as breast cancer would translate to bladder cancer. This has not happened with most adjuvant treatment programmes. This may be because these programmes, which have been used because they are minimally toxic, are also minimally effective. In metastatic disease where the immediate advantages of intensive therapies are more obviously apparent, more intensive treatment schedules have been used with relative enthusiasm and better effect. In this chapter we review chemotherapy for bladder tumours.

THE RESULTS OF CONVENTIONAL THERAPY FOR BLADDER TUMOURS

Radiation

In the UK radiotherapy is the treatment of first choice for invasive bladder tumours. Treatment with radiotherapy is more attractive than cystectomy because the patient is left with a bladder at the end of treatment, usually remains sexually potent, and avoids the operative morbidity of cystectomy.

127

There is great variation in radiotherapeutic techniques, even when treatment is given with curative intent. One preferred schedule involves dosages of approximately 6000 cGy given in 30 fractions over 6 weeks. Treatment is given to a total dosage of 4000 cGy to the whole pelvis and the final 2000 cGy is given to the bladder. The theoretical reason for administering treatment to the whole pelvis is that this includes pelvic lymph nodes. Many radiotherapists feel that there is no point treating the whole pelvis and instead treat the bladder alone. This approach relates to the observation that if pelvic lymph nodes are affected by metastatic malignancy, then it is likely that para-aortic lymph nodes will be affected too. The median survival for patients with para-aortic lymph node metastases is 9 months and therefore, limiting the treatment area to the true pelvis avoids unnecessary bowel toxicity and will not materially affect survival. In addition the chances of sterilizing affected iliac nodes with a dose of 4000 cGy is virtually negligible.

There are two large series of patients treated at one centre by radiotherapy. In the Glasgow series, 709 patients with carcinoma of the bladder were reviewed; these patients had had treatment between 1978 and 1984. A number of different dosage schedules were used to treat these patients and 395 received pelvic nodal radiotherapy. Overall, 24.7% of the patients survived 5 years. When non-cancer deaths were excluded from the analysis, the actuarial 5-year survival rate was 31.1%. Stage survival was 86.9% for the 34 patients with T1 disease, 49.1% for the 189 patients with T2 disease, 21.4% for the 328 patients with T3 disease and 1.8% for the 158 patients with T4 cancer. Histology was an important determinant of 5-year survival and was 41.8% for G1 tumours, 28.3% for G2 tumours and 25.5% for G3 cancers. In this study, nodal irradiation did not positively affect outlook. Those patients receiving nodal radiotherapy did significantly worse and 5-year survival was 26%, as compared with 37% for patients who did not have nodal radiation. Toxicity was significantly higher in patients whose whole pelvis had been irradiated. Late radiation complications occurred in 271 patients. In the Glasgow series, radiotherapy did not prevent local recurrence and 23% of all patients died as a result of local progression of the disease without evidence for metastatic cancer, whilst 46% died with local recurrence and metastases.[1]

In the Edinburgh series, 591 of 889 patients with T1–4 bladder cancer had persistent or recurrent disease after radical radiation. In this series there was a significant morbidity from radiation. Acute symptoms included frequency, dysuria and diarrhoea with associated nausea and tiredness. Severe late radiation morbidity was described in 10% of patients receiving pelvic radiotherapy and 4% of those receiving bladder radiation alone.[2]

Radical surgery

Between 10 and 30% of patients with pT2 tumours have pelvic lymph node metastases, as do between 20 and 65% of patients with pT3 tumours. It has been estimated that lymphadenectomy in addition to radical cystectomy leads to an additional cure rate of only 2% in those patients with pT3 tumours. These awful statistics do not encourage the reader of the literature to expect that cystectomy will cure all patients with invasive bladder cancer. Overall, the 5-year survival rate following radical cystectomy for T2–4 tumours is between 40 and 60%.

These surgical series are obviously highly selected, selection depending upon fitness, patterns of referral and the exclusion of those patients with inoperable disease. The refinement of surgical techniques and the improvement of postoperative care have led to a decrease in the mortality from cystectomy which is now, in centres of excellence, approximately 1% in patients less than 70 years old. The major complications of the procedure are urinary or intestinal fistulae which again have decreased over recent years and occur in between 3 and 10% of patients. Cystectomy is not always locally curative and the incidence of pelvic recurrence is between 6 and 9%. The immediate morbidity, impotence and loss of the bladder are obviously significant sequelae of surgery.[3]

CHEMOTHERAPY FOR INVASIVE BLADDER CANCER

This background of treatments, which are both inadequate in terms of their success rate and suboptimal in terms of their morbidity, provides an extremely substantial basis for the introduction of new treatments for this common cancer. Bladder cancer is a chemotherapy-sensitive tumour. The order of response to single agents is high and is described in Table 8.1. This order of

Table 8.1 Single agents for urothelial tract tumours

	CR + PR/patients	%CR + PR	95% Confidence intervals
Cisplatin			
Single institution	70/206	34	20–40%
Randomized trials	55/315	17	37–55%
Carboplatin	21/186	15	11–19%
CHIP	7/39	18	6–30%
Methotrexate			
'Low' dose	68/236	29	23–35%
'High' dose	16/57	45	37–50%
Adriamycin	47/274	17	13–22%
Vinblastine	6/38	16	4–28%
Cyclophosphamide	30/98	31	22–40%
5-Fluorouracil	22/141	17	11–25%
Mitomycin-C	5/42	13	2–22%
Gallium nitrate	7/26	27	11–48%

CR = Complete response; PR = partial response.
After Arap & Scher.[4]

sensitivity is unusual in solid tumours. As a general principle, the expectation is that the combination of effective single agents should lead to an incremental response rate with their combination. Examples where this has been achieved include the lymphomas and testicular cancer where cure is the expectation when combination chemotherapy is given.

Chemotherapy in bladder cancer has a long history, dating back to the 1960s when methotrexate was used. Methotrexate is an antimetabolite acting to limit nucleic acid synthesis by inhibiting folate metabolism. Responses may be seen in up to 30% of patients with metastatic urothelial cancer. Toxicity is generally limited and may be moderated by folinic acid rescue. Sustained responses are unusual and fewer than 5% of patients with metastatic cancer are alive 1 year from presentation.

The development of cisplatinum and its subsequent investigation in phase II clinical trials in oncology revealed this agent to be one of the most active single therapies for the treatment of bladder cancer. Cisplatinum acts as an alkylating agent crosslinking guanosine residues within DNA and thereby limiting cell division. Approximately 17–40% of patients with bladder cancer respond to cisplatinum chemotherapy. Dosages of cisplatinum effective in producing responses are unfortunately quite toxic. Apart from the immediate toxicity of nausea and vomiting, long-term nephro- and neurotoxicity may be a problem in up to 30% of patients. Unfortunately, as with methotrexate, sustained responses are unusual.

Many other single agents have been used to treat bladder cancer. The data, for the majority, are old and remarkable because of the broad range of activity of many different classes of agents and will not be reviewed further here. There has been interest in a number of new agents, particularly in analogues of methotrexate such as pirotexin which has shown some activity in refractory tumours and requires further investigation in phase II trials in patients who have had no previous chemotherapy.

One of the problems with the use of chemotherapy in patients with invasive bladder cancer is that for the main patients tend to be elderly and frail and unable to tolerate the exigencies of treatment. The development of carboplatin, an analogue of cisplatin, has been greeted with enthusiasm by oncologists and with relief by patients with cancer. The activity of carboplatin is similar to that of cisplatinum. Carboplatin has significant advantages compared to the parent compound and these advantages relate to its lack of toxicity. The main side-effect of carboplatin is myelosuppression; nephrotoxicity and neurotoxicity are unusual. Reports of the activity of carboplatin in bladder cancer have been received with some scepticism. However, as demonstrated in Table 8.1 there are now sufficient patients studied to support the case for its use in this disease.

There is a significant onus for the further investigation of the use of etoposide in urothelial malignancy. The original studies of etoposide showed a low order of activity. Etoposide is a topoisomerase 2 inhibitor. Topo isomerase 2 is a DNA repair enzyme responsible for the maintenance of the topography of DNA. When originally given to patients with cancer, treatment was by intravenous bolus injection. Little activity was seen in chemosensitive diseases such as small cell lung cancer. Many years later, careful investigation of different schedules of administration of etoposide showed that this agent was far more active when given as an oral treatment over many days than as a bolus therapy given in short courses.

This new understanding of the pharmocokinetics of etoposide has led to its re-evaluation in small cell lung cancer, where it is probably the most effective single agent treatment. There is a significant case for reinvestigating the activity of etoposide in urothelial cancer, giving etoposide as an oral treatment rather than as intravenous bolus therapy. We have investigated treatment in patients with advanced disease who have been ineligible for consideration of combination chemotherapy because of their frailty. Responses have been seen which encourage further investigation of etoposide.

COMBINATION CHEMOTHERAPY REGIMENS

The finding that single agents were active in urothelial tumours spurred on the investigation of combination of cytotoxic drugs, in order to reproduce the success of chemotherapy in other malignancies. In many of these trials early promising results have not been reproduced in later, larger investigations.

Two-drug combinations

In early studies the two most active single agents, cisplatin and methotrexate, were combined. The activity of this combination initially appeared to be superior to cisplatin alone but a subsequent large randomized study involving 108 patients with metastatic disease failed to confirm this finding. In this study patients were randomized to receive cisplatinum 80 mg/m^2 or cisplatinum 80 mg/m^2 with methotrexate 50 mg/m^2 on days 1 and 15 of a 3-week treatment cycle. There was no statistically significant difference in overall response (31 versus 45%), or in complete response rates (9 versus 9%), or in median survival (7.2 versus 8.7 months) in those receiving the combination compared with cisplatinum alone.[5] Similarly, cisplatinum and doxorubicin (Adriamycin) combinations have not been shown to be superior to cisplatinum alone, again contrary to expectations from promising phase II trial data.[6] In a study comparing 109 patients randomized to either cisplatinum (70 mg/m^2) with cyclophosphamide (750 mg/m^2) or to cisplatinum alone (70 mg/m^2), response rates [partial response (PR) + complete response (CR)] were 20 versus 11.9% respectively, but this difference was not statistically significant and there was no difference in overall survival.[7]

Three-drug combinations

Oncologists, pursuing a 'more is best' approach, investigated multidrug regimens. More was found to be not much better than less in three randomized studies, all published in 1985, investigating the CAP programme (cisplatinum 600 mg/m^2, Adriamycin 40 mg/m^2 and cyclophosphamide 400 mg/m^2). The South West Oncology Group study (SWOG) compared CAP with amsacrine, a DNA intercalating agent,[8] and The Eastern Cooperative Oncology Group (ECOG) compared CAP with cisplatin alone[9] as did Troner.[10] The MD Anderson Hospital Urological Oncology Group reported their experience of a regimen with the acronym CISCA, in 74 patients. They reported a 70% response rate which included a 39% complete response rate. Some 19% of patients had remissions lasting greater than 2 years and the median survival of the group was over 18 months.[11] This CISCA regimen was slightly different from the standard CAP programme, containing higher dosages of cisplatinum, cyclophosphamide and Adriamycin in a different schedule. In addition, the patient selection criteria were stricter. The MD Anderson study was not comparative and because of this the results were greeted with scepticism. This programme has subsequently been tested against a four-drug regimen in a randomized study of 110 patients with metastatic disease and was found to be inferior in terms of response rates and median survival.[12]

The Stanford University Group reported their experience with CMV (cisplatinum 100 mg/m^2, methotrexate 30–40 mg/m^2 days 1 and 8, and vinblastine 4 mg/m^2 days 1 and 8).[13,14] The first 60 patients entered had a documented complete response rate of 28%. This group of complete responders included partial responders who were surgically downstaged to complete response. Within the CMV programme cisplatin is the drug with the most toxicity. In order to limit toxicity the Medical Research Council Advanced Bladder Cancer Subgroup are coordinating a randomized trial of an altered CMV regimen, with a reduced cisplatinum dosage of 70 mg/m^2, which is compared with MV. It can be argued that the design of this study prejudices response rates at the risk of limiting toxicity.

Four-drug combinations

The four drug combination M-VAC has in certain centres produced spectacular results. Treatment includes methotrexate (30 mg/m^2 days 1 and 15), vinblastine (3 mg/m^2 days 2, 15 and 22), Adriamycin (30 mg/m^2 day 1) and cisplatinum (70 mg/m^2 day 1) and is repeated monthly. M-VAC was developed at the Memorial Sloan Kettering Cancer Centre.[15] In a report of 121 patients with metastatic bladder cancer, 72% patients responded and of these, 26% had a complete response. Treatment was very active and modelled along testicular cancer lines, in that in those patients with residual tumour masses, laparotomies and thoracotomies were performed; resection converted partial into complete response. The median survival for complete responders was >38 months, compared to 14 months for CMV. The overall median survival was 13 months, with an estimated probability of 4-year survival of 18% ($\pm$7%).[16]

This finding has since been investigated in two phase III trials. The first, the multicentre Intergroup Study, compared M-VAC with single-agent cisplatinum in 224 evaluable patients. This study has only been reported in abstract form.[17] An advantage was found for the combination in terms of the overall response rates (34% versus 9%; P = 0.01), complete response rate (13% versus 3%) and overall survival (12.6 versus 8.7 months). However, the complete response rate was half that reported in the original Memorial trial (26%).[15] The second trial compared M-VAC with the MD Anderson CISCA programme, and involved 110 evaluable patients. M-VAC was superior in all respects to CISCA and the median survival time was significantly longer (18.4 versus 9.3 months).[12]

M-VAC remains the only combination protocol which has been shown to be superior to single-agent cisplatin. Although its efficacy has been confirmed, response rates and survival times seem generally lower when reported by authors outside of the acrid air of Manhattan.[18–20] The toxicity of this regimen is considerable; vomiting, variable renal failure, alopecia, neuropathy and deafness occurs in between 30 and 100% of patients, and septic death in 5%.[12,13,16,18]

Reducing toxicities

Although combination chemotherapy is considered standard for the treatment of advanced urothelial tract tumours, the toxicities of standard regimens are serious, occur commonly and require serious consideration. Most patients with urothelial tumours are over 70 years old, and unable to tolerate intensive treatments. We have made a minor modification of the M-VAC programme, attempting to limit toxicity. The Hammersmith treatment protocol has the acronym MVMJ, where mitozantrone is substituted for Adriamycin and carboplatin for cisplatinum. The advantages of this programme are that mitozantrone has significantly less cardiac toxicity than Adriamycin and carboplatin less neuro- and nephrotoxicity than cisplatinum. This regimen causes very little nausea and alopecia is unusual. Hydration and hospital admission are not required, unlike the M-VAC programme. Twenty-one patients with metastatic urothelial cancer were treated. Complete responses occurred in 5 (23%) and partial responses in a further 19% (CR + PR 52% Confidence Intervals (CI; 27–68%).[21] It would seem that MVMJ is equally as effective as M-VAC, at least in terms of response rates achieved outside New York City. More importantly, life quality is better, and toxicity less.

Dosage escalation

Recent clinical trials have examined the value of increasing drug dosage and frequency of treatment in bladder cancer. This has been made possible by the availability of recombinant haemopoietic growth factors. Two approaches have been investigated using growth factor support. The first is to give these agents so that patients receive their scheduled dose at the appropriate intervals without delay. The second is to apply these agents so that higher dosage therapies can be given at the outset. At the Memorial Sloan-Kettering Hospital, treatment with M-VAC given with granulocyte colony-stimulating factor (G-CSF) was compared with M-VAC alone. As a result of G-CSF treatment, therapy was not delayed by leukopenia and there was significantly less mucositis.[22]

A further study in which treatment dosages were escalated with G-CSF support in patients resistant to, or relapsing on M-VAC alone led to impressive complete response rates.[23] These results need to be confirmed.

Biological response modifier

Biological response modifiers are agents which, when given with cytotoxic chemotherapeutic drugs, have the theoretical potential for synergy of effect. Logothetis et al recently reported a 30% response rate in heavily pretreated patients (15–47%; CI: 15–48%) using a combination of 5-fluorouracil and recombinant alpha-2a-interferon.[24] Laboratory data indicate that in cell culture, the metabolism of 5-fluorouracil is modulated by interferon. Interferon may also act in vivo to reduce the renal clearance of 5-fluorouracil, which potentiates the conversion of 5-fluorouracil to its active metabolite. The study was not randomized and we do not know whether 5-fluorouracil alone would give the same results as the two agents.

Current recommendations in advanced disease

Combination chemotherapy should be offered to all patients with a good performance status in the hope of achieving a complete and durable remission. About 10–20% of patients will be long-term survivors. Patients with nodal disease or lung metastases are more likely to respond than patients with bony or liver secondaries. The choice of therapy lies between M-VAC, CMV and MVMJ, the latter regimens showing the least toxicity. A small and highly selected group (about 10–15%) will be downstaged and will benefit from a salvage cystectomy if this is the sole site of residual disease after chemotherapy. About one-third of these patients will be long-term survivors. Some patients with limited pulmonary disease after chemotherapy will similarly benefit from surgery. Partial responses occur in the majority of patients, but provided the treatment regimen chosen is not too toxic, there will be substantial benefit from palliation of distressing symptoms by chemotherapy.

Adjuvant therapy

At presentation, 20–36% of all bladder tumours are at an advanced stage. The treatment of such patients remains controversial because cure is only achieved in a minority of these patients. It has been suggested that treatment fails because of the presence of micrometastases at the patient's presentation.[25] This is supported by data from clinical trials where surgery has been used to stage disease precisely. In these studies 5% of patients with clinical stage pT1 N0 MO bladder cancer have pelvic node involvement. Nodal involvement increases to over 40% in patients with pT4 tumours.[26] Specific categories of patients with a poor outlook can be further defined, thus 40–50% of G3T1 tumours subsequently develop muscle invasion and in these patients the 5-year survival is only 20%.[27]

Bladder cancer, like most malignancies, should be regarded as a systemic disease in the majority of patients at the outset, and systemic diseases can only be cured by systemic therapies.

In this context, adjuvant therapies have been given to patients with poor-prognosis locally advanced bladder cancer. Logothetis et al treated 71 patients with poor-prognosis bladder cancer who had vascular or lymphatic invasion, extravesical tumour extension, or node-position disease with adjuvant CISCA, after radical cystectomy. These patients had a 5-year survival of 70% as compared with 37% in 206 case controls. Vascular and lymphatic invasion defined a poor-prognosis group.[28]

A benefit has been shown in favour of four cycles of adjuvant CAP after radical surgery. The median follow-up of the patients was 3 years. There were significant advantages in terms of median survival (4.25 versus 2.41 years) and the percentage of patients disease-free at 3 years (70 versus 46%; $P = 0.001$). One must err on the side of caution in interpreting these findings: of 453 patients with pT3 and pT4 disease who had surgery, 241 were eligible for entry into the trial but only 91 patients enrolled. Eleven patients randomized to treatment received no chemotherapy and overall only 48% (21 patients) completed all four cycles of treatment.[29]

Neoadjuvant chemotherapy

Neoadjuvant therapy, a term of mixed ontogeny, is used to describe the initial treatment of a bladder tumour with chemotherapy. The advantages of treatment are bladder preservation and the avoidance of radiotherapy with its toxicities and relative lack of efficacy. Primary chemotherapy may have the added advantage of downstaging patients converting an unresectable to a resectable lesion.

There have been two major studies of neoadjuvant combination chemotherapy. In these trials of M-VAC and CMV, chemotherapy has frequently been followed by cystectomy, which rather abrogates one of the most important reasons for treatment, which is the maintenance of normal continence. M-VAC led to downstaging of 70% of 41 patients with stage T2–4 transitional cell cancer as defined by transurethral resection. Thirty patients proceded to cystectomy and, of this group, 33% had no tumour.[30] CMV was given to 32 evaluable patients with metastatic urothelial tumours. In this group 8 patients had disease in the bladder, and were restaged by cystectomy; 7 patients had no pathological evidence of residual disease.[31]

The main disadvantage of neoadjuvant therapy is the likelihood that a significant proportion of patients will be overtreated. This will remain problematical, until our ability to predict tumour behaviour from biological and clinical parameters improves.

CONCLUSIONS

Chemotherapy is effective for metastatic urothelial tumours and sustained responses in a significant proportion of patients are reported. Treatment is currently suboptimal in that the majority of patients eventually have progressive disease. It is clear that bladder cancer is chemosensitive and we await the development of treatments that cure a substantial proportion of our patients. These regimens may involve the rescheduling of agents that are currently in use, along the lines of the programmes that have been developed for small cell lung cancer, or the use of new agents. Only 50% of patients who have muscle-invasive disease are cured by current radical treatment. Future work should aim, as in breast cancer, to identify these patients at risk of disease progression, so that systemic treatment can be given. Currently the optimal timing of adjuvant therapy, choice of agents and duration of therapy are unknown.

KEY POINTS FOR CLINICAL PRACTICE

- Up to two-thirds of patients with muscle-invasive disease will eventually die of distant metastases independent of primary therapy.
- Bladder cancer is sensitive to current combination chemotherapeutic regimes which are platinum-based.
- In advanced disease, chemotherapy can lead to durable remissions in up to one-fifth of patients and should be offered to all such patients deemed medically fit. Symptom relief can be obtained in the majority.

REFERENCES

1   Davidson SE, Symonds RP, Snee MP, Upadhyay S, Habeshaw T, Robertson AG. Assessment of factors influencing the outcome of radiotherapy for bladder cancer. Br J Urol 1990; 66: 288–293
2   Quilty PM, Duncan W, Chisholm GD et al. Results of surgery following radical radiotherapy for invasive bladder cancer. Br J Urol 1986; 58: 396–405
3   Zingg EJ, Studer UE. Radical surgery in locally advanced bladder cancer. In: Waxman J, William G, eds. Urological oncology. London: Edward Arnold, 1992: pp 167–184
4   Arap W, Scher HI. Cytotoxic chemotherapy for locally advanced and metastatic bladder cancer. In: Waxman J, Williams G, eds. Urological oncology. London: Edward Arnold, 1992: pp 185–199
5   Hillcoat BL, Raghavan D, Matthews J et al. A randomized trial of cisplatin versus cisplatin plus methotrexate in advanced cancer of the urothelial tract. J Clin Oncol 1986; 7: 706–709
6   Seidman AD, Scher HI. The evolving role of chemotherapy for muscle infiltrating bladder cancer. Semin Oncol 1991; 18: 585–595

7   Soloway MS, Einstein A, Conder MP et al. A comparison of cisplatin and the combination of cisplatin and cyclophosphamide in advanced urothelial cancer: a national Bladder Cancer Collaborative Group A Study. Cancer 1983; 52: 767–772

8   Al-Sarraf M, Frank J, Smith JA Jr et al. Phase II trial of cyclophosphamide, doxorubicin, and cisplatin (CAP) versus amsacrine in patients with transitional cell carcinoma of the urinary bladder: a Southwest Group Study. Cancer Treat Rev 1985; 69: 189–194

9   Khandekar JD, Elson PF, Dewys WD et al. Comparative activity and toxicity of cisdiammine dichloroplatinum (DDP) and a combination of doxorubicin, cyclophosphamide and DDP in disseminated transitional cell carcinomas of the urinary tract. J Clin Oncol 1985; 3: 539–545

10 Troner MD. Cyclophosphamide (C), adriamycin (A), and platinol (P) in the treatment of urothelial malignancy. Proc Am Soc Clin Oncol 1985; 4: 106–109

11 Logothetis CJ, Dexeus FH, Chong C et al. Cisplatin, cyclophosphamide and doxorubicin chemotherapy for unresectable urothelial tumours: the MD Anderson Experience. J Urol 1989; 141: 33–37

12 Logothetis CJ, Dexeus FH, Finn L et al. A prospective randomized trial comparing M-VAC and CISCA chemotherapy for patients with metastatic urothelial tumours. J Clin Oncol 1990; 8: 1050–1055

13 Hanker WG, Meyers FJ, Freiha FS et al. Cisplatin, methotrexate and vinblastine: an effective chemotherapy regimen for metastatic transitional cell carcinoma of the urinary tract. A Northern California Oncology Group Study. J Clin Oncol 1985; 3: 1463–1470

14 Miller RS, Freiha FS, Reese JH et al. Surgical restaging of patients (pts) with advanced transitional cell carcinoma (TCC) of the urothelium treated with cisplatin (C), methotrexate (M), and vinblastine V (CMV): update of the Stanford University Experience. Proc Am Soc Clin Oncol 1991; 10: 67

15 Sternberg CN, Yagoda A, Scher HI et al. M-VAC (methotrexate, vinblastine, Adriamycin and cisplatin) for advanced transitional cell carcinoma of the urothelium. J. Urol 1988; 139: 461–469

16 Sternberg CN, Yagoda A, Scher HI et al. Methotrexate, vinblastine, doxorubicin and cisplatin for advanced transitional cell carcinoma of the urothelium. Efficacy and patterns of response and relapse. Cancer 1989; 64: 2448–2458

17 Loehrer PJ, Elson D, Kuebler JP et al. Advanced bladder cancer: a prospective intergroup trial comparing single agent cisplatin (CDDP) versus M-VAC combination therapy (INT007). Proc Am Soc Clin Oncol 1990; 9: 132

18 Tannock I, Gospodarowicz M, Connolly J, Jewett M. M-VAC (methotrexate, vinblastine, doxorubicin, and cisplatin) chemotherapy for transitional cell carcinoma: the Princess Margaret Hospital experience. J Urol 1989; 142: 289–292

19 Connor JP, Olsson CA, Benson MC, Rapoport F, Sawczuk H. Long term follow up in patients treated with methotrexate, vinblastine, doxorubicin and cisplatin (M-VAC) for transitional cell carcinoma of the urinary bladder: cause for concern. Urology 1989; 34: 353–356

20 Igawa M, Ohkucki T, Veki T et al. Usefulness and limitations of methotrexate, vinblastine, doxorubicin and cisplatin for the treatment of advanced urothelial cancer. J Urol 1990; 144: 662–665

21 Waxman J, Abel P, James N et al. New combination chemotherapy programme for bladder cancer. Br J Urol 1989; 63: 68–71

22 Gabrilove JL, Jakubowski A, Scher H et al. A study of recombinant human granulocyte colony stimulating factor in cancer patients at risk for chemotherapy induced neutropenia. N Engl J Med 1988; 318: 1414–1422

23 Logothetis CJ, Dexeus FH, Sella A et al. Escalated therapy for refractory urothelial tumours: methotrexate-vinblastine-doxorubicin-cisplatin plus glycosylated recombinant human granulocyte macrophage colony stimulating factor. J Natl Cancer Inst 1989; 82: 667–672

24 Logothetis CJ, Hossan E, Sella A et al. Fluorouracil and recombinant human interferon alfa-2a in the treatment of metastatic chemotherapy — refractory urothelial tumours. J Natl Cancer Inst 1991; 83: 285–288

25 Newman LH, Tannenbaum M, Droller MJ. Muscle invasive bladder cancer: does it arise de novo from pre-existing superficial disease. Urology 1988; 32: 58–62

26 Whitmore WF. Management of invasive bladder cancer: a meticulous pelvic node

dissection can make a difference. J Urol 1982; 128: 34–36
27   Heney NM, Ahmed S, Flanaghan MJ et al. Superficial bladder cancer: progression and recurrence. J Urol 1983; 130: 1083–1086
28   Logothetis CJ, Johnson DE, Chong C et al. Adjuvant cyclophosphamide, doxorubicin and cisplatin chemotherapy for bladder cancer: an update. J Clin Oncol 1988; 6: 1540–1546
29   Skinner DG, Daniels JR, Russell CA et al. The role of adjuvant chemotherapy following cystectomy for invasive bladder cancer. A prospective comparative trial. J Urol 1991; 144: 459–464
30   Scher HI, Yagoda A, Herr HW et al. Neoadjuvant M-VAC (methotrexate, vinblastine, doxorubicin and cisplatin) effect on the primary bladder lesion. J Urol 1988; 139: 470–474
31   Meyers FJ, Palmer JM, Davis CA, Freiha FS, Harker EG, Hannigan J. Fate of the urinary bladder in patients with metastatic bladder cancer (TCC) treated with cisplatin, methotrexate and vinblastine (CMV). J Clin Oncol 1986; 4: 250A

9

Screening for prostate cancer

P. Boyle   F. E. Alexander   B. Standaert   L. Denis

Prostate cancer is the second most common form of cancer in men in most developed countries.[1] In the USA it has even overtaken lung cancer in absolute terms of incidence, although it remains second to lung cancer as a cause of cancer death. Most importantly, given that the increased number of children born in several countries after the Second World War will be in their mid 50s in the early part of the 21st century (at an age when cancer risk is becoming an important consideration), and coupled with the trends in increasing life expectancy, the consequence will be an increase in absolute terms in the number of cases of prostate cancer diagnosed. In the absence of treatment improvements and with prospects of prevention by lifestyle modification remote within our current knowledge, there seems certain to be an increase in the number of deaths from this condition. The situation is intensified by the presence of a temporal trend in risk. For this reason, prostate cancer is of great importance for public health and a major effort is required to reduce the impact of these unavoidable increases. Reduction of mortality by screening has recently been emerging as one possible way to accomplish this.

In this context, screening involves the examination of asymptomatic men in order to classify them as likely or unlikely to have prostate cancer. Men who appear likely to have the disease are investigated further to arrive at a final diagnosis and those who are found to have the disease are treated. The organized application of early diagnosis and treatment activities in large groups is often described as population screening. The goal of screening is to reduce mortality from the disease among the people screened by early treatment of the cases of prostate cancer discovered. Screening calls attention to the likelihood of disease before symptoms appear. Screening in connection with early diagnosis and treatment should be clearly distinguished from other uses of the term in epidemiology and clinical practice. In particular, the term 'screening' is commonly used to describe a series of tests done on a symptomatic patient for whom a diagnosis is not yet established. This type of screening is part of the practice of clinical medicine rather than public health or preventive medicine. Screening procedures may also be used to estimate the prevalence of various conditions without immediate disease-control objectives. Screening may also be used to refer to the identification of people at high risk of a disease but who do not yet have it: this is not yet possible in prostate cancer, given the poor knowledge of risk factors. It is clearly important to know from the outset exactly what is meant, and what is not meant, by screening.

It is also important to distinguish between diagnostic tests and screening tests. Morrison[2] uses the example of diabetes. The glucose tolerance test is considered to be diagnostic, while the (random) blood sugar method may be considered as a screening test. Thus a liver biopsy would be considered a diagnostic test for liver cancer and a biopsy of the prostate lesion a diagnostic test for prostate cancer. It is also important to separate what is meant by screening from case-finding. Screening is aimed at the general population and not merely those who have sought medical attention.

At the present time, the widespread implementation of screening programmes for prostate cancer cannot be recommended: little has changed since the most recent review of the topic by an expert committee of the UICC (International Union Against Cancer) which came to the same conclusion.[3] The main reason is that the available screening modalities have not yet been properly evaluated: it is simply unknown whether screening by whatever combination of available modalities is effective in leading to a reduction in the mortality rate of prostate cancer. This is a necessary prerequisite for embarking on population screening or even screening high-risk groups (even if such a group can be defined for prostate cancer). Screening for prostate cancer at a population level would be expensive and involve a large proportion of the resources available for health: it is essential to have some indication of its effectiveness and efficacy before embarking on such programmes. In the USA alone, there would be 17 million men in the age groups likely to be screened: if the screening tests cost $100 per subject per annum then the cost could be 1.7 billion dollars per annum to screen this population. This is not an inconsiderable sum of money.

However, there is some evidence that tools have been developed which may be useful for screening.[4] Before embarking on trials to evaluate their efficacy there are a number of criteria which should be fulfilled: these were outlined by Wilson and Jungner.[5] Each one of these criteria has been addressed in detail elsewhere[6] and will be summarized below. It must be clear that what is being discussed here is screening and not case-finding: the important distinction lies in the necessity to include as near to every man in the target population as can be identified.

IS PROSTATE CANCER AN IMPORTANT PUBLIC HEALTH PROBLEM?

Prostate cancer is undoubtedly an important public health problem and one which seems set to increase.

In 1980, it was estimated that 235 000 new cases of prostate cancer were diagnosed worldwide and 85 000 new cases in the member states of the

European Community: this latter figure represents 13% of all cancers diagnosed in men (excluding non-melanoma skin cancer).[7] In Europe, prostate cancer is the second commonest form of cancer in men after lung cancer. Prostate cancer accounts for 1 in 10 cancer deaths in men in many countries.

Even if age-specific incidence rates remain stable, the problem of prostate cancer seems sure to increase in absolute terms simply because of the ageing of the population. Life expectancy at birth in many western countries is still increasing and half of all boys born today can expect to reach the age of 80 years.

This has major implications for the future burden of prostate disease, including cancer. Half of the male population can soon expect to attain an age when 88% of them will have histological evidence of benign prostatic hyperplasia (BPH)[8] and at least half will have symptoms compatible with the presence of BPH.[9] Assuming no change in the risk of contracting prostate cancer, the number of cases of prostate cancer in the European Community countries among men aged 65 and over will increase from 79 000 in 1990, to 92 000 in 2000, 102 000 in 2010, reaching 120 000 in 2020: an increase of 50% in 30 years. Comparative figures for Canada reveal increases from 6500 cases in 1990 rising to 13 000 cases in 2020. These estimates are based entirely on applying 1980 incident rates to available population projections: the presence of a temporal trend in risk will only serve to increase further these numbers. At the present time in the European Community[7] there is more than three times the number of prostate cancers than cervical cancer, which is the object of several national screening programmes.

Without a significant improvement in survival following therapy, there will be a corresponding increase in the number of deaths from prostate cancer during the same period. Steps to reduce mortality by primary or secondary prevention [i.e. by preventing disease occurring (primary prevention) or to help advance the stage of the disease diagnosed to an early and curable stage (secondary prevention)] would be important public health measures. As yet there is no identified premalignant lesion of the prostate nor any established cause whose removal could reduce the disease burden, making primary prevention a remote hope at present. Secondary prevention, by detecting the disease at an earlier stage with an associated improved prognosis, seems to be the best hope of reducing prostate cancer mortality.

IS THERE AN EFFECTIVE TREATMENT FOR LOCALIZED DISEASE?

Approximately one-half of patients currently diagnosed with prostate cancer present with locally advanced and/or metastatic disease at the time of first diagnosis. The prognosis of patients with advanced prostate cancer, even with the most aggressive treatment, is poor. Cure is elusive: the median time to progression is 18 months and the median survival of metastatic patients is 24 months.

Locally confined prostatic cancer is usually asymptomatic and is often diagnosed because of symptoms similar to BPH. These tumours (T1a–c), incidental prostatic cancer, are not palpable on rectal examination nor may they be visualized by transrectal ultrasound.[10] Prostate cancer confined to the prostate but palpable on rectal examination or visible on transrectal ultrasound is classified as T2 and may be diagnosed at preventive health check-ups.

Results obtained with either radical prostatectomy or radiotherapy for localized disease are favourable. Median survival has been shown to be longer than 15 years in patients with stage B disease:[11] the observed crude survival rates parallel the normal survival curve.[12]

Thus, the search for early-stage prostate cancer could potentially, if successful, lead to a reduction in the mortality rate from this condition.

ARE FACILITIES FOR FURTHER DIAGNOSIS AND TREATMENT AVAILABLE?

At present, the health services of most countries would be stretched by the increased number of cases, both true cases and false-positives, needing further work-up resulting from the implementation of a population-wide screening programme. An incidental consequence would be in the increased number of men with BPH diagnosed as having a pathological disease: some of these would also consume additional health care resources. Some would need treatment for asymptomatic deterioration of renal function. This concerns only a small group of patients but half of those diagnosed would have symptoms that require medical treatment if they are bothersome. Only the patients operated who reveal incidental carcinoma could jeopardize the conclusions from a population screening study.

However, within the context of a screening trial based within one or two geographical regions of a country, the increased resources necessary to cope with the increased workload resulting from a screening programme could be found. Such an investment could result in longer-term savings.

In addition, as should be evident from the figures presented above, the increases likely in the number of cases of prostate cancer in coming decades will have significant resource implications. There will be, consequently, a need for more urologists, more beds for treatment, more operating room sessions, more diagnostic facilities, etc. Thus general facilities can be anticipated by the time the randomized trials have reported.

IS THERE AN IDENTIFIABLE LATENT OR EARLY SYMPTOMATIC STAGE OF PROSTATE CANCER?

Locally confined prostate cancer is usually asymptomatic and is frequently diagnosed during the course of treatment for BPH: tumours found unexpectedly by the pathologist following prostatectomy for BPH are called incidental prostate cancer. It is frequently observed that between 8 and 14% of all prostatectomy specimens can have evidence of malignancy and the incidence of all early lesions is strongly dependent on age.[13]

Undoubtedly, there is a significant proportion of men who are asymptomatic, leading lives with a natural time course and who have latent prostate cancer. The great majority of such men will have a completely natural life since only 12% progress and 3% die from T1a disease. The pathological grading is important and patients with incidental extensive disease (T1b) or higher histological grades are at high-risk of developing clinical disease. Identification of these lesions, that are neither palpable nor visible (on transrectal ultrasound), can only be made by a blind biopsy. The usual indication for such is an elevated prostate specific antigen (PSA). Restraint in multiple blind biopsies should be exercised to avoid overdiagnosis. While there is no doubt that some of these lesions are prognostically very favourable and do not require any treatment, identifying the men with such lesions who are enrolled within a screening programme and informing them about the diagnosis will cause some psychological trauma.

Recent reports of possible premalignant lesions of the prostate are a hopeful development. These lesions, atypical adenomatous hyperplasia (AAH) and prostatic intraepithelial neoplasia (PIN), have been associated with cancers of the transitional[14] and peripheral zone[15] of the prostate. Identification of a premalignant lesion, particularly one which could be readily identified by a relatively simple test, would be of great consequence to prostate screening. However, there requires much more work to be done before this situation can be confirmed and exploited.

IS THE TECHNIQUE TO BE USED FOR SCREENING EFFECTIVE?

There is a range of possible tests which could be used in screening for prostate cancer covering the entire spectrum of complexity, invasiveness, cost, acceptability and, indeed, efficiency in detecting prostate cancer.[4] These include using a symptom history/score; digital rectal examination (DRE); PSA; transrectal ultrasound; and random biopsy of the prostate.

Use of a symptom score can be discounted almost immediately. The great majority of cancers start in the peripheral zone and have escaped through the prostate gland a long time before any pressure is exerted on the urethra, causing the type of symptoms which can be detected by any scoring system. Symptom scores can usefully draw attention to BPH which in turn can reveal a cancer upon further examination or after treatment. However, this is not an efficient strategy to reduce mortality from prostate cancer. Another test which can be discounted is the use of a random biopsy of the prostate which, as described above, is not a screening test but a diagnostic test.

The performance of screening tests is conventionally assessed in the same way as diagnostic tests using the three basic parameters of sensitivity, specificity and positive predictive value. In screening tests, however, a final 'diagnosis' is not obtained for subjects declared negative at screening. This has no effect on the positive predictive value because diagnosis is available for all subjects screened positive. Since large numbers are involved it has little effect too on specificity, which can be accurately estimated as the percentage presumed healthy who were screened negative. Thus these two parameters can be reasonably accurately measured from the preliminary studies of prostate cancer screening which have been conducted to date.

Sensitivity, or the ability of the test to detect the asymptomatic cases amongst the men screened, is clearly of major importance but much harder to estimate. When long-term follow-up is available for screened persons the best estimates of sensitivity[16] come from observing the ability of the test to prevent those cases which would have arisen in a defined period (conventionally 1 year or the time to the next screen). This is found by comparing the incidence in persons screened negative with the expected incidence. No study to date has provided results from which this estimate of sensitivity can be derived for any of the prostate screening modalities. The alternatives which are usually quoted are more truthfully estimates of relative sensitivity which quantify the ability of the test to detect cancers which were found using multimodality screening. This estimate will be referred to below as sensitivity but we note that increasing the number of latent cases detected by any one modality would increase its sensitivity in this sense, whilst possibly having no impact on either true sensitivity or on prostate cancer mortality.

The DRE is the test which has most often been proposed for prostate cancer screening, with the PSA and transrectal ultrasound later considerations. Prostatic structures such as apex, base, median and lateral sulci and seminal vesicles can be readily palpated transrectally: prostate cancer if it is confined will appear as a discrete induration or nodule (T2). Although the DRE has been available for many years, careful evaluation of this as a screening test has yet to take place. Several observational studies have reported parameter estimates but without appropriate controls and with no adjustment for important biases (lead time or length time). Chodak & Schoenberg[17] performed a study on 811 unselected men aged between 50 and 80 years. Of 43 patients found to have an abnormality on palpation of the prostate, 38 agreed to undergo biopsy. The positive predictive value (i.e. prostate cancer confirmed by biopsy) was found to be 29%. Of the cases of prostate cancer confirmed, 45% were stage B, 6% stage C and 18% stage D. This same group of investigators subsequently found a 25% positive predictive value in a further study, with 68% of the detected tumours clinically localized although in many instances at surgery the tumours were found to extend beyond the gland.[18] A number of other studies have also reported a reasonably high proportion of localized, and hence potentially curable, tumours when detected by routine rectal examination.[4]

The most recent published review of the literature on DRE[19] summarized the characteristics of the DRE as a screening test as sensitivity between 55 and

69%; specificity between 89 and 97%; positive predictive value between 11 and 26%; and negative predictive value between 85 and 96%. Subsequently a detection rate of 1.12% was found in a randomly selected population of men reacting to an invitation.[20] The positive predictive value of a suspect DRE was 30%. The DRE has advantages in being inexpensive, non-invasive and with no measurable associated morbidity. However, the detection rate generally achieved by DRE alone (0.13–1.65%) appears to be too low to recommend use of this test on its own.[4] Furthermore, the value of the test very much depends on the skills of the examiner and it remains to be demonstrated whether routine annual screening by DRE can lead to reductions in prostate cancer mortality. Early assessments have given little encouragement.[21]

Imaging of the prostate gland can be achieved by ultrasound, computed tomography and magnetic resonance imaging.[22] Transrectal ultrasound has been the focus of most attention in a variety of settings: again, unfortunately, there has been no study capable of accounting for the important biases mentioned above. Waterhouse & Resnick[23] summarized the available literature as suggesting that transrectal ultrasound has levels of sensitivity and specificity which are probably too low for a single modality screening test. Sensitivity ranged from 71 to 92% for prostate cancer and from 60 to 85% for subclinical disease. Specificity values ranged from 41 to 79% and reported positive predictive values have frequently been around 30%.

The sensitivity and positive predictive value appear to be better for transrectal ultrasound than for DRE, although the relatively low specificity, the invasiveness and the cost of the test are powerful arguments against widespread use of transrectal ultrasound as a single modality screening test.

PSA has recently emerged as a test with promise in screening although, once again, the characteristics of the test as a screening tool have yet to be investigated satisfactorily. The estimated sensitivity appears to be around 70% and the positive predictive values between 26 and 52%. These, of course, can be optimized by changing the cut-off levels of the definition of normal in the test.

The PSA has both advantages and disadvantages as a screening test. On the positive side the test is simple, lacks real invasiveness and its relatively inexpensive (especially when compared to transrectal ultrasound or even DRE if the specialist's time is included in the cost). However, there are great discrepancies demonstrated in the results of the test between the commonly used kits to assay PSA,[24] and PSA is not a specific marker of prostate cancer since it can also be elevated in BPH: it is essentially a product which should be ejected in the ejaculate but, in an enlarged prostate, finds its way into the serum. This means that the PSA could identify an excessive number of false positives (men selected as likely to have prostate cancer at screening but found to be free of the disease on further assessment). This is likely to be exacerbated by the somewhat arbitrary selection of 10 and 4 as cut-off points of normal and the lack of concordance between tests, resulting in a value of 3.0 having different meanings (for disease likelihood) depending on which kit was used to perform the analysis.[24]

Catalona et al[25] used PSA as a first-line screening modality in an asymptomatic population, using a cut-off value of 4.0 µg/l. If an abnormal PSA was found (>4.0 µg/l) the measurement was repeated and DRE, transrectal ultrasound and biopsy followed if the PSA remained abnormal. In 10% of men the PSA was between 4 and 10 µg/l and was greater than 10 µg/l in a further 2%. Of a total of 422 men with a PSA between 4 and 10 µg/l, in 304 a second PSA resulted in a value of greater than 4. In 240 men, transrectal ultrasound-guided biopsy was performed and 58 men (nearly one-quarter) were found to have prostate cancer; in three-quarters it was locally confined. In 78 men with a PSA >10 µg/l, 47 (60%) men had prostate cancer with only 1 in 3 found to be confined to the prostate. The detection rate was 2.45% and the positive predictive value was found to be 33%.

The PSA can be improved, as noted above, by altering the definitions of the normal range. It is also possible when investigating men with large prostates to utilize a correction factor known as the PSA density. When the volume of the prostate is known by ultrasound, correction of elevated PSA levels is thought to be possible by dividing the PSA level by the estimated volume. However, the limited information available about this comes uniquely from clinical studies of symptomatic patients and cannot be applied to (asymptomatic) screening populations: the value of PSA for screening, whether adjusted for volume or otherwise, will require to be calculated in this same population (of asymptomatic men from the general population).

It seems that a combination of screening tests could be most appropriate for prostate cancer. Each of the three tests discussed assesses a different aspect of the prostate: the DRE for induration; transrectal ultrasound for hypoechoic lesions, and PSA for elevated levels of an enzyme that should only be present in ejaculate. There have been two observational studies reported[26,27] using the three tests. Both studies were in good agreement regarding the low rate of prostate cancer detected in men who had a normal DRE and PSA but a positive transrectal ultrasound. This does not appear to support the performance of transrectal ultrasound on all men as a screening test. Given the financial implications alluded to earlier, good financial management would lead investigators to consider the possible efficacy of screening initially with DRE and PSA and performing transrectal ultrasound only on those men found to be suspicious on one examination.

ARE THE TESTS ACCEPTABLE TO THE POPULATION?

It is difficult to quote reliable, global estimations of acceptance/compliance in prostate screening studies: none has really been conducted so far. However, some information is available from the pilot programme undertaken in Antwerp (Denis L and Standaert B, personal communication, 1993) which looked at DRE, PSA and transrectal ultrasound.

Each selected candidate is visited at home by a social nurse who explains the nature of the study, including the randomization procedure. Those who agree to participate are then randomized into two groups. Group A is invited to the screening centre to receive the three screening tests. Group B receives a letter mentioning that the participant has not been allocated to the screening group but that he can consult his general practitioner if he wishes. After visiting the screening centre, a randomly selected sample of Group A (1 in 3) is interviewed at home regarding the acceptability of the screening tests.

After the first 6 months of the Antwerp pilot programme, 7766 men from the age group 60–74 were identified as potential study participants. It was surprising to the organizers that 1732 (22.3%) could not be contacted after two home visits. A total of 2286 (37.9%) men who were contacted agreed to participate in the study, with equal numbers allocated to both groups.

As of May 1992, 857 men of group A had been investigated. Of these, 285 men had received a second visit at home and had been interviewed concerning their feeling on the acceptability of the test and the level of discomfort perceived during the examination. The interviews were conducted by a social nurse (community nurse) who asked approximately 20 questions.

Of those interviewed, 23% expressed to having experienced some anxiety prior to the examination regarding positive findings. Only 13% were concerned about pain or discomfort prior to the examination. Some 22% reported experiencing some pain during the transrectal ultrasound examination, 56.8% reported experiencing some discomfort but 87.4% were prepared to participate in further examinations within 2 years.

Despite the uncomfortable nature of the examination, the high proportion of men who agreed to be screened again is very reassuring.

IS THE NATURAL HISTORY OF PROSTATE CANCER KNOWN?

This is a crucial question which must be addressed. Specifically for prostate cancer this relates to the biological development of the asymptomatic lesions detected by screening. Some of these will on clinical assessment be infiltrating and requiring therapy, yet might never have caused any morbidity during the subject's natural life span. Others will be more conventionally classifiable as latent or preinvasive. Some of both categories might regress if left untreated. All of the above are examples where screening confers no benefit. At present there is an inadequate understanding of the factors which influence transition from latent and/or slow-growing disease to more aggressive forms with the potential to reduce life expectancy. Reports from screening studies suggest detection rates at initial screening can be close to 3% in general populations, yet if other causes of mortality are ignored, only 3% of a population of men aged 50–74 might die from prostate cancer before their 85th birthday. Since a substantial, though unknown, proportion of these would be undetectable at the single screening, these figures suggest that a large proportion of cases detected at screening would not have surfaced clinically during the remaining life span.

The situation begins, as ever, with a normal epithelial cell. Recently it has been suggested that AAH may be a premalignant lesion for the transitional zone of the prostate and PIN a premalignant lesion of the peripheral zone of the prostate,[14,15] although this is controversial and remains to be proved. It is certainly clear, however, that PIN can be described when there is dysplasia in a prostate but its precise significance is not yet clear. Therefore, the change from a normal cell to a focal carcinoma may possibly have an identifiable intermediate state but this has not been proved. Focal carcinoma is a much less advanced disease than adenocarcinoma which is hormone-dependent, which in its turn is not so aggressive as adenocarcinoma which is hormone-independent.

However, it is not entirely clear that the transformation of PIN to focal carcinoma occurs and whether the transformation from focal carcinoma to infiltrating adenocarcinoma takes place.[6] There is some rationale for considering that focal carcinoma may be a different disease, particularly in that the incidence does not demonstrate geographical variability compared to the 120-fold variation which exists in the incidence rate of prostate cancer.[28]

Thus, simply, it cannot be predicted on an individual basis which, if any, AAH or PIN lesions will progress to focal carcinoma (or indeed directly to infiltrating carcinoma) or which incidental focal carcinomas may progress to infiltrating adenocarcinomas. It is important to recall the findings of Lowe and Listrom,[29] who calculated that the median time of progression for T1a lesions was 13.5 years and for T1b lesions was 4.75 years: in other words, very few patients seemed to live long enough to die from prostate cancer, although being elderly, the death rate from intercurrent disease was high. Blute et al[30] observed that there was a higher rate of progression and death from prostate cancer in younger men in their series, although this was not subsequently confirmed.[29]

It cannot, at present, be excluded that screening may upset this balance through diagnosing more cases of early prostate cancer, leading to more men being treated and to more deaths resulting from complications from the surgery either in the short or medium term.

IS THERE A STRATEGY FOR DETERMINING WHICH PATIENTS SHOULD AND SHOULD NOT BE TREATED?

The only group of patients who can safely be excluded from treatment on the basis of a pretreatment evaluation are those who have well-differentiated small-volume focal prostate carcinoma.

Use of transrectal ultrasound (as a diagnostic procedure) is now making it increasingly possible at the present time to preselect patients with localized, palpable disease and the possibility of overtreatment in this particular group, which could not be excluded in the immediate past, is now decreasing. This is an important advance in the development of screening tests for prostate cancer.

IS THE COST OF SCREENING ACCEPTABLE?

It is true to say that the costs involved in an evaluation of prostate screening in a large, randomized trial are much less than those which would be incurred—and squandered—if an unevaluated methodology which was ineffective became commonly accepted and implemented as a screening procedure by the medical profession. This is particularly true for transrectal ultrasound and PSA.

The recent finding that two-thirds of members of the American Urological Association used PSA as a screening test in men up to the age of 80 is of considerable concern. It remains unknown if using PSA as a screening test will lead to a reduction in mortality from prostate cancer and the costs of the test, including the significant costs of working up those false positives, would eat up a significant proportion of the entire health budget in many countries with an ageing population. Calculations of the likely cost of diagnosing each new case of prostate cancer are much higher than those for screening for cervix cancer.

IS EFFECTIVE TREATMENT AVAILABLE AND DOES MANAGEMENT OF CASES IN THE EARLY STAGES HAVE A FAVOURABLE IMPACT ON PROGNOSIS?

Radical prostatectomy and radiation therapy are clearly effective forms of treatment to cure tumours limited to the prostate for appropriately selected patients. Unfortunately, no evidence yet exists from randomized studies indicating that patients with localized prostatic cancer benefit from early treatment in terms of overall mortality and cancer-related mortality.[29,31]

It is clear that the majority of the criteria of Wilson & Jungner[5] can be met, although there are some important doubts. Principally, the present uncertainties about the natural history of PIN and focal carcinomas are disturbing and there is evidence suggesting that screening could cause excess morbidity through 'over-diagnosis'. Secondly, the true sensitivities of the screening modalities are unknown. We do not consider these to be weighty arguments against the establishment of large randomized trials to determine whether screening can indeed reduce mortality for prostate cancer. Indeed, these trials are timely since public and clinical attention is already being directed towards screening. There is a danger of this public health measure being introduced without scientific evaluation to an extent where randomized trials would be impractical and/or unethical.

These trials will in addition provide some insight into the relative performance of the screening modalities and the natural history of the disease by, for example, reporting the true incidence rate of disease and its stage distribution in men undergoing regular screening. Complementary studies of disease natural history will also be required.

It is also clear that the criteria of Wilson and Jungner[5] do not mention whether screening adds positive value to the quality of the participants life. This point is very difficult to evaluate but may be of particular interest for prostate cancer since many men with prostate cancer will die from other causes.

Principles of screening trials

There are a number of important considerations which should be taken into account before undertaking even trial of screening for prostate cancer.

The increased demand for services created by the screening programme should not be underestimated. Men with positive screening tests will need rapid further assessment as anxiety is created by the screening test. The decision of whether they are considered to have prostate cancer or not should be arrived at as soon as possible. Most of the workload from a screening programme is likely to come from men who are positive at the screening test but who do not have prostate cancer (the false positives). The proportion of those screened without prostate cancer who are positive at the screening test will be determined by the specificity of the screening test used. However, it is likely that one single test will not be adequate for prostate cancer screening and it seems at present that a series of tests will require to be evaluated: DRE, PSA and transrectal ultrasound. The order of the tests is of importance: if the tests are given in the order of decreasing false-positive rate (i.e. the test with the highest false-positive rate first) then the overall false-positive rate will be minimized. The likeliest order would be DRE, PSA and then transrectal ultrasound (with biopsy of hypoechogenic lesions) on men who were not negative on both DRE and PSA. (Note that this is true if a series of decision rules apply, including certain negative results precluding application of the next test.)

Thus, an important prerequisite to any trial would be to have adequate information about the specificity and relative sensitivity of the screening tests.

It is also important that the management of prostate cancer does not differ between the screened and the unscreened group since it would be difficult to separate the benefits of treatment and screening between the two groups. A protocol for treating patients entered into the trial would be a major advantage: this may be standard clinical practice.

During the course of the screening examinations, there will undoubtedly be a proportion of men found to have asymptomatic BPH. The temptation to treat these men should be resisted since surgical treatment could have two implications. Men could be found to have latent carcinoma (10% upon histological examination of the surgical specimen) which could not be detected by the screening examination. Furthermore, men could have a prostatectomy and no carcinoma found. The net effect would be to leave the trial in balance for 'men-at-risk', but not balanced regarding 'prostates-at-risk'.

The requirements of a study to assess whether, for example, transrectal ultrasound is better than DRE as a screening test are different from a study designed to assess whether transrectal ultrasound and DRE in combination is an effective screening procedure. The study aims and hypotheses must be agreed clearly before embarking on a study.

The only conclusive end-point for the evaluation of a screening test for prostate cancer is a significant reduction in prostate cancer mortality in the screened population compared to the control group. In this comparison, the screened group must include all men offered screening, not merely all those who are screened. Other possible end-points are susceptible to the effects of lead time bias, length time bias or selection bias: these terms are explained by Morrison.[2]

COMPARISON OF SCREENING FOR BREAST AND PROSTATE CANCER

It is always important to learn from previous experience in related areas. A good comparison would be of the current situation in prostate cancer with that in breast cancer around the period when mammography was being developed in the 1960s.

Breast cancer shares with prostate cancer the characteristic of (essential) restriction to one sex for which it has major public health importance. Although lung cancer rates occasionally exceed it, breast cancer is the most common cancer in females—using either incidence or mortality rates— in many parts of the world, including most of Europe and the USA.[32] The cause of the disease is poorly understood[33] and therapeutic improvements in the last 30 years have led to the use of less aggressive and damaging therapy rather than to survival benefit, although the use of adjuvant therapy by, in particular, tamoxifen is a recent and notable exception.[34]

However, survival for smaller and early-stage tumours was (and is) known to be better than for more advanced disease (at least in the first decade post-diagnosis). Thirty years ago screening tests were already available[35] which satisfied the Wilson & Jungner[5] criteria and offered the possibility of reduction in mortality from breast cancer through secondary prevention. The Health Insurance Plan (HIP) trial of breast cancer screening was the first randomized controlled trial of cancer screening.[36]

It is appropriate to make two comparisons of prostate and breast cancer: firstly at the time when the screening trials were first being introduced (i.e. the 1990s for prostate cancer, 1965 for breast cancer) and secondly, at the present time.

The pretrial situations are similar in many respects: there is above all a need to determine whether the existing favourable signs for prostate cancer will be proved to be correct, with the confirmation that mortality can be reduced and a tension between those who appreciate the need for large, expensive studies avoiding bias and those who would prefer to use simpler, though incorrect analyses (e.g. survival in cases detected by screening). There is concern regarding the possible costs of work-up for those people found positive on screening and the potential for over-diagnosis. It was not clear for breast cancer in the late 1960s which test (mammography or physical examination) would be most suitable and the HIP trial used the two independently. Four important factors were different:

1. The age-incidence pattern of disease and hence the age of the population to be screened (screening for breast cancer was initially for women 40–64 years of age since 41% of deaths from breast cancer are associated with cases diagnosed 35–49 years and 38% with cases diagnosed at ages 50–64 years).[37]
2. Partly as a consequence of this, overall acceptance rates of offers of breast cancer screening are rarely below 65%.
3. Screen detection rates for breast cancer are of the same order of magnitude as the population incidence rate (for HIP, they were 2.73/1000 women screened and 1.87/1000 women years); the ratio of these two is a crude estimate of lead time and the 10-fold excess for prostate cancer combined with the age of the population provides evidence for possible major over-diagnosis.
4. The vast majority of breast cancers detected by the screening tests were of favourable stage (i.e. operable, localized disease), thus almost all cases detected by screening could potentially receive some benefit from early treatment and it was anticipated that mortality improvement would be observed within 5 years of follow-up (since many of the asymptomatic cases of prostate cancer are already metastatic, much longer periods of follow-up may be required).

Now, in the 1990s, four randomized trials of breast cancer screening have been reported (involving some 280 000 women) and there is a consensus that screening (at least for women aged 50–64 years) does lead to mortality benefit;[38] this is part of public health policy in many countries and is believed to be cost-effective. The best estimates for the mortality reduction are around 20%, although 10-year results from the HIP[39] and more recent results from Sweden[16] reported 30% reductions. Often the results of individual trials have not been statistically significant, power calculations having been based on a 30% reduction. Acceptance rates in the context of trials (where scepticism regarding benefit must prevail) have varied from 65% to over 90%[16] but, critically, have shown a marked reduction with increasing age. Results from the HIP study[39] have shown that over-diagnosis was not then a problem, since cumulative incidence rates in the two arms of the trial were identical 4 years after the end of screening. The HIP trial did not—and could not, since both screening modalities were involved in selecting people for diagnostic procedures—provide clear guidance on screening modality; this has developed gradually and, in any event, modern mammography is technically far superior to that used by HIP. None of the studies conducted to date has succeeded in answering the important question of whether screening women under 50 years is beneficial. These lessons provide a total vindication of policy of evaluating screening through properly conducted randomized trials while at the same time emphasizing that they will never be a panacea providing all the answers we require. It also reminds current investigators of the need for size, both in the numbers entered into the studies and in terms of years of follow-up.

SUMMARY AND CONCLUSIONS

The number of deaths from prostate cancer in many western countries is set to increase with the ageing population: more men will live to older age, when prostate cancer is more frequent. There are currently no great hopes of major advances in outcome due to therapy, and prospects for prevention are remote: risk factors for prostate cancer are poorly understood. Advances in tools introduced to diagnose prostate cancer without the need for biopsy have resulted in hopes that they could be successfully employed as screening procedures.

At present there is not enough evidence to advocate the implementation of widespread screening programmes: the screening tests available, alone or in combination, have not been properly characterized in terms of sensitivity and specificity and none has been tested to determine whether their routine application can lead to a reduction in the mortality rate of prostate cancer. However, the current situation goes a long way to meeting the criteria established by Wilson & Jungner[5] to judge whether screening can be advocated, at least on a trial basis. There remains an urgent need for more information and a clearer understanding of the natural history of AAH and PIN lesions and focal carcinoma and the conversion from hormone-dependent to hormone-independent adenocarcinoma.

Before a screening trial of prostate cancer can be initiated, the sensitivity and specificity of the proposed screening test (or their combination) must be assessed. A protocol for treatment of diseases of the prostate must be agreed upon prior to the study: this may simply be existing standard clinical practice but it must be the same in the screened and the unscreened groups.

It is essential that some element of randomization of individuals forms the basis of the evaluation of the screening. Randomization of individuals is just as necessary in the present context as in clinical trials of cancer therapy.

To avoid bias it is essential that screening trials are analysed on an intention-to-treat basis. Thus an intervention group offered screening is compared with a control group not offered screening. The mortality experience of the two groups of men from their date of randomization is compared. In order to maximize the statistical power of the trial it is necessary both to screen as many men as possible in the intervention group and to discourage men in the control group from having screening outside the trial. The result of this action leads to a very significant dilution effect[40] and a dramatic decrease in the power of any study. This is particularly problematic in the USA where so many urologists screen with PSA in men up to the age of 80.

Once the choice of design of the screening trial is made, a small, feasibility study must be undertaken to get satisfactory estimates of response rates, sensitivity and specificity for screening tests and other important variables. In particular, it needs to be sure that there is a follow-up system in place to obtain notification of deaths in both groups and cancers diagnosed between screens in both groups. For an open-ended study a stopping rule must also be agreed in advance.

It is clear that at present, the need is for randomized trials of prostate cancer screening: it must be shown that the screening tests can reduce mortality from the disease. The analogy with the situation of breast cancer in the mid 1960s is apposite and the lessons learned from breast cancer screening should be borne in mind when designing studies of prostate cancer. Principally these include the need to design trials so that individual tests or policies can be evaluated; the need for large studies; and the necessity not to be too optimistic when estimating the proposed benefit of screening in terms of mortality reduction. With these lessons learned and incorporated into large, coordinated randomized trials, it will hopefully prove possible to turn any screening advantage for prostate cancer into a public health measure in less time than the 25 years taken from mammography development to its use in national programmes.

GLOSSARY OF TERMS

Measures of accuracy of binary classification

It is always valuable to have a quantitative estimate of the accuracy (validity) of any measurement. This is particularly important when evaluating the accuracy of the result of a binary classification (disease/not disease) such as that given as a result of a screening test. It is also impossible to know the true disease status ($+$ve/$-$ve) for those found to be negative on screening.

Classification	Number of cases
Screen $+$ve, disease $+$ve	a
Screen $+$ve, disease $-$ve	b
Screen $-$ve, disease $+$ve	c
Screen $-$ve, disease $-$ve	d
disease $+$ve	$a + c$
disease $-$ve	$b + d$
False-positive rate $= b/(a + b)$	
Positive predictive value $= a/(a + b)$	

When working with such a classification of outcome there are two distinct aspects of the accuracy of measurement.

Sensitivity is the proportion of those who truly have the disease who are correctly classified as having it by the screening test.

Specificity is the proportion of those who truly do not have the disease who are correctly classified as not having it by the screening test.

Sensitivity = $a/(a + c)$
Specificity = $d/(b + d)$

Note that c and d cannot be known at the time of screening but since $c \ll d$ the assumption that $c = 0$ permits accurate estimation of specificity.

The screening test is only perfect when both sensitivity and specificity are 1.0. In the case where sensitivity is equal to 1 minus the specificity then the screening test is no better than an entirely random means for classifying individuals.

Possible biases in screening studies

There are two possible effects of screening that may result in a higher survival among screen-detected cases than in routinely diagnosed cases: these effects are biases since they are not separated readily from the therapeutic effect of early treatment.

Patients whose disease is detected by screening gain *lead time*: the diagnosis of their disease is earlier than the time the clinical diagnosis would have occurred. Even if the time of death is unchanged, the proportion of cases that survive for some specified period after diagnosis (and the proportion of earlier-stage cases) will increase as a result of earlier diagnosis alone.

Screening may also tend to identify cases destined to have a relatively benign course even if there is no lead time or reduction in mortality from early treatment. This prognostic selection would occur if screening programmes attract volunteers who are relatively healthy and who will tend to have a favourable clinical course (i.e. selection bias). It is also the situation that screening itself preferentially identifies disease with a long preclinical phase: this phenomenon is referred to *length-biased sampling*. Patients with such disease may also have a long clinical phase, i.e. with a favourable survival. Comparisons of survival are likely to suggest a benefit even if none exists and may greatly exaggerate the size of the true benefit as it would be reflected in the mortality rate of the screened population.

The interested reader is referred to Morrison[2] for more substantial discussion of these and other methodological and practical aspects of screening.

REFERENCES

1   Muir CS, Waterhouse JAH, Powell J, Mack T, Whelan S. (eds) Cancer incidence in five continents, vol V. IARC scientific publication 88. Lyon: IARC, 1988
2   Morrison AS. Screening in chronic disease. New York: Oxford University Press, 1985
3   Miller AB. Issues in screening for prostate cancer. In: Miller AB, Chamberlan C, Day NE, Hakama M, Prorock PC, eds. Cancer screening. Cambridge: UICC, Cambridge University Press, 1991

4   Bentvelsen FM, Schroder FH. Modalities available for screening for prostate cancer. Eur J Cancer 1993; 29A: 804–811

5   Wilson JMG, Jungner G. Principles and practice of screening for disease. Public health paper no 34. Geneva: WHO, 1969

6   Schroder FH, Boyle P. Screening for prostate cancer–necessity or nonsense? Eur J Cancer 1993; 29A: 656–661

7   Jensen OM, Esteve J, Moller H, Renard H. Cancer in the European Community and its members states. Eur J Cancer 1990; 26: 1167–1256

8   Boyle P. Epidemiology of benign prostatic hyperplasia. Prospectives 1990; 1: 1–4

9   Guess H. Population studies in benign prostatic hyperplasia. Prospectives 1992; 2: 1–4

10 Hermanek P, Hutter RVP, Sobin LH. Prognostic grouping – the next step in tumour classification. J Cancer Res Clin Oncol. 1990; 116: 513–516

11 Gibbons RP. Total prostatectomy for clinically localized prostate cancer: long-term surgical results and current morbidity.Natl Cancer Inst Monograph 1988; 7: 123–126

12 National Cancer Institute Consensus Development Conference on the management of clinically localized prostate cancer. Bethesda: NIH, 1988 (NCI Monograph 7)

13 Schroeder FH. The natural history of incidental prostatic carcinoma. Proc Symp Incidental Prostatic Cancer 1993; (in press)

14 Bostwick DG, Srigley JR. Premalignant lesions. In: Bostwick DG, ed. Pathology of the prostate. New York: Churchill Livingstone, 1990: pp 37–59

15 Mostofi FK, Davis CJ, Sesterhenn I. Pathology of carcinoma of the prostate. Cancer 1993; 70: 235–253

16 Tabar L, Fagerberg G, Duffy SW, Day NE. The Swedish two county trial of mammographic screening for breast cancer: recent results and calculation of benefit. J Epidemiol Community Health 1989; 43: 107–114

17 Chodak GW, Schoenberg HW. Early detection of prostate cancer by routine screening. JAMA 1984; 252: 3261–3264

18 Chodak GW, Keller P, Schoenberg HW. Assessment of screening for prostate cancer using the digital rectal examination. J Urol 1989; 141: 1136–1138

19 Resnick MI. Editoral comments. In: Rattiff TL (eds) Genitourinary cancer. Boston: Martinus Nijhoff, 1987: pp 94–99

20 Pederson KV, Carlsson P, Varenhorst E, Lofman O, Berglund K. Screening for carcinoma of the prostate by digital rectal examinations in a randomly selected population. Br Med J 1990; 300: 1041–1044

21 Friedman GD, Hiatt RA, Quesenberry CP, Selby JV. Case-control study of screening for prostate cancer by digital rectal examination. Lancet 1991; 337: 1526–1529

22 Rifkin MD, Daehnert W, Kurtz AB. State of the art: endorectal sonography of the prostate gland. Am J Roentgenol 1990; 154: 691–700

23 Waterhouse RL, Resnick MI. The use of transrectal prostatic ultrasonography in the evaluation of patients with prostatic carcinoma. J Urol 1989; 141: 233–239

24 Turkes A, Nott JP, Griffith K. Prostate-specific antigen: problems in analysis. Eur J Cancer 1981; 27: 650–653

25 Catalona WJ, Smith DS, Ratliff TL et al. Measurement of prostate-specific antigen in serum as a screening-test for prostate cancer. N Engl J Med 1991; 324: 1156–1161

26 Cooner WH, Mosley BR, Rutherford CL et al. Prostate cancer detection in a clinical urological practice by ultrasonography, digital rectal examination and prostate specific antigen. J Urol 1990; 143: 1146–1154

27 Lee F, Torp-Pedersen ST, Littrup PJ et al. Hypoechoic lesions of the prostate: clinical relevance of tumour size, digital rectal examination and prostate-specific antigen. Radiology 1989; 170: 29–33

28 Zaridze DG, Boyle P. Cancer of the prostate: epidemiology and aetiology. Br J Urol 1987; 59: 493–503

29 Lowe BA, Listrom MB. Incidental carcinoma of the prostate: an analysis of predictors of progression. J Urol 1988; 140: 1340–1344

30 Blute ML, Zincke H, Farrow GM. Long-term follow-up of young patients with stage A adenocarcinoma of the prostate. J Urol 1988; 140: 1340–1344

31 Whitmore WF. Overview: historical and contemporary. Natl Cancer Inst Monograph 1988; 7: 7–11

32 Boyle P. Breast cancer epidemiology. Baillieres Clin Oncol 1988; 2: 1–59

33 Miller AB, Bulbrook RD. UICC multidisciplinary project on breast cancer: the epidemiology, aetiology and prevention of breast cancer. Int J Cancer 1986; 37: 173–177

34 Early Breast Cancer Trialists Collaborative Group. Systematic treatment of early breast cancer by hormonal, cytotoxic or immunetherapy. Lancet 1992; 1: 1–17

35 Gershen-Cohen J, Helmel MB, Berger SM. Detection of breast cancer by periodic x-ray examination: a five-year survey. JAMA 1961; 176: 1114–1116

36 Shapiro S, Strax MD, Venet L. Periodic breast cancer screening in reducing mortality from breast cancer. JAMA 1971; 215: 1777–1785

37 Shapiro S. Evidence on screening for breast cancer from a randomized trial. Cancer 1977; 39: 2772–2782

38 Wald N, Frost C, Cuckle H. Breast cancer screening: the current position.Br Med J 1991; 302: 845–846

39 Shapiro S, Venet W, Strax P, Venet L, Roeser R. Ten- to fourteen-year effect of screening on breast cancer mortality. J Natl Cancer Inst 1982; 69: 349–355

40 Zelen M. Are primary cancer prevention trials feasible? J Natl Cancer Inst 1988; 80: 1442–1444

10

Optimal therapy for metastatic prostate cancer

F. J. Mayer   E. D. Crawford

In the USA, prostate cancer is the most frequently diagnosed neoplasm in men and the second leading cause of cancer death. It has been estimated that 132 000 new cases would be diagnosed in 1992, and 35 000 men will die of prostate cancer this year. The public is becoming increasingly aware of the disease, to the point where American men are bypassing their primary physician and presenting directly to the urologic specialist and requesting 'a screening exam for prostate cancer'. A recent American periodical went so far as to pronounce that while the most common topic of discussion in elderly (65 years old and older) male quarters these days is still politics, prostatic diseases is running a close second place. Already this public is starting to ask some exceedingly difficult questions regarding the diagnosis and treatment of prostate cancer—questions for which urologists do not always have good answers.

Several factors make prostate cancer a difficult disease to study. While the autopsy incidence of prostate cancer in men 50–90 years old is roughly 30–40%, only about 8% of men will ever develop 'clinically significant prostate cancer', that is, a cancer which presents a mortal threat.[1] Thus, the majority of men with microscopic prostate cancer will never require treatment, but at the same time we have no differential test which can reliably determine which men are at risk for developing potentially lethal disease. Once a cancer is clinically evident, it will progress. Additionally, prostate adenocarcinoma is an inherently slow-growing tumor, with a doubling time of roughly 6 months to 2 years. Therefore, studies which attempt to show a survival advantage between competing therapies in prostate cancer must have rather extensive follow-up periods before a significant survival difference may be observed. In a world where results are often rushed to publication before the data have matured, invalid conclusions are sometimes drawn regarding optimal treatment of prostate cancer, solely due to short follow-up periods. Finally, the variability in response to androgen withdrawal among prostate tumors mandates that a large study population be provided so as to avert potential sampling errors and to assure equality among study arms. If one wishes to conduct a prospective, multiarmed trial in prostate cancer, the number of subjects required to assure adequate statistical power can be quite large—and virtually impossible to obtain except through the efforts of a

159

well-run cooperative group. The above impediments must be considered during the design of a clinical trial for metastatic prostate cancer to ensure that valid conclusions are drawn.

While metastatic prostate cancer may be an inherently difficult disease to study, this is not due to a lack of available subjects. Greater than 50% of men with newly diagnosed prostate cancer will have metastatic disease revealed upon completion of their staging protocol. Two recent studies quantify the magnitude of the problem. In an extensive study of men with clinically localized prostate cancer (stage A or B) who were subjected to staging pelvic lymphadenectomy, 30% were found to harbor pelvic lymph node metastases.[2] In a population-based study of over 600 Swedish subjects undergoing a standardized staging protocol, 24% of the men presented with osseous metastases as disclosed by bone scintigraphy.[3] Thus, using traditional means of diagnosing prostate cancer we can expect to cure fewer than half of all men diagnosed with prostate adenocarcinoma. Clearly the majority of men presenting with prostate cancer will not be candidates for radical prostatectomy, but rather will be treated in a palliative sense. While there has been only modest improvement in survival since the landmark work of Huggins and Hodges,[4] there is still considerable interest in this arena, and the thrust in research may soon be toward better palliation of the many men with metastatic disease and away from early, aggressive treatment of occult or localized prostate cancer.

EARLY ANDROGEN ABLATION

In the 20 years after the publication of the first Veterans Administration Co-operative Urological Research Group study (VACURG 1),[5] most men in the USA with advanced or metastatic prostate cancer were managed on an observation protocol and only treated with androgen ablation at the first sign of symptomatic progression. The study failed to show enhanced overall survival when patients were begun on diethylstilbestrol (DES) 5 mg/day or received orchiectomy at diagnosis, as compared to a placebo group who were allowed to cross-over to either therapy at symptomatic progression.[5] The study can be faulted due to its failure to stratify the results by cause-specific mortality, as cancer-specific survival did appear to be improved slightly if instituted at diagnosis and not in delayed fashion. The increased rate of cardiovascular mortality in the patients receiving DES seemed to be responsible for the equivalence in survival of the DES and placebo arms.[6] In the second Veterans Administration Co-operative study (VACURG 2), patients with advanced or metastatic disease who were randomized to DES 1 mg/day experienced improved overall survival compared to the placebo group, though the survival curves only diverged after 2 years and did not stratify for cancer-specific mortality.[7]

More compelling data for the advantages of early androgen withdrawal comes from the placebo-controlled trial of leuprolide with or without flutamide in patients with D2 prostate cancer (National Cancer Institute protocol 0036). In the subgroup of patients with good performance status and minimal osseous metastases (low volume of disease), the progression-free survival was considerably greater when compared to the subgroup with more numerous bone lesions and similar performance status.[8] With these studies, the rationale for allowing prostate cancer to proceed unfettered until large volumes of metastatic deposits caused severe symptoms was effectively abandoned.

CANCER CELL HETEROGENEITY

Fifty years of experience with hormonal treatment for metastatic prostate cancer has generated a few well-known facts regarding the natural history of the disease. While medical or surgical castration ensures a roughly 80% initial response rate, uniformly 20% of patients treated appropriately will never respond to androgen deprivation. Of the patients experiencing a remission or stabilization of their disease, nearly all will eventually show progression of the cancer and die from the disease. If relapsing patients are treated with secondary attempts at androgen ablation—exchanging medical castration for surgical castration, adding an antiandrogen, medical or surgical adrenalectomy, etc.—the results are predictably poor.[9] The above facts are tacit evidence for the existence of androgen-unresponsive cell lines in prostate cancer. These clones may be present in the nascent tumor or arise as mutations due to selective environmental pressures induced by androgen withdrawal.

An alternate hypothesis holds that in any given prostate cancer cell population there exists subpopulations of cells which demonstrate variable responsiveness to androgen withdrawal, some populations being exquisitely sensitive to androgen ablation, while others are only marginally sensitive or even insensitive to withdrawal. The Shionogi mouse mammary tumor, a dihydrotestosterone-responsive cancer, has demonstrated this phenomenon in elegantly performed basic science studies.[10] Finally, prostate cancer cells can be successfully cultured in a synthetic medium devoid of androgens.[11]

STAGE D0 DISEASE

The presence of a persistently elevated serum enzymatic acid phosphatase level during preoperative staging (so-called D0 disease) is an ominous finding for the patient with prostatic adenocarcinoma. Generally speaking, 60–100% of men with this predicament will have incurable disease. In a study of patients with elevated serum enzymatic acid phosphatase levels who were subjected to staging pelvic lymphadenectomy (25 subjects), 60% of patients were found to have metastases to the pelvic lymph nodes. Of the group without metastases to the lymph nodes, the majority (70%) developed bone scan evidence of metastatic disease within 2–3 years. Overall, 20 of 22 men available for follow-up demonstrated systemic disease during the observation period.[12] Of note, in the group of men without pelvic lymph node metastases, most had the prostate gland left in situ, and the bone metastases detected during follow-up may have been attributable to the extant tumor and were not present at the time of lymphadenectomy. Recently, the M.D. Anderson Cancer Center reviewed its result of staging pelvic lymph node dissection in prostate cancer, finding metastases to the pelvic lymph nodes in all 18 patients with preoperative clinical stage D0 disease.[13] Clearly, a majority of patients with clinically localized prostate cancer but persistently elevated serum enzymatic acid phosphatase levels will have systemic disease at presentation.

Nevertheless, strict management guidelines for the patient with D0 prostate cancer have not been formulated. Most patients with presumed stage D0 disease will indeed harbor pelvic lymph node metastases and should be managed as though they have D1 disease. However, a small percentage of men with D0 disease will have clinically localized prostate cancer on digital rectal exam and would have negative pelvic lymphadenectomy results (and negative bone scan results) upon completion of surgical staging. Treating these men as though they have systemic cancer may be a disservice to the group. At the present time, prospective trials are underway to evaluate this group, utilizing staging pelvic lymphadenectomy, and neoadjuvant androgen blockade for 3–6 months followed by radical prostatectomy. By necessity, follow-up in this study should be upwards of 10 years before definitive recommendations may be made, owing to the indolent nature of prostate cancer and the possibility of prolonged survival in 'low-volume' metastatic disease. Thus, we will likely be well into the next century before this question is adequately answered. Further, until the results of this study are available, we must recommend that patients be managed in this manner only as part of a carefully designed clinical trial. At present, no cogent plan for managing the rare patient with true stage D0 prostate cancer has been presented.

STAGE D1 DISEASE

In the USA, approximately 20% of all men diagnosed with prostatic carcinoma will have stage D1 disease at presentation. However, it is the authors' opinion that this percentage is decreasing. Nevertheless, there is still tremendous controversy regarding the appropriate management of patients with this stage of disease. To date, nearly every possible combination of surgery, radiotherapy, chemotherapy, and hormonal therapy has been attempted in efforts to provide long-term palliation in men with pelvic metastases, with no clear consensus resulting from these studies. Most of the trials in the literature which address management of stage D1 disease are retrospective, non-randomized, contain too few subjects to gain statistical significance, or have a follow-up which is relatively short—thus rendering their conclusions specious.

Furthermore, stage D1 prostate cancer presents a spectrum of diseases—from a solitary, pelvic lymph node micrometastasis diagnosed during staging for radical prostatectomy to bulky pelvic adenopathy on computed tomography scanning—with clearly different survival at either end of the spectrum. Finally, with recent evidence indicating that tumor ploidy may independently impact survival in stage D1 prostate cancer, should we substratify patients enrolled in our protocols by their ploidy status and should we report our results according to the ploidy status? When the above variables are considered, it is easy to understand how no management consensus has evolved for stage D1 prostate adenocarcinoma.

External beam radiotherapy fails to cure patients with biopsy-proven pelvic lymph node metastases from prostate cancer.[14] Patients who received extended-field radiation therapy to include the hypogastric, external iliac, and common iliac lymph node chains may experience improved survival when compared to an identically selected cohort who receive therapy to the periprostatic area only. Nevertheless, in patients with biopsy-proven stage D1 prostate cancer, external beam radiotherapy as monotherapy is associated with only a 50% actuarial 5-year survival. Androgen ablation does not improve survival when added to definitive external radiotherapy.[14]

Radical prostatectomy with pelvic lymphadenectomy, likewise, fails to cure patients with stage D1 prostate cancer. However, with radical prostatectomy alone, crude survival should exceed 5 years in most patients (roughly 75%).[15] Early androgen ablation enhances slightly the overall survival of patients undergoing radical prostatectomy for low-volume D1 disease, with roughly 90% of patients surviving 5 years.[15,16] Adjuvant radiotherapy offers nothing to the patient undergoing radical prostatectomy with pelvic lymph node metastases.[17,18]

To date, no chemotherapeutic regimen has shown even modest effectiveness in treating systemic prostate cancer. The lengthy tumor cell doubling time makes prostate adenocarcinoma inherently resistant to most cytotoxic chemotherapeutic agents, which attack the rapidly dividing cells foremost. However, rarely does a patient receive chemotherapy for prostate adenocarcinoma until he has failed androgen withdrawal and his tumor has achieved its maximum malignant potential.

Early androgen ablation seems to offer excellent chances for 5-year progression-free survival to most men with stage D1 prostate cancer (roughly 75%).[19,20] No large-scale, prospective, randomized trial has been performed yet to prove the benefits of early androgen ablation at this stage. Though yet to be proven, early androgen ablation may be as efficacious as radical prostatectomy with adjuvant hormonal therapy—though this point may be contentious, as the Mayo Clinic has shown enhanced survival if the prostate gland is removed along with the institution of early androgen withdrawal.[21] When one considers the potential morbidity of radical prostatectomy, early hormonal therapy may seem attractive to many patients with stage D1 disease.

In summation, although 20% of all patients with prostate cancer will have isolated pelvic lymph node metastases at diagnosis, we have yet to see a well-performed, randomized, prospective trial answering the question of which mode of therapy is superior. The Mayo Clinic data on radical prostatectomy with early androgen ablation are compelling, yet should be carefully subjected to further trial before one adopts this aggressive approach. When cost factors and quality of life issues are factored into the equation, simple orchiectomy may be the treatment of choice for stage D1 disease.

STAGE D2 DISEASE

The demonstration of the androgen sensitivity of prostate adenocarcinoma by Huggins & Hodges in 1941 was met with considerable optimism, as it was hoped that androgen deprivation by orchiectomy or the administration of pharmacologic doses of estrogen may cure prostate cancer.[4] They soon realized that androgen withdrawal by orchiectomy or estrogen therapy did not cure patients of their cancer, and most eventually progressed and died of their disease. Recognizing that the adrenal androgens may have been responsible for the progression of the cancer, Huggins & Scott then attempted to treat relapsing patients with bilateral adrenalectomy. Their efforts were hindered by the fact that adrenal hormone replacement therapy was inadequate at the time, and no patient survived longer than 4 months.[22] Nevertheless, in this short span of time, these pioneers laid the basic groundwork for all the studies which would follow, including the basic concepts of surgical and medical castration and the potentially important role of the adrenal androgens in the progression of prostate cancer.

The vast majority of circulating androgens in the male arise from the testicular production of testosterone. This steroidal hormone easily penetrates the cell membrane of hormonally sensitive cells and is converted to dihydrotestosterone (DHT) by the intracellular enzyme 5-alpha-reductase. It is believed that DHT is the primary intracellular messenger responsible for stimulating transcription of new messenger RNA and ultimately for the translation of proteins necessary for the maintenance of the hormone-sensitive cell.

Leydig cell production of testosterone is under pituitary control through the actions of leutinizing hormone (LH, aka interstitial cell secreting hormone; ICSH). The ultimate control of the entire cascade rests in the hypothalamus, where LH-releasing hormone (LHRH) is released in pulsatile fashion and flows through the hypothalamic–pituitary portal venous system to reach the anterior pituitary gland. Negative feedback inhibition by circulating testosterone ensures that relatively normal levels of testosterone are maintained.

Roughly 5–10% of circulating androgens in the intact male arise from the adrenal gland as the considerably less potent hormones androstenedione and dehydroepiandrosterone (DHEA). The adrenal cortex is also under anterior pituitary control via the hormone adrenocorticotrophic hormone with ultimate control once again seated in the hypothalamus through its messenger, corticotropin-releasing factor (CRF). While the adrenal androgens are considerably less potent than DHT, it is believed that they play an important role in the growth of prostate cancer and their neutralization forms the basis for the rationale of complete androgen blockade.

For over 40 years hormonal monotherapy was the primary means of managing metastatic prostate cancer, with orchiectomy and estrogens (DES) utilized almost exclusively. At the close of the Veterans Administration Co-operative studies, several facts became exceedingly clear. First, the combined rate of objective response and disease stabilization for either therapy was roughly 80% with a mean duration of response of 20 months. Neither therapy yielded superior survival, and switching from one therapy to the other at the first sign of relapse was useless.[7] At doses of 3 mg/day or greater, DES was associated with a prohibitive cardiovascular and thromboembolic complication rate—as high as 25–30%.[23] However, while often failing to produce castrate levels of serum testosterone, DES at 1 mg/day yielded results equal to the higher doses of DES.[7]

Orchiectomy remains the treatment of choice in cases of ureteral obstruction or impending spinal cord compression. Castrate levels of serum testosterone are achieved in 3 days or less. Obviously, it is the treatment of choice in the non-compliant patient. Side-effects, other than the psychologic aspects of castration, are minor and reasonably well-tolerated (loss of libido, impotence, vasomotor hot flashes). The main attractiveness of DES or orchiectomy in today's market is the relatively low cost on a per-day basis of either therapy when compared to the alternate therapies.

After the isolation and amino acid coding of the LHRH peptide, analogs to the molecule became readily available for pharmacologic use. At the pituitary level, the highly potent LHRH analogs cause a generalized desensitization of the pituitary due to the disruption of the normally pulsatile release of native LHRH. The result is a rapid diminution of LH release by the pituitary (after an original 72-hour surge of pituitary stimulation). In the absence of circulating LH, the Leydig cells of the testes fail to produce testosterone. Castrate levels of testosterone are reliably produced after 28 days of LHRH analog administration. The peptide is rapidly degraded in the gastrointestinal tract, requiring a parenteral mode of delivery. Two daily parenteral formulations, leuprolide (Lupron) and goserelin (Zoladex), have gained widespread support due to their favorable side-effects profile and ease of administration.

In 1984 in the USA, the Leuprolide Study Group reported their results of a randomized prospective trial of 200 men with stage D2 prostate adenocarcinoma treated with daily subcutaneous injections of leuprolide or DES 3 mg orally per day. There were no statistically significant differences in subjective or objective responses, time to first objective progression, or survival. The cardiovascular toxicity of DES was once again observed.[24] In the UK, a multicenter, randomized, phase III trial compared a depot preparation of

Zoladex (3.6 mg subcutaneously/28 days) to DES 1 mg t.i.d. and orchiectomy. Accrual of subjects exceeded 600 men. Overall, subjective and objective response, time to treatment failure, and survival were generally equivalent among the three arms.[25] The Zoladex Prostate Study Group confirmed the equivalence of Zoladex and orchiectomy in a separate trial.[26] When combining the results of the above studies, the safety and efficacy of LHRH analogs became readily apparent. The flare phenomenon, denoted as increased bone pain or increased difficulty with micturition due to exacerbation of the prostate cancer by early testosterone stimulation, was observed in fewer than 5% of cases. Roughly 80% of men suffered decreased libido and erectile difficulties, and 50–60% experienced vasomotor hot flashes.[24–26]

As the 1980s came to a close, much activity in the field of hormonal monotherapy for prostate cancer left the patient with considerable choice for treating metastatic prostate cancer. Depot formulations of Zoladex and Lupron were available for monthly injection, were well-tolerated, and were found to be equivalent to orchiectomy or DES. Recognizing the adverse cardiovascular and thromboembolic side-effects profile of DES, the LHRH analogs became the treatment of choice for patients desiring medical over surgical castration.

As stated earlier, valid concerns over the role of the adrenal androgens in the progression of metastatic prostate cancer were expressed as early as 1945, when Huggins & Scott[22] first attempted bilateral adrenalectomy for hormone-refractory disease. Two separate studies added to the concern, as Labrie et al demonstrated that as much as 50% of intraprostatic DHT remains after surgical or medical castration,[27] and Harper et al showed that the adrenal androgens were responsible for roughly 20% of the total intraprostatic DHT.[28] These data, when combined with the hypothesis of tumor cell heterogeneity and the variability of hormonal sensitivity of prostate cancer cells, form the scientific basis for combined androgen blockage in treating metastatic prostate cancer.

The search for a safe and effective means of ablating or blocking the adrenal androgens ended with the introduction of the non-steroidal antiandrogens, nilutamide (Anandron) and flutamide (Eulexin). Aminoglutethimide was one of the first therapies to suppress adrenal steroid production by potently inhibiting several P450-mediated hydroxylation steps. Its use required the co-administration of physiologic doses of hydrocortisone to avert adrenal escape of suppression by pituitary override. A number of patients treated with this regimen for hormone-refractory prostate cancer had to discontinue therapy due to its side-effects of lethargy, nausea, vomiting, and ataxia.[29,30] The side-effects profile, while acceptable in the patient with hormone-refractory prostatic carcinoma, would be less than optimal in the good-performance status patient with recently diagnosed prostate cancer. The oral antifungal, ketoconazole, at supratherapeutic doses also inhibited several cytochrome P450-requiring steps in adrenal steroidogenesis but also had an unsatisfactory gastrointestinal side-effect profile, which limited its utility in the otherwise asymptomatic prostate cancer patient. The steroidal antiandrogens, cyproterone acetate and megestrol acetate, demonstrated both central (suppression of LH release) and peripheral (target cell inhibition of androgen binding to receptors) effects, but never seemed to gain favor in the USA, possibly due to the required co-administration of DES to avert eventual pituitary escape of central inhibitory effect. With experience with the non-steroidal antiandrogens came the realization that they represented the ideal agent for utilization in total androgen blockade regimens.

The synthetic non-steroidal antiandrogens exert their effect at the cellular level of the androgen-dependent cell. They block cytosolic or nuclear receptor binding, preventing androgens from stimulating production of new messenger RNA. They do not cause a medical castration, as serum testosterone levels are normal or increased. For this reason, they have not been approved in the USA for monotherapy of prostate cancer and may only be used along with an LHRH analog. The side-effects of flutamide are primarily gastrointestinal in nature: nausea, vomiting, diarrhea. Nilutamide causes impaired adaptation to darkness in up to 90% of patients (less than 5 min in duration) and rarely causes interstitial pneumonitis.[31]

In the early 1980s, Labrie et al reported their results with combination therapy for stage C and D prostate cancer, demonstrating a remarkably enhanced survival time in patients treated with combination therapy.[32-34] The trials lacked appropriate control arms as comparisons were made to historic controls. Nevertheless, the trials generated considerable interest and several groups set out to test their hypothesis.

In the USA a prospective, randomized, double-blind, placebo-controlled trial was initiated under the auspices of the National Cancer Institute in order to test the concept of total androgen ablation. The multicenter cooperative protocol was simple in its design, comparing leuprolide 1mg s.c./day plus placebo to leuprolide 1 mg s.c./day plus flutamide 250 mg t.i.d. in patients with stage D2 disease documented on bone scintigraphy. Cross-over from placebo to flutamide was allowed at signs of first progression. Over 600 subjects were enrolled, with results stratified according to severity of disease at presentation. Presently, the data are sufficiently mature to comment on all subgroups of the protocol. Overall, median progression-free survival favored the group receiving flutamide (16.5 versus 13.9 months) as did overall survival (35.6 months for the flutamide arm versus 28.3 months for the placebo arm). In the subset analysis, patients with good performance status and minimal disease on bone scan who were treated with flutamide at diagnosis (41 patients in each arm) experienced a longer time to objective progression (48 months for the flutamide arm, 19 months for the placebo arm) and prolonged overall survival (median, 61 versus 42 months). The majority of patients fit into the category of good performance status but severe disease (241 patients in each arm). In this group, median time to progression was prolonged 3 months by the addition of flutamide at enrollment (16 versus 13 months) and overall survival was enhanced by 6 months in the combination

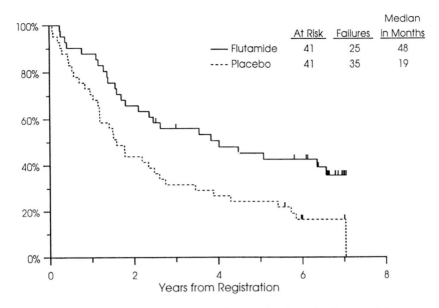

	At Risk	Failures	Median in Months
—— Flutamide	41	25	48
---- Placebo	41	35	19

Fig. 10.1   Progression-free survival of the good-prognosis subset of patients receiving leuprolide with flutamide or placebo, as at September 1992: National Cancer Institute intergroup protocol 0036.

therapy group. Diarrhea was the only significant side-effect reported more frequently by the flutamide group (13.6% of subjects). Recently, Denis reported improved cancer-specific survival in a group receiving combined androgen blockade (overall 7 months greater with combination therapy), lending support to the concept of total androgen ablation.[35]

Other studies have yet to demonstrate improved survival with combined androgen blockade. A large, prospective, randomized trial comparing Zoladex (3.5 mg s.c./month) and flutamide to orchiectomy alone failed to show any significant difference in subjective response rate, time to disease progression, or overall survival in the 571 evaluable subjects after a median follow-up of 2 years.[36] A similar study with 591 patients also compared Zoladex and flutamide to orchiectomy alone.[37] The study failed to show any significant difference in overall survival, although time to objective progression or death from prostate cancer was delayed by the institution of combination therapy. Median follow-up was fairly short—2 years. While the results of the above studies have not shown prolonged survival with total androgen blockade at interim analysis, a survival advantage may be demonstrated as the data mature. In both studies, the median follow-up had just reached 2 years, and the advantages of combined blockade may be masked by this short follow-up. Certainly, if patients are stratified according to extent of disease and performance status, then the groups with minimal disease and good perfor-

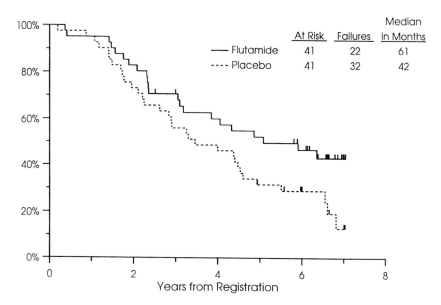

	At Risk	Failures	Median in Months
—— Flutamide	41	22	61
---- Placebo	41	32	42

Fig. 10.2 Overall survival rate of the good-prognosis subset of patients receiving leuprolide with flutamide or placebo, as at September 1992: National Cancer Institute intergroup protocol 0036.

mance status should not have approached 50% mortality by 2 years and will definitely require longer follow-up before final conclusions may be entered. It is doubtful that the failure in showing improved survival in the Zoladex arm is due to the use of the depot formulation instead of a daily preparation, since reliable castrate levels of serum testosterone have been shown with depot Lupron. However, the data may be confounded by the comparison of surgical castration to medical castration in these studies, although general equivalence is usually assumed between the two forms of treatment.

It has been suggested that the enhanced survival with combined androgen blockade is due to the ability of the antiandrogens to neutralize the transiently elevated testosterone levels seen in the first week after initiation of LHRH analog therapy. As stated previously, the flare phenomenon is clinically apparent in fewer than 10% of patients receiving an LHRH analog alone and would be expected to occur in less than 30 subjects in the placebo arm of the National Cancer Institute protocol. Though it is possible that early adverse effects from tumor stimulation by high testosterone levels in these patients could be responsible for the differences in survival, the hypothesis seems tenuous. Due to the durability of the survival advantage exhibited in the trial it seems unlikely that an event which occurs in the first week of therapy would be responsible for survival differences 4–5 years later. At the present time, the Southwest Oncology Group in the USA is conducting a large-scale, multi-

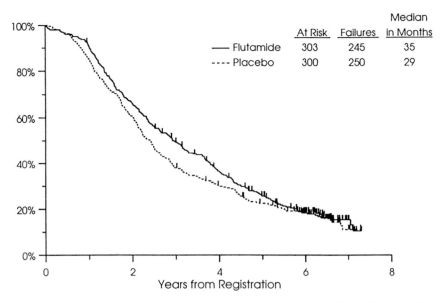

Fig. 10.3   Overall survival rate of all patients receiving leuprolide with flutamide or placebo, as at September 1992: National Cancer Institute intergroup protocol 0036.

institutional trial comparing orchiectomy plus placebo to orchiectomy plus flutamide. Since the flare phenomenon is not observed after orchiectomy, any enhanced survival with flutamide must be related to its neutralization of the adrenal androgens and not due to the avoidance of tumor flare. It is hoped that this simple trial will answer the question of whether the flare phenomenon is clinically deleterious to survival.

Regarding the optimal treatment of patients with stage D2 prostate cancer, the data appear to favor the early institution of total androgen blockade. An antiandrogen should be employed to neutralize the adrenal contribution to circulating androgens. At the present time, studies are underway to test the safety and efficacy of a once-daily preparation (Casodex) which could greatly simplify the patient's medical regimen. While it is generally assumed that medical castration with an LHRH analog is equivalent to surgical castration, the efficacy of combined androgen blockade with orchiectomy is yet to be proved in a large-scale study. This question should be answered as the data from the Southwest Oncology Group's trial become available.

D3 disease

Progression of metastatic prostate cancer which had previously been rendered quiescent with androgen ablation is a uniformly poor prognostic finding. Median survival in patients escaping androgen blockade ranges from 6 to 9 months and is rarely prolonged with aggressive therapy. A multitude of

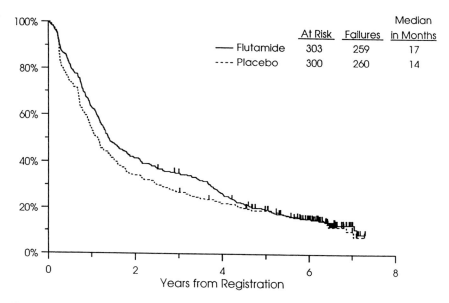

Fig. 10.4   Progression-free survival of all patients receiving leuprolide with flutamide or placebo, as at September 1992: National Cancer Institute intergroup protocol 0036.

chemotherapeutic and secondary hormonal ablative approaches have been employed in the endocrine-resistant prostate cancer patient, with no therapy proving to be superior. In all approaches, objective responses are rarely encountered and disease stabilization is infrequently seen. Subjective responses and symptomatic palliation are possible, however.

In the USA, no single chemotherapeutic agent and no drug combination has demonstrated efficacy in combating hormone-resistant prostate cancer.[38] Objective responses (complete and partial; CR + PR) average 8% overall, with an additional 8% having 'stable disease' for a period of at least 3 months. In this arena, response criteria are often nebulous and disease stabilization may simply represent the natural history of the patient's disease. Most studies are not controlled so any response may be artifactual.

Patients have shown some mild subjective improvement (28%) or disease stabilization (17%) with estramustine phosphate—an estrogenic compound with nitrogen mustard[39,40] Short-term disease stabilization has been observed with cis-platinum and doxorubicin, either alone or in various combinations, also.[38]

Certainly it is true that the majority of patients who receive chemotherapy for prostate cancer do so after their tumor has escaped from hormonal withdrawal and this may represent a select group with an overly aggressive tumor. Ostensibly, the tumor volume at this stage is greater than at the time when the patient is first diagnosed with metastatic disease. While it might be expected that tumor response to chemotherapy may be better if chemotherapy is instituted at the time of diagnosis, two randomized studies by the National Prostate Cancer Project refute this contention.[41,42] Patients were treated with standard androgen withdrawal alone (orchiectomy or DES 3 mg/day), or DES with Cytoxan, or DES with Cytoxan and estramustine phosphate. Chemotherapy was begun within 3 months of diagnosis in all cases. Median survival of roughly 90 weeks was obtained—similar to the historical survival duration for patients receiving hormonal monotherapy.[42] Objective response rates, response duration, and overall survival were not enhanced by the addition of chemotherapy.[41] Although these studies were sound in their logic, they were primarily hindered by the lack of a chemotherapeutic agent with activity toward prostatic adenocarcinoma.

Secondary androgen ablative attempts are also usually futile. In the National Cancer Institute protocol, delayed institution of flutamide therapy (placebo recipients crossing over to flutamide therapy at progression) did not appreciably prolong survival,[8] although data to the contrary have been presented.[43] A large, prospective, non-controlled, randomized trial of estramustine phosphate versus flutamide in patients relapsing after orchiectomy yielded no responses, 26–31% disease stabilization, and a median survival of 48 weeks.[44] The oral antifungal, ketoconazole, when used at supratherapeutic doses (600–1200 mg/day) can block adrenal and gonadal androgen synthesis. In one recently reported trial, roughly 15% of patients experienced short-term remission with a mean duration of 27 weeks.[45] Aminoglutethimide inhibits several steps in the P450-mediated conversion of cholesterol to sex steroids and has been used quite extensively in hormone-refractory patients.[29,30,46] Partial objective improvement is seen in up to 18% of cases and symptomatic improvement is seen in better than half the subjects. Co-administration with hydrocortisone (40 mg/day) is required to avert pituitary over-ride of adrenal cortical inhibition.

In the USA, the National Institutes of Health is currently conducting a phase 2 trial with the antiparasitic agent suramin in patients with hormone-refractory prostate cancer. Suramin acts in an inhibitory manner toward several tumor growth factors while showing considerable activity in hormone-refractory disease. The trial is currently enrolling patients and the early results are encouraging.

In all likelihood, the next major breakthrough in the management of metastatic prostate cancer will be through the discovery of novel drugs or innovative drug delivery systems. With the ability effectively to neutralize the entire hormone-responsive component of the prostate tumor, some means of ablating the hormone-unresponsive component must be developed if survival is to be improved. Immunomodulatory drugs will likely be attempted in efforts to enhance the body's natural defenses. Monoclonal antibodies directed against prostate-specific cell antigens and tagged with radioisotopes or cytotoxic agents should be available in the future and may represent the breakthrough that is so sorely needed. Until that time, it can be assumed that the number of men diagnosed annually with metastatic prostate cancer will continue to increase, and the mortality due to the disease to increase in concert.

KEY POINTS FOR CLINICAL PRACTICE

- With increasing public awareness of prostate cancer and more vigorous screening for prostate cancer, the number of cases diagnosed is sure to increase and the number of cases with metastases at diagnosis should increase commensurately.
- The current trend is toward early institution of androgen withdrawal in patients with metastatic disease. The majority of patients with D0 disease will have pelvic metastases if taken to staging lymphadenectomy. Thus, patients with D0 disease should be managed, at present, as though they have stage D1 disease. Patients with clinically organ-confined prostate cancer but few pelvic lymph node micrometastases may benefit by radical prostatectomy combined with early androgen withdrawal. Another option would be simple androgen ablation alone.
- Combined androgen blockade appears to offer improved survival in patients with stage D2 disease, when compared to hormonal monotherapy.
- Patients with minimal disease and good performance status benefit the most by combined androgen blockade. Extrapolation of the data from patients with stage D2 disease to patients with D0 and D1 disease is rational, although in a strict sense has yet to be demonstrated in clinical trials.
- Patients with hormone-refractory disease continue to present a management challenge. Novel drug delivery systems or a chemotherapeutic breakthrough are sorely needed if we are to have an impact on survival time at this stage.

REFERENCES

1   Stamey TA, McNeal JE. Adenocarcinoma of the prostate. In: Walsh PC, Retik AB, Stamey TA, Vaughan ED, eds. Campbell's urology. 6th edn. Philadelphia: WB Saunders, 1992
2   Donohue RE, Mani JH, Whitesel JA et al. Guide to patient management in clinically locally confined adenocarcinoma of the prostate. Urology 1982; 20: 559–565
3   Johansson JE, Adani MD, Andersson SO et al. Natural history of localized prostate cancer. Lancet 1989; 1: 799–803
4   Huggins C, Hodges CV. Studies on prostate cancer I: the effect of castration, of estrogen and of androgen injection on serum phosphatase in metastatic carcinoma of the prostate. Cancer Res 1941; 1: 293–297
5   Veterans Administration Co-operative Urologic Research Group. Treatment and survival of patients with cancer of the prostate. Surg Gynecol Obstet 1967; 124: 1011–1017
6   Sarosdy MF. Do we have a rational treatment plan for stage D1 carcinoma of the prostate? World J Urol 1990; 8: 27–33
7   Byar DP, Corle DK. Hormonal therapy for prostate cancer: results of the VACURG studies. Natl Cancer Inst Monogr 1988; 7: 165–170
8   Crawford ED, Eisenberger MA, McLeod DG et al. A controlled trial of leuprolide with and without flutamide in prostatic carcinoma. N Engl J Med 1989; 321: 419–424

9   Crawford ED, Nabors WL. Total androgen ablation: American experience. Urol Clin North Am 1991; 18: 55–63

10 Labrie F, Veilleux R. A wide range of sensitivities to androgens develops in cloned Shionogi mouse mammary tumor cells. Prostate 1986; 8: 293–300

11 Chan SY. A chemically defined medium for the propagation of rat prostatic adenocarcinoma cells. Prostate 1981; 2: 291–298

12 Whitesel JA, Donohue RE, Mani JH et al. Acid phosphatase: its influence on the management of carcinoma of the prostate. J Urol 1984; 131: 70–72

13 McDowell GC, Johnson JW, Tenney DM, Johnson DE. Pelvic lymphadenectomy for staging clinically localized prostate cancer. Urology 1990; 35: 476–482

14 Bagshaw MA. Radiation therapy for cancer of the prostate. In: Skinner DG, Lieskovsky G, eds. Diagnosis and management of genitourinary cancer. Philadelphia: WB Saunders, 1988

15 Zinke H. Combined surgery and immediate adjuvant hormonal treatment for stage D1 adenocarcinoma of the prostate: Mayo Clinic experience. Semin Urol 1990; 8: 175–183

16 Stein A, DeKernion JB. Adjuvant endocrine therapy after radical prostatectomy for stage D1 prostate carcinoma, Semin Urol 1990; 8: 184–189

17 Lange PH, Reddy PK, Medini E et al. Radiation therapy as adjuvant treatment after radical prostatectomy. Natl Cancer Inst Monogr 1988; 7: 141–149

18 Bahnson RR, Garnett JE, Grayhack JT. Adjuvant radiation therapy in stages C and D1 prostatic adenocarcinoma: preliminary results. Urology 1986; 27 403–406

19 Van Aubel O, Hoekstra WJ, Schroeder FH. Early orchiectomy for patients with stage D1 prostate carcinoma. J Urol 1985; 134: 292–294

20 Kramolowsky EV. The value of testosterone deprivation in stage D1 carcinoma of the prostate. J Urol 1988; 139: 1242–1244

21 Myers RP, Therneau TM, Zinke H et al. Radical prostatectomy and the influence of early endocrine therapy for stage D1 prostate cancer: long term follow-up study. In: Multidisciplinary analysis of controversies in the management of prostate cancer. New York: Plenum Press, 1988

22 Huggins C, Scott WW. Bilateral adrenalectomy in prostate cancer. Ann Surg 1945; 122: 1031–1041

23 Glashan RW, Robinson MRG. Cardiovascular complications in the treatment of prostate cancer. Br J Urol 1981; 53: 624–627

24 The Leuprolide Study Group. Leuprolide versus diethylstilbestrol for metastatic prostate cancer. N Engl J Med 1984; 311: 1281–1286

25 Peeling WB. Phase III studies to compare goserelin (Zoladex) with orchiectomy and with diethylstilbestrol in treatment of prostatic carcinoma. Urology 1989; 33 (suppl): 45–52

26 Soloway MS, Chodak G, Vogelzang NJ et al. Zoladex versus orchiectomy in treatment of advanced prostate cancer: a randomized trial. Urology 1991; 37: 46–51

27 Labrie F, Luthy I, Veilleux R et al. New concepts of the androgen sensitivity of prostate cancer. Progr Clin Biol Res 1987; 243A: 145–172

28 Harper ME, Pike A, Peeling WB et al. Steroids of adrenal origin metabolized by human prostate tissue both in vivo and in vitro. J Endocrinol 1984; 60: 117

29 Worgul TJ, Santen RJ, Samojlik E et al. Clinical and biochemical effect of aminoglutethimide in the treatment of advanced prostatic carcinoma. J Urol 1983; 129: 51–54

30 Drago JR, Santen RJ, Lipton A et al. Clinical effect of aminoglutethimide, medical adrenalectomy, in treatment of 43 patients with advanced prostatic carcinoma. Cancer 1984; 53: 1447–1450

31 Crawford ED, Smith JA, Soloway MA et al. A randomized controlled clinical trial of leuprolide and anadron versus leuprolide and placebo for advanced prostate cancer. J Urol 1990; 143: 221A

32 Dupont A, Labrie F, Giguere M et al. Combination therapy with flutamide and [D-trp 6] LHRH ethylamine for stage C prostatic carcinoma. Eur J Cancer Clin Oncol 1988; 24: 659–666

33 Labrie F, Dupont A, Belanger A et al. New approaches in the treatment of prostatic cancer: complete instead of partial withdrawal of androgens. Prostate 1983; 4: 579–591

34 Labrie F, Dupont A, Giguere M et al. Combination therapy with flutamide and castration (orchiectomy or LHRH agonists): the minimal therapy in both treated and

previously treated patients. J Steroid Biochem 1987; 27: 525–532

35   Denis LJ. Treatment of M1 prostate cancer: update of the EORTC trials. Special report, Plenary Session I, American Urological Association Scientific Meeting 1992, Washington DC

36   Lunglmayr A and The International Prostate Cancer Study Group. A multicenter trial comparing the LHRH analog Zoladex, with Zoladex plus flutamide in the treatment of advanced prostate cancer. Eur Urol 1990; 18 (suppl 3); 28–29

37   Iversen P, Suciu S, Sylvester R et al. Zoladex and flutamide versus orchiectomy in the treatment of advanced prostate cancer: a combined analysis of two European studies EORTC 30853 and DAPROCA 86. Cancer 1990; 66: 1067–1073

38   Eisenberger MA, Bezerdjian L, Kalash S. A critical assessment of the role of chemotherapy for endocrine-resistant prostatatic carcinoma. Urol Clin North Am 1987; 14: 695–706

39   Jonsson G, Hogberg B, Nilsson T. Treatment of advanced prostatic carcinoma with estramustine phosphate. Scand J Urol Nephrol 1977; 11: 231–238

40   Veronessi A, Zattoni F, Frustacci S et al. Estramustine phosphate treatment of T3-T4 prostatic carcinoma. Prostate 1982; 3: 159–164

41   Gibbons RP, Beckley S, Brady MF et al. The addition of chemotherapy hormonal therapy for treatment of patients with metastatic carcinoma of the prostate. J Surg Oncol 1983; 23: 133–142

42   Murphy GP, Beckley S, Brady MF et al. Treatment of newly diagnosed metastatic prostate cancer patients with chemotheraphy agents in combination with hormones versus hormones alone. Cancer 1983; 51: 1264–1272

43   Labrie F et al. Benefits of combination therapy with flutamide in patients relapsing after castration. Br J Urol 1988; 61: 341

44   deKernion JN, Murphy GP, Priore R. Comparison of flutamide and emcyt hormone-refractory metastatic prostate cancer. Urology 1988; 31: 312–317

45   Eichenberger T, Trachtenberg J. Effects of high dose ketoconazole in patients with androgen-independent prostatic cancer. Am J Clin Oncol 1988; 11 (suppl 2): S104–S107

46   Crawford ED et al. Aminoglutethimide in metastatic adenocarcinoma of the prostate. In: Prostate cancer, part A: research, treatment and histopathology. New York: Alan R. Liss, 1987

11

The pharmacological management of benign prostatic hyperplasia

R. S. Kirby

Benign prostatic hyperplasia (BPH) is the commonest pathological process to affect the ageing male. More than 70% of 70-year-old men have histological evidence of BPH.[1] However, a lesser proportion of patients are actually troubled by symptoms due to the presence of this disease. A recent population survey from Stirling in Scotland revealed an incidence of either symptoms of bladder outflow obstruction or reduced uroflow in 43% of men over 65.[2] It is clear that although a considerable number of prostatectomies are performed each year (over 400 000 per annum in the USA and about 35 000 in the UK), this represents only a small proportion of the total number of patients afflicted by this condition, and many of these individuals might consider a pharmacological agent for the management of their symptoms, provided that it was shown to be both safe and reasonably effective.

The concept of a pharmacotherapy for bladder outflow obstruction due to BPH or 'a pill for the prostate' has always been an alluring one for both patients and their doctors. From ancient times up to the end of the 19th century and beyond, a great variety of supposed remedies for bladder and prostatic disturbances have been advocated. These have included hemlock, strychnine and a considerable variety of other plant extracts, a not inconsiderable number of which are still in common use in western Europe and other parts of the world. There is little doubt, however, that the main effect of these medications was, and is, as a placebo.

BPH is a condition the symptoms of which naturally wax and wane[3] and which is not always progressive.[4] Partly because of this its manifestations are particularly prone to a placebo effect, although once outflow obstruction is present it seldom resolves spontaneously. Since the turn of the 20th century, prostatectomy has gradually taken on a dominant role as the optimum method of management of patients with BPH. However, although the procedure is effective and safe, there is a small but significant incidence of morbidity and mortality which, together with the need for reoperation of something like 2% of patients per annum, has led to a considerable endeavour directed towards developing a medical form of management of this most prevalent condition.

Because of the very pronounced placebo response the clinical evaluation of any compound used for the management of BPH must include a careful study of its efficacy by comparison of its performance with an identical placebo in a double-blind manner. Moreover, the studies must be set up with sufficient statistical power to enable assessment of the ability of a drug to perform better than placebo in improving both subjective and objective parameters and the efficiency with which bladder outflow obstruction is relieved. In addition, the study must also document and quantitate the likelihood of patients suffering side-effects from any medications employed and the longer-term outcome of therapy. Unfortunately not all the studies mentioned below fulfil these criteria and the results of small uncontrolled investigations of pharmacotherapy for BPH must be interpreted with considerable caution and some scepticism.

THE MOLECULAR MECHANISMS UNDERLYING BPH AND THE RATIONALE FOR THE USE OF MEDICAL THERAPY

The prostate requires the presence of adequate levels of circulating testosterone in order to develop and grow.[5] The decapeptide luteinizing hormone-releasing hormone (LHRH) is released in a pulsatile fashion from the hypothalamus and stimulates the pituitary to secrete luteinizing hormone (LH). LH then acts directly on Leydig cells within the testes, stimulating them in turn to secrete 95% of the 6–7 mg of testosterone produced in the body each day. The remaining 5% of daily testosterone production is either directly synthesized by the adrenal gland or produced by peripheral metabolism.

In the plasma, 98% of circulating testosterone is bound to a variety of proteins: the most important of these are human serum albumin and sex hormone-binding globulin (SHBG).[6] As a consequence, only 2% or so of free testosterone is available to enter prostatic cells and does so by a process of simple diffusion. Once within the cell, testosterone is rapidly metabolized by a series of prostatic enzymes. Over 90% is irreversibly converted to the main prostatic androgen, dihydrotestosterone (DHT) by a nicotinamide-adenine dinucleotide phosphate (NADP)-dependent enzyme localized predominantly on the nuclear membrane and named 5-alpha-reductase. The 5-alpha-reduced metabolite DHT is considerably more potent as an androgen within the prostate than testosterone itself, by virtue of its greater affinity for androgen receptors located within the nucleus. Binding of DHT to these androgen receptors produces a conformational change in the chromatin that facilitates transcription of specific sequences of DNA into messenger RNA. This sets off a complex but orderly series of events including signal-transducing protein synthesis, ribosomal RNA production and finally DNA synthesis and cell replication.[7]

Ageing has a gradual but profound effect on both testicular function and androgen metabolism. Hypothalamic pituitary responsiveness is maintained— LH levels remain within normal limits and there is no loss of pulsatile diurnal variation in the ageing male—but there is a decreased responsiveness of the testes to bioactive LH. In addition, there is an increased binding capacity of SHBG due to an increase in free plasma oestradiol levels, which stimulates synthesis of binding proteins by the liver. The consequence of these changes is an age-related decrease in free testosterone, while free oestradiol levels are maintained, producing an increase of up to 40% in the ratio of free oestradiol to free testosterone.

Following the separate demonstrations by Bruchovsky & Wilson[8] and Anderson & Liao[9] that DHT is the major intracellular androgen in the prostate, several workers reported a three- or fourfold increase in DHT levels in BPH tissue compared with controls.[10] However, subsequent work by Walsh et al[11] has cast doubt on these observations. Walsh's group in Baltimore demonstrated that differences between BPH and control tissue were the result of the fact that the control material was obtained at autopsy, while BPH tissues were all fresh surgical specimens. Subsequently, it was shown that incubation of prostatic tissues at 37°C for several hours will result in a marked decrease of intracellular DHT levels as a result of cell autolysis.

Although DHT levels may not be supranormal in BPH, 5-alpha-reductase activity has been demonstrated to be greater in BPH tissue compared with controls. Moreover, there is evidence to suggest that androgen receptor levels are elevated in BPH,[12] although the accurate measurement of these is still dogged by methodological problems. The sum of these changes may make the ageing prostate progressively more supersensitive to androgen stimulation.

In the dog, oestrogens have also been shown to be involved in induction of androgen receptors, and the canine prostate contains abundant quantities of high-affinity oestrogen receptors.[13] Experimental hyperplasia of the prostate in young castrated dogs cannot be induced by androgens alone, but does occur following administration of oestradiol and DHT in combination.[14] In humans, however, although oestrogen receptors are present in BPH tissue, their levels are considerably lower than those found in other peripheral tissues. As a consequence, although the alterations in the oestrogen : testosterone ratio associated with ageing remain an attractive hypothesis for the causation of BPH, other additional factors almost certainly play a role.

It has long been known that BPH tissue contains a considerable amount of fibromuscular stroma, and Franks & Barton[15] were the first to suggest that epithelial cells may be stimulated in some way by prostatic stroma to induce growth. This has been termed 'epithelial reawakening'. Subsequently, Cunha,[16–18] in an impressive series of experiments, recombined isolated mouse urogenital sinus mesenchyme (the embryonic prostatic stroma) with adult mouse bladder epithelium and transplanted these combined tissues beneath the capsule of the kidney of the nude mouse. With the testes intact the epithelial cells differentiated and developed into mouse prostatic epithelium, an effect not seen when the nude mice were castrated. When similar recombinations were made using the same urogenital sinus mesenchyme, but epithelium from mice with testicular feminization syndrome (i.e. tissue deficient in androgen receptors), the epithelial tissue still differentiated and grew in intact nude mice. No development of prostatic epithelium occurred, however, if embryonic stroma from mice with testicular feminization syndrome was combined with normal bladder epithelium.

These experiments elegantly demonstrate that differentiation and development of prostatic epithelium are indirectly controlled by androgens, through androgen-dependent mediators of stromal origin. Extensive research is currently directed towards the identification of these mediators— paracrine growth factors produced by stromal cells which exert an influence on the physiological process within the epithelial cells—as they could hold the key to the abnormal growth processes that characterize BPH, and perhaps also prostatic cancer.

The stromal mediators involved in the paracrine, and possibly autocrine, control of growth within the prostate are still to be identified. However, results from a number of institutions have confirmed that neither testosterone nor DHT has much effect on prostatic epithelial cell growth in culture. By contrast, epidermal growth factor (EFG),[19] insulin-like growth factor (IGF) and fibroblast growth factor (FGF)[20] have all been shown to have increased gene expression in BPH and exert a marked mitogenic effect on prostatic epithelial cells in vitro. Not all of these factors are stimulatory; transforming growth factor-beta (TGFβ) may inhibit mitotic activity or modulate the effects of other growth factors.[21] In addition EGF receptors, which also have affinity for transforming growth factor-alpha (TGFα), have been clearly demonstrated to be localized on the surface of prostatic epithelial cells.

The nodular hyperplasia produced by these mechanisms appears in both the transition zone and the periurethral zone of the prostate. Transition zone hyperplasia consists of large amounts of glandular tissue which arises by budding and branching from pre-existing prostatic ducts while periurethral zone hyperplasia is more stromal in nature. BPH tissue in general contains a greater percentage of smooth muscle within its stroma (approximately 60%) than normal prostate (around 40%) and its has been suggested that this increase in the quantity of smooth muscle is an important factor in the development of obstruction in BPH. Furthermore, studies with the electron microscope have shown a threefold increase in the number of intracellular organelles including rough endoplasmic reticulum, mitochondria and Golgi apparatus within the smooth muscle cells of prostatic adenomata as compared with normal prostatic tissue.[22] The autonomic innervation of the prostate has been investigated by neurohistochemical studies, radioligand binding and organ bath experiments. Both adrenergic and cholinergic nerves have been demonstrated within the prostate.[23] Muscarinic cholinergic fibres are mainly located within the glandular tissue and probably have a secretor-motor function. Adrenergic fibres release noradrenaline which stimulates receptors of two types, alpha$_1$ and alpha$_2$ adrenoceptors. Radioligand binding suggests that both types of adrenoceptor are present within the prostate.[24]

Stimulation of adrenergic receptors within the smooth muscle element of the prostate by addition of agents such as noradrenaline, an alpha$_1$- and alpha$_2$-agonist, and phenylephrine, a selective alpha$_1$-agonist, has been shown to lead to an increase in the muscle tone in in vitro prostate strip experiments.[25] The contraction of smooth muscle within the prostate is inhibited by the addition of the alpha$_1$-specific antagonist prazosin, but not greatly suppressed by the alpha$_2$-specific agonist, rauwolscine.[26] The findings suggest that the alpha-adrenoceptors on prostatic smooth muscle which mediate contraction are predominantly of the alpha$_1$ subtype.

The functional significance of the alpha adrenoceptors within the smooth muscle of the prostate was highlighted by Furuya et al,[27] who demonstrated that almost 40% of bladder outflow obstruction due to BPH consisted of a dynamic (i.e. reversible) component. This not only suggested that the static, mechanical aspect of prostatic outflow obstruction was not the overwhelming factor, but also offered an explanation for the well-recognized fluctuation in symptoms of voiding dysfunction in BPH.

These insights into the underlying causes of BPH have stimulated the development of pharmacotherapy for the condition.

PHARMACOLOGICAL MODIFICATION OF ANDROGEN STIMULATION TO THE PROSTATE

Clearly there are a number of ways in which the androgen drive to the prostate can be modified, each with its own implications therapeutically and in terms of toxicity; in this chapter these will be considered in turn.

Bilateral orchidectomy

John Hunter in 1786[28] was able to demonstrate that the prostate required normally functioning testes for its growth and development. It was not until 1895, however, that White[29] developed this concept as a form of therapy for the benignly enlarged prostate. He reported a series of more than 100 men with presumed BPH who had undergone castration and noted a diminution in prostatic size in nearly 90% of patients and 'a return to local conditions not far removed from normal' in 46% of these individuals. One year later Cabot[30] gathered information on 79 patients who survived the operation, performed by 27 different surgeons. Retention of urine was relieved in 27 patients following orchidectomy and overall symptoms of outflow obstruction were noted to have been improved in the great majority. It is not entirely clear, however, whether either of these series in fact included some patients suffering from malignant rather than benign enlargement of the prostate.

In spite of these results, bilateral orchidectomy for BPH never gained wide acceptance, largely because, as is still the case, the majority of patients were unwilling to sacrifice their potency and libido, or suffer the other adverse symptoms and signs of hypogonadism, in exchange for the relief of symptoms of prostatism. In addition, around the turn of the century, techniques for surgical removal of obstructing prostatic tissue were beginning to be popularized and refined.

A more recent study of the effect of castration on patients with BPH was reported by Schroder et al[31] who used transrectal ultrasonography (TRUS) with volume measurements of the prostate to assess response. This group from Holland reported an average reduction in prostatic volume of 31% in 4 out of 5 patients with BPH; however, at 3 months there was little improvement in urodynamic parameters.[32] In fact, as early as 1940 the Nobel prize winner Charles Huggins had provided some insight into the mechanism of the effect of androgen deprivation by castration on the prostate. In his histological study of the prostate in 3 patients castrated for BPH,[32] it was apparent that significant epithelial atrophy occurred only after 90 days following androgen withdrawal. Moreover, there was apparently little change in prostatic stroma. Subsequently, Wendel et al[33] confirmed that castration acts mainly to reduce the epithelial rather than the stromal component of BPH tissue present in the prostate glands of men suffering from prostatic cancer.

Steroidal antiandrogens

Cyproterone acetate is a synthetic antiandrogen with additional progestational activity that has been shown to inhibit prostatic growth in experimental animals.[34] In addition to its major action as a competitive androgen receptor, this compound also inhibits the release of both gonadotrophins and adreno-corticotrophic hormone (ACTH) from the pituitary. Therefore, cyproterone acetate not only blocks androgen action directly, but also reduces the production of androgens from the Leydig cells in the testes. As a consequence of this, serum testosterone levels are reduced.

After the efficacy of cyproterone had been demonstrated in patients suffering from prostatic cancer, Scott & Wade undertook a phase II evaluation of the efficacy of this compound in BPH. In their small and uncontrolled study, 13 men were treated for up to 15 months.[35] Uroflowmetry was reported to have increased in 9 of the 13 patients and symptoms of bladder outflow obstruction improved in nearly all of them. Because the study was uncontrolled however, the extent of a placebo effect in these cases is unquantifiable. Prostatic biopsies taken before and during treatment did reveal a reduction in the height of the cells lining the acini of the prostate. Surprisingly, only 4 men in this study were reported to have developed impotence, although in current clinical practice cyproterone acetate seems to induce impotence in nearly every patient treated.

Progestational agents

Progestational agents have an effect on the benignly enlarged prostate by decreasing gonadotrophin secretion from the pituitary, thereby decreasing circulating androgen concentrations. They also have some direct antiandro-genic effect by interfering with the binding of testosterone and DHT with androgen receptors in the prostate. An early report by Geller et al[36] suggested that hydroxyprogesterone caproate resulted in some prostatic regression. Subsequently, the same group studied the effect of a similar compound, megestrol acetate, in a double-blind, placebo-controlled study of 61 patients who were maintained on therapy for 20 weeks.[37] Subjective symptom improvement occurred in 78% of treated patients, but in only 57% of the placebo group. Statistically significant flow rate improvements were also apparent by 14 weeks, although these were modest. Donkervoort et al[38] reported rather similar results in men treated with compound for 16 weeks. In both of these studies loss of libido and impaired potency occurred in more than 70% of patients in the active treatment arms; however this side-effect was reversible on discontinuing the medication.

Flutamide

Flutamide is a non-steroidal antiandrogen that is effective orally and is metabolized within the body to a hydroxylated derivative that competes directly with both testosterone and DHT for androgen-binding sites.[39] Although the compound has been clinically available for more than two decades, there has been a recent revival of interest in it, largely as a result of the demonstration that flutamide used in combination with an LHRH analogue in patients with metastatic prostate cancer results in a longer time to progression and survival than LHRH monotherapy (see Chapter 10). As flutamide does not have any antigonadotrophic or progestational effects, plasma testosterone levels are not depressed: in fact, testosterone levels tend to rise with this compound to compensate for the pituitary androgen receptor feedback blockade.

In dogs, flutamide has been shown to induce regression of the hyperplastic prostate.[40] Subsequently, Caine et al[41] treated 30 patients in one of the first double-blind placebo-controlled studies of any drug therapy in BPH. A statistically significant improvement in flow rate was reported by this group, but prostatic biopsies failed to reveal evidence of either glandular or stromal regression. However, these samples were taken after only 12 weeks of therapy. The major side-effect was the development of nipple tenderness and gynaecomastia, presumably because of the unopposed action of oestrogens resulting from peripheral aromatization of testosterone to oestradiol. In addition, a significant proportion of patients developed diarrhoea, but impotence was not reported as a side-effect of this compound.

More recently, Stone et al[42,43] reported the results of a larger multicentre study of flutamide in patients with BPH. After 3 months there was a 23% reduction of prostate volume as measured by TRUS, compared with little change in the placebo group. A small number of patients who continued to receive the drug in an open uncontrolled protocol for a total of 6 months were reported to have experienced a 42% reduction in prostatic volume. At 3 months in the double-blind study maximum uroflow rates increased from 9 to

10.1 ml/s with flutamide and there was a statistically significant improvement in symptom score. In the small cohort previously mentioned who were continued on this compound in an open protocol for a further 3 months, additional improvement in uroflow parameters were reported. Toxicity, however, was a major problem; the incidence of gynaecomastia was 54%, with nearly half of the patients complaining of gastrointestinal side-effects, particularly diarrhoea. Only 1 patient in the active treatment arm reported erectile dysfunction, but gynaecomastia was a considerable problem.

Currently several other non-steroidal antiandrogens are in development. The ICI compound ICI 176334 (Casodex) looks promising; however the majority of the research to date on this compound has been directed towards its activity against prostatic cancer rather than BPH. It does, however, appear to have some potential for the treatment of benign prostatic enlargement. Moreover its side-effect profile looks considerably better than that of flutamide.

LHRH analogues

A number of LHRH analogues are now available that act by transiently stimulating and then blocking pituitary receptors controlling the secretion of LH, thereby reducing testicular androgen secretion to castrate levels. Recent formulations of both goserelin and leuprolide now permit administration by once-monthly subcutaneous injections and 3-monthly depot injections are pending. Peters & Walsh[44] reported 9 patients with bladder outlet obstruction resulting from BPH who were treated for 6 months with nafarelin acetate, another LHRH analogue, in a small uncontrolled study. Impotence occurred as expected in all patients and there was also a reduction in prostatic volume as measured by TRUS. The mean gland shrinkage was 24% and this appeared to stabilize after 4 months of therapy. Within a few months of discontinuing therapy the prostate volume returned to pretreatment values. In spite of prostatic shrinkage, only 33% of patients noted improved symptoms or enhanced uroflow; however the study period was rather short. Morphometric analysis of prostatic biopsies before and after treatment did confirm a 40% reduction in epithelial cell volume as well as some stromal reduction, which was in the order of 20%.

Bosch et al[45] also reported 30% prostatic volume reductions in patients with BPH treated with either an LHRH analogue or cyproterone acetate in a small number of cases in an open protocol. Like Peters & Walsh, they showed rebound prostatic enlargement to pretreatment values on stopping the medication.

5-Alpha-reductase inhibitors

The fundamental disadvantage of all the hormonal remedies for BPH described above is the inevitable hypogonadism that they almost all induce.

The recent development of a new class of drugs however—the 5-alpha-reductase inhibitors—now permits, for the first time, a blockade of androgen stimulation of the prostate without the associated loss of androgen-dependent muscle strength, libido and potency.

It has been known since 1968[48] that within the prostate testosterone undergoes metabolism to DHT. Shimazaki et al[46] later characterized the enzyme responsible and named it 5-alpha-reductase, also showing it to be dependent on NADP. It is now appreciated that there are two subtypes of 5-alpha-reductase enzyme: 5-alpha-reductase-1, and 5-alpha-reductase-2.[47] The function of 5-alpha-reductase-1 is not yet clear; however the behaviour of 5-alpha-reductase-2, which has been localized to chromosome 2, indicates that it could encode the major isoenzyme in genital tissue. On the basis of experiments in rats two groups of workers, Bruchovsky & Wilson[48] and Andersen & Liao,[49] simultaneously reported that DHT rather than testosterone itself was the main androgen modulating prostatic growth.

The pivotal role of DHT in inducing and maintaining prostate growth was subsequently confirmed by the studies of Imperato-McGinley et al[50] who investigated 12 families from the Dominican Republic consisting of 24 men suffering from congenital 5-alpha-reductase deficiency with consequently very low DHT levels. The females in these families are apparently unaffected, but the males, being unable to metabolize testosterone to DHT, are born with features of ambiguous genitalia, including a labia-like scrotum, a microphallus, a blind-ending vaginal pouch, as well as a very underdeveloped prostate gland. Cryptorchid testes are usually palpable on examination. As testosterone levels rise with the onset of puberty in these individuals, several masculine features develop including penile enlargement, scrotal rugae with hyperpigmentation, typical male pubic hair, a noticeable increase in muscle bulk as well as testicular descent. Despite these remarkable changes in phenotype, the prostate gland remains vestigial, only minimal beard growth occurs and male-pattern balding does not occur. Testicular biopsies in these patients have demonstrated intact Leydig cells and complete spermatogenesis. These patients have slightly elevated serum testosterone levels and markedly sub-normal serum levels of DHT.

The recognition of this differential sensitivity of the prostate to 5-alpha-reduced androgens compared with other tissues and the important role of DHT in maintaining prostatic growth has led to a flurry of activity directed towards developing compounds which will selectively inhibit 5-alpha-reductase, thereby decreasing DHT levels but maintaining testosterone-dependent functions.

The first group of this new class of drugs to be identified and evaluated clinically were the 4-azasteroids of which only one, finasteride (Proscar), has so far undergone extensive clinical evaluation in BPH. Animal experiments have demonstrated that in dogs suffering from spontaneous BPH finasteride can significantly reduce the size of the prostate gland (Fig. 11.1).[51] Finasteride was first administered to man in 1986:[52] in single-dose studies plasma DHT

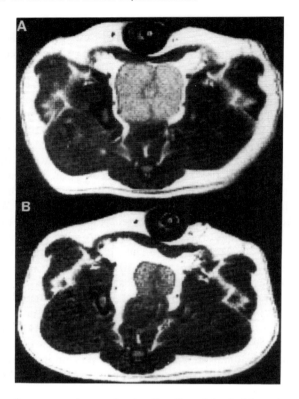

Fig. 11.1   Magnetic resonance images showing the effect of the 5 alpha reductase inhibitor, finasteride, in spontaneous canine benign prostatic hyperplasia. **A.** Pre-treatment transaxial MR image (SE 1 500/30), a pelvis of dog. **B.** Image of a corresponding section measured after administration of finasteride 5 mg/kg/day for 12 weeks.

levels were significantly reduced for up to 5 days with doses as low as 0.5 mg of the compound.[53] To determine the effect of finasteride on DHT production within the prostate itself men with BPH were treated with finasteride 7–10 days before prostatectomy. Tissue obtained at surgery showed that intraprostatic DHT was decreased by a mean of 92% to levels of 0.18 ng/g (± 0.11), while intraprostatic testosterone levels rose substantially from 0.26 ng/g (± 0.18) to 1.91 ng/g (± 1.19).[54]

The clinical effects of finasteride at a dosage of 5 mg/day have been carefully evaluated in two large double-blind, placebo-controlled studies, one in the USA,[55] the other internationally. Taken together, results are now available concerning the effects of this compound over 12 months on more than 1500 patients. In addition, extension studies in an open-label protocol in a subset of patients are now available up to 36 months.

Suppression of DHT was well-maintained. Prostatic shrinkage by a mean of 19% was evident (Fig. 11.2) with continued shrinkage up to 3 years.

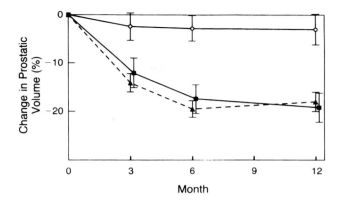

Fig. 11.2 Median change (± 95% confidence interval) in prostatic volume in men with benign prostatic hyperplasia during treatment with placebo (○), 1 mg finasteride (▲) or 5 mg finasteride (■). Month 0 = baseline. Reprinted, by permission of the *New England Journal of Medicine* (327; 1185–1191, 1992).[55]

Prostate-specific antigen (PSA), a glycoprotein secreted exclusively by prostatic epithelial cells, which is measurable in the serum, also declined to about 50% of its pretreatment value in response to 1 year's finasteride therapy, presumably in line with involution of prostatic glandular epithelium. In line with prostate volume reduction there is at first a modest improvement of symptoms and uroflow, with a mean increase of 1.6 ml/s ($P < 0.001$; Figs 11.3 and 11.4). By 1 year nearly 50% of patients have an improvement of urinary flow of more than 3 ml/s. Although this uroflow increase is not as considerable as the greater than 100% flow rate improvement seen after transurethral resection of the prostate (TURP), it has been estimated that the mean flow rate decline with ageing in males (presumably mainly due to developing BPH) is 0.2 ml/year.[56] One year's therapy with finasteride

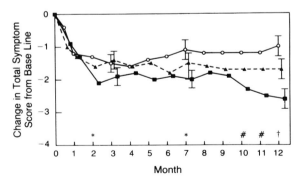

Fig. 11.3 Mean (± s.e.) change in the total symptom score in men with benign prostatic hyperplasia during treatment with placebo (○), 1 mg finasteride (▲) or 5 mg finasteride (■). Asterisks ($P<0.05$), hash symbols ($P<0.01$) and the dagger ($P<0.001$) indicate significant differences between the finasteride-treated groups and the placebo group. Month 0 = baseline. Reprinted, by permission of the *New England Journal of Medicine* (327; 1185–1191, 1992).[55]

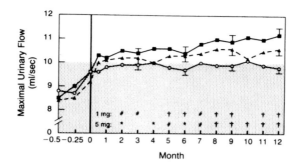

Fig. 11.4 Mean (±s.e.) maximal urinary flow rates in men with benign prostatic hyperplasia during treatment with placebo (○), 1 mg finasteride (▲) or 5 mg finasteride (■). The stippled area indicates the range in which unrinary flow was considered to be obstructed. Month 0 = baseline. Values before month 0 were obtained during the 2-week placebo run-in period. The asterisks ($P<0.05$), hash symbols ($P<0.01$) and daggers ($P<0.001$) indicate significant differences between the finasteride-treated groups and the placebo group. Reprinted, by permission of the *New England Journal of Medicine* (327; 1185–1191, 1992).[55]

therefore may reverse nearly 8 years' progressive flow rate decline due to prostate outflow obstruction.

Symptoms of prostatism as measured on a symptom score system modified from Boyarsky et al[57] responded to finasteride to a significantly greater extent than to placebo (P < 0.001). As might be expected, those patients with higher symptom scores and lower flow rates at baseline appeared to respond better than the moderately or minimally obstructed groups. This symptom score improvement is well-maintained up to 36 months in the extension study. The urodynamic effects of finasteride have been reported in a smaller phase II study,[58] with similar improvement in flow rate and a trend towards reduced voiding pressures at 3 months. Longer-term therapy appears to normalize voiding pressures and maximum urinary flow rates in those patients who respond to therapy.

Other 5-alpha-reductase inhibitors are currently in development including the SmithKline Beecham product SKB 105657. Early results suggest that this agent may have some activity against prostatic cancer,[59] and an action on BPH would also be anticipated.

ALPHA ADRENOCEPTOR BLOCKING AGENTS

Professor Marco Caine was the first to demonstrate the therapeutic possibilities of alpha-adrenoceptor antagonists in BPH. A number of studies from Israel confirmed that phenoxybenzamine, a combined alpha$_1$-and alpha$_2$-adrenoceptor blocker, reduces prostatic urethral pressure profile and significantly improves both symptoms of prostatism and urinary flow rates.[60] However, in other studies side-effects including orthostatic hypotension, dizziness, tiredness and nasal stuffiness occurred in more than 30% of patients, leading to frequent discontinuation of therapy.[61] Phenoxybenzamine is chemically related to nitrogen mustard and binds irreversibly to alpha-adrenoreceptors. The drug has also been shown to induce gastrointestinal tumours in rats and is mutagenic in mouse tissue cultures and for these reasons is no longer generally available. Some of its undesirable side-effects in man may have been due to its activity against $alpha_2$-adrenoceptors. These are largely prejunctional in location and are concerned with noradrenaline reuptake into the sympathetic nerve endings. Blockade of these receptors by phenoxybenzamine therefore results in a generalized rise in circulating noradrenaline levels, probably contributing to the undesirable side-effect profile.

The first $alpha_1$-selective adrenoceptor blocker used clinically in BPH was prazosin. In a double-blind placebo-controlled urodynamic study of prazosin 2 mg b.d. of 4 weeks' duration, Kirby et al[62] demonstrated both improvement in symptoms and enhanced uroflow. A subsequent 12-week study confirmed these findings[63] and also found there was a statistically significant fall in maximum detrusor pressure during voiding but little improvement in residual urine volumes, at least at this dosage. Since then a number of other alpha-blocking agents requiring twice-a-day dosage have been evaluated against the performance of placebo, including indoramine,[64] alfuzosin[65] and the Yamanuchi product YM 617.[66] Their relative efficacies as judged from published data are rather similar. Almost all the studies involving alpha-blockers in BPH show a significant dropout rate, with side-effects in the active treatment arm outnumbering those of patients randomized to placebo. These side-effects are the result of blockade of the numerous $alpha_1$-adrenoceptors elsewhere in the body—most notably in the blood vessels and brain—and are most prominent soon after commencing therapy with these agents.

In an attempt to reduce cardiovascular and other side-effects, newer alpha-blockers have been developed which take longer to reach peak plasma concentrations. This confers the dual advantage of a smoother onset of action and allows a once-a-day dosage regime to be used. Most experience in BPH so far has been gained with terazosin where the early reports of efficacy in open-label dose titration studies[67] have now been confirmed by larger placebo-controlled studies over longer durations.[68]

A mean flow rate improvement of slightly more than 30% has been reported, together with a statistically significant reduction in symptom score. Although gradual incremental dose increase from 1 mg to as high as 10 mg has been suggested by Lepor, most patients seem to obtain benefit without much in the way of side-effects at 5 mg/day, which is now the recommended dosage.

A recent multicentre study of another second-generation alpha-blocker doxazosin at a final dose of 4 mg/day achieved after incremental increase from 1 mg/day revealed symptom improvement (Fig. 11.5), a statistically significant improvement in uroflow (Fig. 11.6), together with significant reductions in maximum voiding pressures (Fig. 11.7).[69] The usual side-effects associated

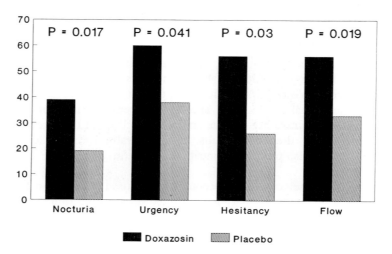

Fig. 11.5   Symptom improvement in patients treated with doxazosin 4 mg/day.

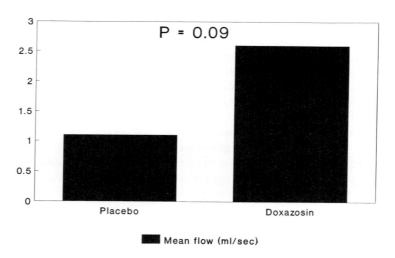

Fig. 11.6   Flow rate improvement in patients treated with doxazosin 4 mg/day.

with alpha-blockers—tiredness, nasal stuffiness and dizziness–were seen more frequently in the patients treated with active drug, but many patients at the end of the trial opted to stay on medication rather than undergo TURP. As with other alpha-blockers, titration of dosage will improve efficacy (Fig. 11.8) but also increase the incidence of side-effects. Currently 4 mg/day is the recommended dose but some patients may benefit from 8 mg/day.

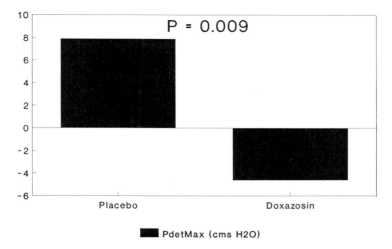

PdetMax (cms H2O)

Fig. 11.7   Voiding pressures after 3 months' treatment with doxazosin 4 mg/day.
PdetMax = maximum detrusor pressure.

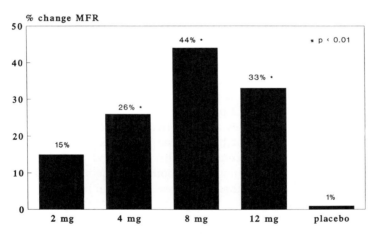

Fig. 11.8   Dose titration of doxazosin showing dose-related enhancement of uroflow in
patients with benign prostatic hyperplasia. MRF = maximum flow rate.

AROMATASE INHIBITION AND ANTIOESTROGENS

Aromatase is a cytochrome P450-dependent enzyme complex responsible for
the conversion of androgens to oestrogens and which is widely distributed
in the reproductive tissues of both sexes in many species. In the human
male oestrogen production occurs mainly by extratesticular aromatization of
androstenedione to oestrone and of testosterone to oestradiol in peripheral
tissues such as subcutaneous fat. Immunocytochemical studies[70] have

identified a predominant localization of oestrogen receptors in the stroma and ductal epithelium of the periurethral zone of normal canine prostate. Moreover, it has been reported that aromatase activity in the human prostate is also greatest in the periurethral zone[71] where the stromal form of BPH especially appears to develop. Experimental studies in both dogs and monkeys have also indicated that prostatic stromal proliferation, induced by the administration of androstenedione, can be antagonized by the administration of an aromatase inhibitor.

The best known and most widely used aromatase inhibitors are aminoglutethimide and ketoconazole. However, neither of these agents was originally developed as an aromatase inhibitor. Ketoconazole is much more widely used as an antifungal agent and in most countries has been withdrawn as therapy for endocrine disorders. Aminoglutethimide is also sometimes used as a treatment for carcinoma of the prostate, with some clinical success, although there is disagreement over the precise mechanism of action of the drug. Lassitude, depression and gynaecomastia have all been associated with the use of aminoglutethimide and it has been argued that the adverse effects are too hazardous and severe to justify continued use of the compound, especially in a benign condition like BPH. Ketoconazole has also been used in the treatment of carcinoma of the prostate, but again side-effects have been troublesome: the most serious toxicity is hepatitis, which is usually reversible on discontinuation of the therapy, but occasionally may be fatal.

Neither aminoglutethimide nor ketoconazole is a selective inhibitor of aromatase. A range of more selective agents is now under investigation; however experience in BPH is still limited. Tunn & Schweikert[72] reported some prostatic shrinkage in 13 patients treated in an uncontrolled study with testolactone 200 mg/day. They also reported that preliminary results with a new aromatase inhibitor 1-methyl-androsta-1, 4-diene-3, 7-dione (1-methyl-ADD) were rather more encouraging; the compound produced significant reductions in plasma concentrations of both oestrone and oestradiol. However, Oesterling[73] reported that aromatase inhibition was not an effective treatment for BPH in the dog, the only species other than humans in which BPH occurs spontaneously.

Perhaps a more logical approach is to block the effects of oestrogens at the level of the prostate by means of antioestrogen therapy (i.e. an oestrogen receptor antagonist). One report of the use of tamoxifen at a dose of 80 mg/day for 4 weeks demonstrated no useful effect; however, tamoxifen itself has some agonist activity as a weak oestrogen, and moreover 4 weeks' treatment is probably too short a period in which to detect an effect on the prostate. However, ICI have a new antioestrogen, ICI 183720, which is considerably more potent as an oestrogen receptor blocker than tamoxifen and has no oestrogenic agonist properties. No reports of its use in BPH are available yet but it does seem possible that it may have some useful activity, especially perhaps if used in combination with a 5-alpha-reductase inhibitor such as finasteride.

PHYTOTHERAPY

Plant extracts have been used since ancient times in the treatment of BPH. In Germany, Austria, Switzerland and to a lesser extent France, they are still widely prescribed. Indeed in 1986 in West Germany alone sales of the 16 most popular phytotherapeutic drugs were valued at 131 million Deutschmarks per annum. The manufacturers suggest that the effects of these various phytotherapeutic products are based on their content of phytosterols, of which it is claimed that the sitosterols are the most important. However there are almost no reliable data to inform us of the pharmacological mechanisms by which sitosterols exert their supposed effects in BPH. None the less, the following hypothetical mechanisms have been proposed:

1. Sitosterols may interfere with prostaglandin synthesis in the prostate, thereby producing an anti-inflammatory effect.
2. They may have an action in the liver to reduce the production of SHBG.
3. They may exert some obscure cytotoxic effect on hyperplastic prostatic cells.
4. It has been claimed, without a great deal of supporting data, that compounds like Permixon may have a weak 5-alpha-reductase inhibitory effect, as well as some androgen receptor-blocking action.[74]

A considerable number of studies have investigated the effects of various phytotherapeutic agents on the symptoms of BPH and subjective responses in terms of symptom improvement of between 50 and 100% have been reported.[75] Unfortunately the vast majority of these studies have been undertaken in small numbers of patients without placebo controls and with little in the way of objective evaluation by uroflowmetry, urodynamics or prostate volume measurements. Those few controlled studies that have been performed have usually involved few patients and unrealistically large doses of the agent concerned. Long-term studies have not often been undertaken.

At the present state of knowledge, the use of phytotherapy in BPH must be considered a relatively expensive way of administering placebo.

THE POTENTIAL FOR COMBINATION THERAPIES

Since the two major tissue components of the prostate—stroma and epithelium—have potentially different susceptibilities to drug therapies (antiandrogens and 5-alpha-reductase inhibitors act mainly on epithelium; alphablockers, aromatase inhibitors and antioestrogens affect largely the stromal component of BPH) there is a good theoretical basis for testing combination therapies in BPH. Only one small study of this nature has been reported to date—a combination of an antiandrogen and the antioestrogen tamoxifen[76] with reportedly enhanced results from the use of two agents compared with either as a single agent. Another combination already mentioned, that of an alpha-blocker and a 5-alpha-reductase inhibitor, has obvious theoretical appeal: the former agent acts rapidly to relieve symptoms, while the 5-alpha-reductase inhibitor has the potential to relieve the underlying disease process. Studies in the USA and in Europe are currently being commenced to evaluate this combination. As new agents and new classes of drugs active in BPH appear, combination therapy for this condition seems a fertile area for further research and development.

THE PROBLEM OF OCCULT CARCINOMA OF THE PROSTATE

A potential problem of any non-surgical therapy for BPH is the lack of tissue available for histological evaluation. It is well-established that around 10% of patients undergoing TURP for presumed BPH are subsequently found to harbour unsuspected foci of histological adenocarcinoma. The management of these patients is still controversial however. Study of the residual tumour volume in radical prostatectomy specimens from patients with stage A disease has revealed that the A1–A2 subclassification (A1 = <5% TUR chippings involved; A2 = >5% chippings involved or any prostatic tumour which is less than well-differentiated) does not always accurately reflect the volume of residual adenocarcinoma present, and may therefore be misleading in terms of prognosis.[77] Very small-volume (<0.3 ml) well-differentiated lesions in the transition zone are probably simply the latent histological disease identified by Franks[78] which may have little or no impact on survival. Larger-volume lesions, especially those extending into the peripheral zone, are more dangerous in younger patients and attempts should be made to identify these before medical or surgical treatment is commenced. To this end a PSA measurement is advisable: however, BPH may itself result in an elevation of PSA (around 25% of BPH patients have a PSA > 4 ng/l) and not all stage A carcinomata have an elevated PSA. In order to help distinguish BPH from localized adenocarcinoma two techniques have recently been described:

1. *Volume-corrected PSA*: since PSA rises by 0.3 ng/l per g of BPH tissue (and nearly 10 times this for each gram of cancer tissue), a correction can be made for the volume of BPH tissue present. Patients with PSA levels above the expected value may be at risk of occult adenocarcinoma and should undergo TRUS and systematic prostatic biopsy.[79]

2. *Sequential PSA estimations*: a recent report from Carter et al[80] has revealed that in BPH patients there is only a very gradual increase in PSA with time. By contrast, in patients with prostatic cancer serum PSA levels increase progressively as the tumour enlarges. A cut-off value of 0.75 ng/l per year has been suggested. Patients with PSA values increasing by more than this amount annually might therefore be considered for TRUS and guided as well as systematic prostatic biopsy, although the consistency of PSA assay results must also come into the equation.

To add to the complexity of the situation, 5-alpha-reductase inhibitors reduce serum PSA values by almost 50% over the first year of therapy, by producing glandular involution of benign tissue. However, from repeated PSA measurements on patients entered into the double-blind trials of finasteride with subsequently discovered carcinoma of the prostate, it would appear that in malignant prostatic disease finasteride produces an initial PSA decline followed by an exponential PSA rise that in most cases led to identification of the lesion.

CONCLUSIONS

We are currently entering a new era in the treatment of BPH. It now seems likely that the dramatic increase in the number of individuals undergoing TURP will level off and perhaps fall somewhat, but the need for prostatectomy will certainly still exist for those with severe obstruction, complications of BPH and patients presenting with urinary retention. Pharmacological therapy seems set to be used more widely, especially in earlier stages and in some of the 80% or more of mildly symptomatic patients who currently never come to surgery. 5-Alpha-reductase inhibitors, perhaps in combination with longer-acting, second-generation alpha-blockers, seem the most promising agents at present, but in this fast-moving field, even more potent 5-alpha-reductase inhibitors, increasingly selective alpha-blockers and new and more potent antioestrogens and antiandrogens are all in development. In the final analysis all these agents must be judged in a blinded fashion in their performance against placebo, not only in terms of symptom improvement, but also their ability to relieve prostatic obstruction and reverse the secondary changes in the bladder in the longer term. Only if they can be shown to achieve this reliably and safely in a reasonable proportion of patients will pharmacotherapy seriously challenge surgery in the treatment of this most prevalent condition of elderly men.

REFERENCES

1 Berry SJ, Coffey DS, Walsh PC, Ewing LL. The development of human benign prostatic hyperplasia with age. J Urol 1984; 132: 474–479
2 Garraway WM, Collins GN, Lee RJ. High prevalence of benign prostatic hypertrophy in the community. Lancet 1991; 338: 469–471
3 Birkhoff JD, Wiederhorn AR, Hamilton ML, Zinsser HH. Natural history of benign prostatic hypertrophy and acute urinary retention. Urology 1976; 7: 48–52
4 Ball AJ, Feneley RCL, Abrams PH. The natural history of untreated "prostatism". Br J Urol 1981; 53: 613–616
5 Isaacs JT, Coffey DS. Changes in DHT metabolism associated with the development of canine benign prostatic hyperplasia. Endocrinology 1981; 108: 445–453
6 Vermeulen A. The endocrine function of the human testis, vol 1. New York: Academic Press, 1973: p 157
7 Coffey DS. The endocrine control of the normal and abnormal growth of the prostate. In: Rajfer J ed. Urologic endocrinology. Philadelphia: WB Saunders, 1986: pp 170–193
8 Bruchovsky N, Wilson JD. The conversion of testosterone to 5-alpha-androstan-17

beta-ol-3-one by rat prostate in vivo and in vitro. J Biol Chem 1968; 243: 2012–2021

9 Anderson KM, Liao S. Selective retention of dihydrotestosterone by prostate nuclei. Nature 1968; 219: 227–279

10 Siiteri PK, Wilson JD. Dihydrotestosterone in prostatic hypertrophy. J Clin Invest 1970; 49: 1737–1745

11 Walsh PC, Huggins AM, Ewing LL. Tissue content of dihydrotestosterone in human prostatic hyperplasia is not supra-normal. J Clin Invest 1983; 72: 1772–1777

12 Barrack ER, Bujnovsky P, Walsh PC. Subcellular distribution of androgen receptors in human normal benign hyperplastic and malignant prostatic tissues: characterization of nuclear salt-resistant receptors. Cancer Res 1983; 43: 1107–1116

13 Trachenberg J, Hicks LL, Walsh PC. Androgen and estrogen receptor content in spontaneous and experimentally induced canine prostatic hyperplasia. J Clin Invest 1980; 651: 1051–1059

14 Walsh PC, Wilson JD. The induction of prostatic hypertrophy in the dog with androstanediol. J Clin Invest 1976; 72: 1772–1777

15 Franks LM, Barton AA. The effects of testosterone on the ultrastructure of the mouse prostate in vivo and in organ culture. Exp Cell Res 1960; 19: 35–50

16 Cunha GR. Tissue interactions between epithelium and mesenchyme of urogenital and integumental origin. Anat Rec 1972; 172: 529–542

17 Cunha GR. Epithelio-mesenchymal interactions in primordial gland structures which become responsive to androgenic stimulation. Anat Rec 1972; 172: 179–196

18 Cunha GR. The role of androgens in the epitheliomesenchymal interactions involved in prostatic morphogenesis in embryonic mice. Anat Rec 1973; 175: 87–96

19 Davies P, Eaton CL. Binding of epidermal growth factor by normal, hypertrophic and carcinomalous prostate. Prostate 1989; 14: 123–132

20 Mori H, Maki W, Oishi K, Jaye M, Igarashi K, Yashida O. Increased expression of genes for basic fibroblast growth factor and transforming growth factor type beta 2 in human benign prostatic hyperplasia. Prostate 1990; 16: 71–80

21 Martikainen P, Kypriandu N, Issacs JN. Effect of transforming growth factor beta on proliferation and cell death of rat prostatic cells. Endocrinology 1990; 127: 2963–2968

22 Bartsch G, Frick J, Ruegg I et al. Electron microscopic stereological analysis of the human prostate and of benign prostatic hyperplasia. J Urol 1979; 122: 481–486

23 Dunzendorfer U, Jonas D, Weber W. The autonomic innervation of the human prostate. Histochemistry of acetyl-cholinesterase in the normal and pathological state. Urol Res 1976; 4: 29–31

24 Lepor H, Shapiro E. Characterization of alpha-1 adrenergic receptors in human benign prostatic hyperplasia. J Urol 1984; 132: 1226–1229

25 Lepor H, Gup DI, Bauman M, Shapiro E. Laboratory assessment of terazosin and alpha-1 blockade in prostatic hyperplasia. Urology 1988; 32: 21–26

26 Hedlund H, Andersson KE, Larsson B. Alpha receptors and muscarinic receptors in the isolated human prostate. J Urol 1985; 134: 1291–1298

27 Furuya S, Kumamoto Y, Yokoyama E, Tsukamoto T, Izumi T, Abiko Y. Alpha adrenergic activity and urethral pressure in prostatic zone in benign prostatic hypertrophy. J Urol 1982; 128: 836–839

28 Hunter J. Observations on certain parts of the animal oeconomy. In: Bibliotheca osteriana. London: 1786: pp 38–39

29 White JW. The results of double castration in hypertrophy of the prostate. Ann Surg 1895; 22: 1

30 Cabot AT. The question of castration for the enlarged prostate. Ann Surg 1896; 24: 265–301

31 Schroder FH, Westerhof J, Bosch RJ, Benign prostatic hyperplasia treated with cyproterone acetate. J Urol 1969; 101: 81

32 Huggins C, Stevens RA. The effect of castration on benign hypertrophy of the prostate in man. J Urol 1940; 43: 705

33 Wendel EF, Brannen GE, Putong PB. The effect of orchiectomy and estrogens on benign prostatic hyperplasia. J Urol 1972; 108: 116

34 Sufrin G, Coffey DS. A new model for studying the effect of drugs on prostatic growth. 1. Antiandrogens and DNA synthesis. Invest Urol 1973; 11: 45

35   Scott WW, Wade JC. Medical treatment of benign prostatic hyperplasia with cyproterone acetate. J Urol 1969; 101: 81
36   Geller J, Bora R, Roberts T. Treatment of benign prostatic hypertrophy with hydroxyprogesterone caproate: effect on clinical symptoms, morphology, and endocrine function. JAMA 1965; 193: 121
37   Geller J, Nelson CG, Albert JD, Pratt G. Effect of megestrol acetate on uroflow rates in patients with benign prostatic hyperplasia. Urology 1979; 14: 467
38   Donkervoort T, Sterling AM, Van Ness J. Megestrol acetate in treatment of benign prostatic hyperplasia. Urology 1975; 6: 580
39   Sufrin G, Coffey DS. Flutamide: mechanism of action of a new steroidal antiandrogen. Invest Urol 1975; 13: 429
40   Neri RO, Monahan M. Effects of a novel non-steroidal antiandrogen. Invest Urol 1972; 10: 123
41   Caine M, Perlberg S, Gordon R. The treatment of benign prostatic hypertrophy with flutamide (Sch 13521): a placebo controlled study. J Urol 1975; 114: 564–568
42   Stone NN, Clejan S, Ray PS et al. A double blind randomized study of the effect of flutamide on benign prostatic hypertrophy. Side-effects and hormonal changes. J Urol 1989; 141: 307A
43   Stone NN, Ray PS, Smith JA et al. A double blind randomized study of the effect of flutamide on benign prostatic hypertrophy: clinical efficacy. J Urol 1989; 141: 240A
44   Peters CA, Walsh PC. The effect of nafarelin acetate, a luteinizing-hormone-releasing hormone agonist, on benign prostatic hyperplasia. N Engl J Med 1987; 317: 599
45   Bosch RJ, Griffiths DJ, Blom JHM. Treatment of benign prostatic hyperplasia by androgen deprivation: effects on prostate size and urodynamic parameters. J Urol 1989; 141: 68
46   Shimazaki J, Kurihara H, Ho Y, Studa K. Testosterone metabolism in the prostate. Gunma J Med Sci 1965; 14: 313–333
47   Andersson S, Berman DM, Jenkins EP, Russell DW. Deletion of steroid 5 alpha reductase 2 gene in male pseudohermaphrodism. Nature 1991; 354: 159–161
48   Bruchovsky N, Wilson JD. The conversion of testosterone to 5-alpha-androstan-17beta-ol-3-one by rat prostate in vivo and in vitro. J Biol Chem 1968; 219: 227–279
49   Andersen KM, Liao S. Selective retention of dihydrotestosterone by prostatic nuclei. Nature 1968; 219: 227–279
50   Imperato-McGinley J, Guerrero L, Gautier T, Petersen RE. Steroid 5-alpha reductase in man: an inherited form of male pseudohermaphrodism. Science 1974; 186: 1213–1215
51   Cohen SM, Taber KH, Malatesta PF et al. Magnetic resonance imaging of the efficacy of specific inhibition of 5 alpha reductase in canine spontaneous benign prostatic hyperplasia. Magnetic Resonance Med 1991; 21: 55–70
52   Stoner E. The clinical development of a new 5-alpha reductase inhibitor, finasteride. J Steroid Biochem 1990; 37: 375–378
53   Rittmaster RS, Stoner E, Thompson DL. Effect of MK906, a specific 5-alpha reductase inhibitor on serum androgens and androgen conjugates in normal men. J Androl 1989; 10: 259–262
54   Geller J. Effect of finasteride, a 5-alpha reductase inhibitor, on prostate tissue androgens and prostate specific antigen. J Clin Endocrinol Metab 1990; 71: 1552
55   Gormley GJ, Stoner E, Bruskevitz RC et al. The effect of finasteride in men with benign prostatic hyperplasia. N Engl J Med 1992; 327: 1185–1191
56   Drach GW, Layton TN, Binard WJ. Male peak urinary flow rate: relationships to volume voided and age. J Urol 1979; 122: 210–214
57   Boyarsky S, Jones G, Paulson DF, Prout GR. A new look at bladder neck obstruction by the Food and Drug Regulators: guidelines for the investigation of benign prostatic hypertrophy. Trans Am Assoc Genitourin Surg 1977; 68: 29–32
58   Kirby RS, Bryan J, Eardly I et al. Finasteride in the treatment of benign prostatic hyperplasia—a urodynamic evaluation. Br J Urol 1992; 70: 65–72
59   Lamb JC, Levy MA, Johnson RK, Issacs JT. Response of rat and human prostatic cancer to a novel 5 alpha reductase inhibitor SK and F 105657. Prostate 1992; 21: 15–34
60   Caine M, Perlberg S, Meretyk S. A placebo-controlled double-blind study of the effect of

phenoxybenzamine in benign prostatic obstruction. Br J Urol 1978; 50: 551–554

61   Abrams PH, Shah PJR, Stone R, Choa RG. Bladder outflow obstruction treated with
     phenoxybenzamine. Br J Urol 1982; 54: 527–530

62   Kirby RS, Coppinger SW, Corcoran MO, Chapple CR, Flanigan M, Milroy EJG.
     Prazosin in the treatment of prostatic obstruction: a placebo-controlled study. Br J Urol
     1987; 60: 136–142

63   Chapple CR, Christmas TJ, Milroy EJ. A 12 week placebo-controlled study of prazosin
     in the treatment of prostatic obstruction. Urol Int 1990; 45 (suppl 1): 47–55

64   Gower R, Wells P. Low dose indoramin, an alpha adrenoceptor antagonist in the
     management of benign prostatic hypertrophy. Neurourol Urodyn 1988; 7: 216–217

65   Jardin A, Bensadoun H, Delauche-Cavallier MC et al. Alfuzosin for treatment of benign
     prostatic hypertrophy. Lancet 1991; 337: 1457–1461

66   Kawabe K, Ueno A, Takimoto Y, Aso Y, Kato HU. Use of an alpha 1 blocker YM617 in
     the treatment of benign prostatic hypertrophy. J Urol 1990; 144: 908–912

67   Dunzendorfer U. Clinical experience: symptomatic management of BPH with terazosin.
     Urology 1988; 32: (suppl) 27–31

68   Brawer M, Epstein H, Adams G, Henry D, Clifton G. Efficacy and safety of terazosin in
     patients with benign prostatic hyperplasia. J Urol 1992; 147: 365A

69   Chapple CR, Carter P, Christmas TJ et al. A three month double-blind placebo
     controlled study of Doxazosin on prostatic bladder outflow obstruction. J Urol 1992; 147:
     366A

70   Schulze H, Barrack ER. Immunocytochemical localization of oestrogen receptors in
     spontaneous and experimentally induced BPH. Prostate 1987; 11: 145–162

71   Stone NN. Oestrogen formation in the human prostate from patients with and without
     BPH. Prostate 1986; 9: 311–318

72   Tunn UW, Schweikert HU. Aromatase inhibitors in the management of benign prostatic
     hyperplasia. In: Ackermann R, Schroeder FH, eds. Walter de Gruyter Prostatic
     hyperplasia. Berlin: 1989: pp 139–149

73   Oesterling JE. Aromatase inhibition in the dog. Effect on growth, function and pathology
     of the prostate. J Urol 1988; 139: 832–839

74   Champault G, Patel JC, Bonnard AM. A double blind trial of an extract of the plant
     serenoa repens in benign prostatic hyperplasia. B J Clin Pharmacol 1984; 18: 461–462

75   Dreikorn K, Richter R. Conservative non hormonal treatment of patients with benign
     prostatic hyperplasia. In: Ackermann R, Schroeder FH, eds. Prostatic hyperplasia. Berlin;
     Walter de Gruyter 1989: pp 109–121

76   Tenaglia R, Di Silverio F. Management of benign prostatic hyperplasia with
     antiandrogens and anti estrogens—clinical results In: Ackermann R, Schroeder FH, eds.
     Prostatic hyperplasia Berlin; Walter de Gruyter, 1989: pp 123–130

77   Voges GE, McNeal JE, Redwine EA, Freiha FS, Stamey TA. Predictive significance of
     substaging stage A prostate cancer for volume and grade of total cancer of prostate. J
     Urol 1992; 147: 858–863

78   Franks LM. Latent carcinoma of the prostate. J Pathol Bacteriol 1954; 68: 603–616

79   Benson MC, Whang IS, Olsson CA, McMahon DJ, Cooner WH. Use of prostate specific
     antigen density to enhance predictive value of intermediate levels of serum prostate
     specific antigen. J Urol 1992; 147: 817–821

80   Carter BH, Pearson JD, Metter J et al. Longitudinal evaluation of prostate specific
     antigen levels in men with and without prostate disease. JAMA 1992; 267: 2215–2220

12

Management of posterior urethral injuries

G. D. Webster   S. A. MacDiarmid

Significant injuries to the posterior urethra occur in approximately 10% of pelvic fractures, most commonly as a result of automobile or occupational accidents.[1,2] The urethral injury may be devastating, having the potential to cause significant long-term morbidity especially when not managed appropriately.

The following chapter will discuss the initial and long-term management of urethral injuries following pelvic fractures and update its controversies. It will detail the treatment of choice of post-traumatic distraction defects, a versatile one-stage perineal end-to-end anastomotic repair, and will also highlight recent advances in endourologic techniques.

SPHINCTER ANATOMY OF THE POSTERIOR URETHRA

In order to understand the functional significance of posterior urethral injuries one must have a working knowledge of the anatomy of the posterior urethral sphincter mechanisms.

The entire posterior urethra in the male is sphincter-active and any injury in this area will always alter sphincter function to some degree. Gosling describes the sphincter mechanism as consisting of both proximal and distal mechanisms and these may be considered to be functioning independently.[3] The proximal sphincter consists of a collar of smooth muscle, predominantly around the bladder neck, and it alone can maintain passive continence. This sphincter opens only when the detrusor contracts, whether voluntarily or involuntarily.[4] The distal or external sphincter has two parts—an intrinsic and extrinsic component both comprising striated musculature. The intrinsic component lies within the wall of the membranous urethra from the level of the verumontanum to the bulbar urethra. It consists of slow-twitch muscle fibers capable of sustained contraction and maintaining passive continence (Fig. 12.1a). The extrinsic component consists of fast-twitch fibers that only abut the membranous urethra posteriorly and posterolaterally and insert into the perineal body (Fig. 12.1b). These fibers are capable of interrupting the voided stream momentarily by compressing the urethra from behind but they do not add to passive continence. Contrary to most anatomic descriptions, it

199

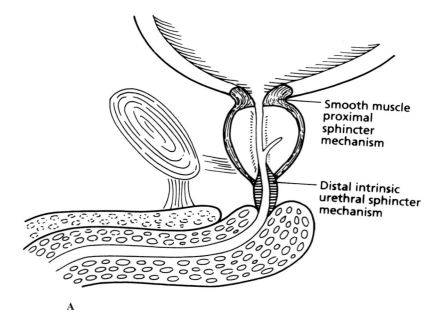

Smooth muscle
proximal
sphincter
mechanism

Distal intrinsic
urethral sphincter
mechanism

A

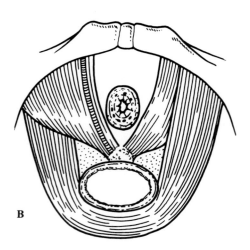

B

Fig. 12.1   The male urethral sphincter mechanism. **A** The intrinsic component of the distal sphincter mechanism resides within the wall of the membranous urethra. **B** The extrinsic component abuts on the membranous urethra posteriorly and laterally only. Reproduced with permission from Webster et al.[33]

has been shown that a 'urogenital diaphragm' perforated by the urethra does not exist.[5]

Pelvic fracture injuries of the membranous urethra and their subsequent repair invariably destroy or severely compromise the intramural distal sphincter and therefore continence after an open urethroplasty relies primarily upon a functioning bladder neck. Every effort must be made to preserve its integrity and in the event that it has been previously injured or surgically ablated, its reconstruction may be necessary as part of the urethroplasty.

URETHRAL INJURY FOLLOWING PELVIC FRACTURE

During pelvic fracture urethral injuries the bladder base and prostatic urethra tend to behave as a single unit, so that the urethra is torn in the membranous area distal to the prostate.[6] The urethra is most often injured in pelvic fractures that disrupt the anterior pelvic ring, particularly if both superior and inferior rami are fractured bilaterally.[7]

Depending upon the magnitude of injury the urethra can be contused, partially torn, or totally disrupted, resulting in what Turner-Warwick refers to as a 'urethral distraction defect'.[8]

Urethral contusion generally does not result in urethral stricture but may damage the distal intrinsic sphincter mechanism. This injury is likely to go unnoticed if the proximal urethral sphincter is intact but it may result in incontinence later on in life if the bladder neck is subsequently ablated by prostatectomy.[6]

In approximately one-third of urethral injuries following pelvic fracture the urethra is only partially torn and continuity is maintained. Partial tears may heal without stricture or with only a short stricture manageable by either dilatation or direct-vision internal urethrotomy. These injuries should be managed acutely by suprapubic urinary diversion since transurethral instrumentation carries with it the risk of further urethral disruption and introduction of infection.

In the majority of cases total urethral transection occurs, resulting in a urethral distraction defect. Separation of the urethral ends depends upon the size of the pelvic hematoma and the intactness of the fascial attachments between the vesicoprostatic unit and the pelvic floor and pubis. Usually the separation is minor, and with the passage of time the bladder will descend as the pelvic hematoma is resorbed, further shortening the urethral defect.

The most devastating injury occurs when a urethral distraction defect is associated with injury to other local structures including the bladder, rectum, and integument. These are referred to by Turner-Warwick as complex injuries and result in 'complex strictures'.[8] They often require different initial management, and the ultimate urethroplasty will invariably be more difficult.

DIAGNOSIS OF URETHRAL INJURY

History and physical

In multitrauma involving the abdomen or perineum or in patients with pelvic fractures, a high index of suspicion is required in order to make an early diagnosis of posterior urethral injury, especially if the patient is unconscious.

The majority of patients with posterior urethral injuries are unable to void. Patients with partial tears may complain of painful bloody urination often associated with swelling in the perineum due to urinary extravasation during voiding.

The signs of posterior urethral injury have been previously well-described and include blood at the urinary meatus, a high-riding or ill-defined prostate with a boggy prostatic bed, and bruising and swelling in the scrotum and perineum, its spread limited by Colles fascia.[9] One must suspect a concomitant bladder tear, especially when the bladder is impalpable after fluid resuscitation, and a rectal tear must be ruled out by careful circumferential rectal examination.

RADIOGRAPHIC EXAMINATION

All suspected urethral injuries require a retrograde urethrogram using sterile technique with or without the aid of fluoroscopy. Approximately 10 ml of water-soluble contrast should be injected under gentle pressure with the patient in the oblique position in order to visualize the entire urethra. Retrograde injection of contrast around the catheter is recommended for those patients arriving with an indwelling Foley catheter. All patients also require an intravenous pyelogram (IVP) and a retrograde or intravenous cystogram (from the cystogram phase of the IVP) to rule out concomitant renal and bladder injury.

ENDOSCOPY

Endoscopy is *not* routinely recommended in the immediate evaluation of post-traumatic posterior urethral injuries since it adds little new information and it may cause further urethral injury, infection, and fluid extravasation.

THE ACUTE MANAGEMENT OF POSTERIOR URETHRAL INJURIES

The acute management of traumatic posterior urethral injuries remains controversial. Many urologists believe that insertion of a suprapubic cystostomy tube at the time of injury followed by delayed urethroplasty of the resulting stricture is the preferred treatment and results in the lowest morbidity. Others feel that immediate primary realignment of the injured urethra over a stenting catheter, with or without suture ligatures, is an excellent alternative and in experienced hands gives equal results.

A number of primary realignment techniques have been described. The conventional method comprises immediate retropubic exploration with evacuation of hematoma and realignment of the torn urethra over a catheter.[10] Downward traction on the Foley catheter helps maintain urethral reapproximation but carries with it the risk of ischemia to the bladder neck jeopardizing continence, and should be avoided.[11,12] An acceptable alternative is the use of prostatic traction sutures brought out through the perineum or sutured to the endopelvic fascia.[13,14] Less invasive procedures avoid this widely criticized dissection of the perivesical/periprostatic space by operating through a vertical cystostomy and delivering the Foley catheter with the aid of urethral catheters or Davis interlocking sounds.[15,16] An endourologic technique using a Goodwin sound and urethroscopy has been described and offers the potential advantage of realigning the urethra under direct vision.[17]

Primary repair of urethral tears has been criticized for exposing the severely traumatized and unstable patient to further surgical risks; it may also introduce infection and/or aggravate bleeding. Critics also believe, but have not proven, that the incidence of impotence and incontinence is higher in these patients and is a result of excessive periprostatic and perivesical dissection. In 1972, Morehouse et al spearheaded the opposition against primary repair by reporting excessively high impotence and incontinence rates in patients referred after failed attempts at immediate repair when compared to their own patients managed by suprapubic cystostomy and delayed urethroplasty.[18] Webster et al summarized the available literature in 1983, and similarly concluded that continence and potency rates were higher in patients managed with suprapubic cystostomy and elective urethroplasty.[19] They noted an average potency rate of 88% and continence rate of 98% for delayed repair, while these same rates were only 56 and 80% for patients managed by primary realignment. In contrast, more recent series of primary repairs by Follis et al[15] and Patterson et al[16] have documented potency and continence rates equal to those of delayed repair, emphasizing the advantage of the newer less traumatic techniques over the conventional primary repairs once popular.

Currently, the most commonly accepted philosophy is that impotence and incontinence are a result of the primary injury and not of the surgery itself, as long as one avoids extensive perivesical/periprostatic dissection and traction on the stenting catheter. Also, most authors who advocate primary repair discourage suture reanastomosis and repeated unsuccessful attempts to place catheters that will not pass easily. In addition, most believe that suprapubic cystostomy and delayed repair form the treatment of choice in patients critically unstable and in cases where the physician lacks the experience or expertise required to do a primary repair.

Advocators of primary repair believe that the incidence of postinjury strictures and the need for urethroplasty are decreased by initial realignment management. The incidence of strictures after primary realignment varies greatly in the literature but in recent series ranges from 38 to 54%:[16,20] these require further management by urethral dilatation, direct-vision internal urethrotomy, or by urethroplasty. Not uncommonly these patients require long-term repeated urethral dilatations or urethrotomies in order to maintain urethral patency. Though nearly 100% of complete tears managed by suprapubic cystostomy will require a formal urethroplasty, the cure rate of this group in experienced hands is arguably much higher and approaches 95%.

These authors manage the majority of posterior urethral distraction defects by suprapubic cystostomy and delayed repair, but individualize their approach depending upon the degree of injury and whether injury to other local structures exists.[18] In our opinion there are three situations that require immediate exploration with pelvic hematoma evacuation and urethral realignment (Fig. 12.2):

1. The 'pie-in-the-sky' bladder exists when the bladder and prostatic urethra are widely separated from the pelvic floor as the bladder floats on a large pelvic hematoma. This severe prostatourethral dislocation often results in considerable distraction of the urethral ends separated by dense pelvic floor fibrosis, significantly complicating the ultimate urethroplasty.

2. A concomitant tear of the rectum requires immediate rectal repair and defunctioning sigmoid colostomy to prevent infection of the pelvic hematoma. During pelvic dissection it is advisable to reapproximate the torn urethra over a stenting catheter.

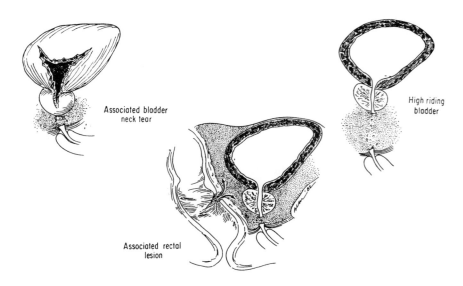

Associated bladder neck tear

High riding bladder

Associated rectal lesion

Fig. 12.2 Primary indications for early intervention in cases of posterior urethral injury after pelvic fracture. Reproduced with permission from Webster et al.[33]

3. Simultaneous injury to the bladder occurs in 18% of patients with urethral disruptions and is identified from extravasation seen on the excretory urogram.[21] Since the bladder neck maintains continence after disruption of the distal sphincter, any tears through the bladder neck should be debrided primarily and repaired. Injuries to the bladder neck alone often can be repaired intravesically without disturbing the pelvic hematoma. However, tears through the bladder neck generally require more extensive mobilization and hematoma evacuation to insure an anatomic repair, and the urethra should be aligned at the same time. The repair should be wrapped with omentum to facilitate re-exploration later and to preserve functional mobility in this area.

A final management option of pelvic fracture distraction defects is initial insertion of a suprapubic tube followed by delayed primary repair 7–21 days following the injury. Its primary advantage is the elective restoration of urethral continuity in a stable patient by an experienced urologist and avoiding the risks of additional surgery in the acutely injured patient. Mundy describes evacuation of the pelvic hematoma followed by suture repair of the severed urethra over a Foley catheter[22] while Herschorn et al[20] and Cohen et al[23] have used various endoscopic techniques, all with reasonable success.

Unfortunately the controversies surrounding these different therapeutic approaches are likely to persist indefinitely since without a randomized prospective study valid comparisons between the various treatments and their outcomes cannot be made with accuracy.

THE DELAYED MANAGEMENT OF POSTERIOR URETHRAL INJURIES

In patients managed by initial suprapubic cystostomy, elective urethroplasty is recommended 3–6 months after the injury. This allows ample time for resorption of the pelvic hematoma and descent of the bladder and prostatic urethra to a more anatomic position. Fortunately in the majority of cases the resulting urethral distraction defect is short (<2 cm) and easily amenable to urethroplasty.

The options for subsequent reconstruction include urethroplasty via perineal, abdominal transpubic, or combined routes, as well as innovative endourologic techniques.

ENDOUROLOGIC MANAGEMENT

As previously mentioned, urethral dilatation or direct-vision internal urethrotomy is the preferred treatment of non-obliterative urethral strictures following partial urethral tears. Unfortunately, in many cases these non-operative techniques are not curative and can cause further worsening of the spongiofibrosis, sometimes leading to an open urethroplasty.

There continues to be enthusiasm for the use of various endoscopic techniques for the re-establishment of urethral continuity in post-traumatic obliterative distraction defects in an attempt to spare the patient an open urethroplasty. Various 'cut for the light' techniques using either a urethrotome or small resectoscope have been described,[24–27] as have newer innovative procedures involving small trocars and balloon dilators.[28] Urethral continuity is often obtained with these procedures but patients commonly require long-term urethral dilatation or repeated urethrotomies, and, in some, eventual urethroplasty. Endoscopic treatment has potential risks, especially if performed by inexperienced hands. Reported complications include development of false passages into the bladder base; rectal injury resulting in urethrorectal fistula; and injury to remaining sphincteric and/or cavernosal nerve function.[24–27]

The role of these techniques in the management of posterior urethral distraction defects is controversial and remains to be established by long-term follow-up of large series of cases. Until then, these authors caution against overenthusiasm with these procedures, and believe the current treatment of choice is open urethroplasty.

SURGICAL MANAGEMENT

The one-stage combined abdominoperineal transpubic bulboprostatic reanastomotic repair with omental pedicle support was popularized by Turner-Warwick and used for complex strictures and when the bulboprostatic anastomosis could not be achieved by a perineal approach alone.[6] It is these authors' opinion that only rare and extremely complex strictures require this combined aproach and its overzealous use exposes the patient to unnecessary difficult retropubic dissection, potentially increasing the incidence of pelvic bleeding and postoperative impotence.[29]

Although there is no panacea, these authors believe that the optimal repair of nearly all obliterative defects irrespective of length is a one-stage primary anastomotic repair approached through the perineum.[30,31] This repair has proven remarkably versatile, successfully bridging defects up to 7 cm in length.

PROGRESSIVE PERINEAL APPROACH FOR THE REPAIR OF POSTERIOR URETHRAL DISTRACTION DEFECTS

In the late management of pelvic fracture distraction defects, urethroplasty is delayed for approximately 3–6 months. All patients preoperatively undergo simultanenous cystogram and retrograde urethrogram to evaluate the complexity and length of the urethral defect; the competence of the bladder neck; and the normality of the anterior urethra. Antegrade and retrograde endoscopy is used preoperatively if verification of radiographic findings is required and intraoperatively in all cases to rule out bladder stones, present as a result of long-term catheterization.

The patient is positioned in the lithotomy position and both the abdomen and perineum are prepared in case combined retropubic access is required intraoperatively. Excellent exposure of the posterior urethra is attained by a midline perineal incision bifurcated posteriorly and division of the bulbospongiosus muscle in the midline (Fig. 12.3A). The bulbar urethra is then circumferentially mobilized as far proximally as the obliterated segment where it is transected, and distally to a few centimeters distal to the crura (Fig. 12.3B). The anterior urethra is in essence converted to a urethral flap depending upon collateral retrograde blood supply from the corpora cavernosa and glans. Previous anterior urethral surgery or strictures and significant hypospadias may jeopardize the blood supply to the flap, precluding this mobilization and dictating an alternative repair.

Through the suprapubic tract a urethral sound is then carefully negotiated through the prostatic urethra until its tip can be palpated in the perineum and a vertical incision is then made through the perineal scar on to its tip. Adequate exposure is obtained with a nasal speculum inserted retrogradely into the membranoprostatic urethra, allowing one to spatulate the membranous urethra at 6 o'clock as far proximally as the verumontanum. The bulbar urethra is similarly spatulated to ensure a 40F sized bulboprostatic anastomosis.

At this point it will become apparent whether a simple tension-free anastomosis is possible or whether further lengthening procedures are required. These further maneuvers are carried out in a progressive stepwise fashion as the need for further lengthening is required.[30] In order, these maneuvers are:

1. *Further circumferential mobilization to the suspensory ligament:* Careful dissection is required to avoid dissection into the spongy tissue which could jeopardize the blood supply of the flap. Mobilization should not proceed beyond the suspensory ligament to avoid penile chordee (Fig. 12.3C). Up to 3 cm of lengthening can be obtained by this maneuver due to the elasticity of the healthy bulbar urethra.

2. *Separation of the proximal corporal bodies:* If the urethra is allowed to course between the separated corporal bodies rather than over them, up to 1–2 cm of apparent urethral lengthening can be achieved. The proximal 4–5 cm of the corporal bodies can be separated by careful sharp dissection along a relatively avascular plane in the midline (Fig. 12.3D). Beyond this point the corporal bodies are more intimately connected, making further separation too difficult.

3. *Inferior pubectomy:* The above two maneuvers achieve a tension-free anastomosis in more than 55% of cases. A further 1–2 cm can be gained by redirecting the urethra through a bony channel excised from the inferior pubic bone using an osteotome and bone rongeur (Fig. 12.3E), facilitating the

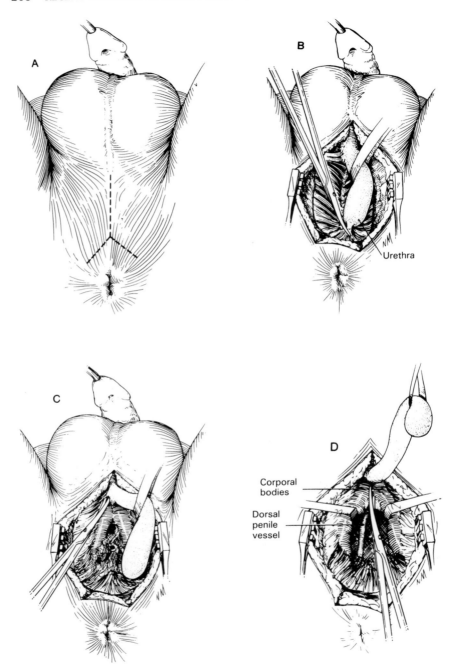

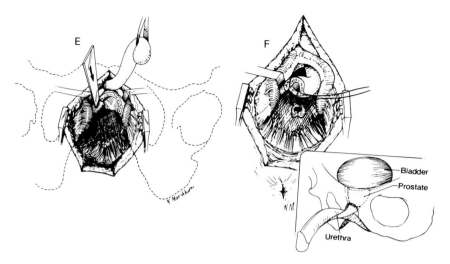

Fig. 12.3   Perineal repair of pelvic fracture urethral distraction defects. **A** A midline perineal incision is bifurcated posteriorly. **B** After dissecting the bulbospongiosus muscle from the bulbar urethra, it is circumferentially mobilized proximally to the obliterative defect. Incision of the posterior urethral attachments (with scissors) facilitates mobilization. **C** Once transected posteriorly, the urethra is mobilized distally as far as the suspensory ligament of the penis, if necessary. **D** Penile corporal bodies are separated, right from left, from the crus distally for 5–7 cm. The dorsal penile vesels dorsal to the corpora lie beneath the inferior ramus of the pubic above. **E** A channel is excised from the inferior ramus of the exposed pubis between the separated corporal bodies using bone osteotome and/or bone rongeur. **F** The corporal body is circumferentially dissected and the mobilized urethra rerouted around it and through the resected bony defect. The mobilized bulbar urethra is spatulated dorsally for anastomosis to the posteriorly spatulated prostatomembranous urethra. (Inset) Supracrurally rerouted urethra shown traversing resected inferior bony defect to facilitate bulboprostatic anastomosis.

anastomosis in an additional 30% of cases. In an attempt to preserve the laterally situated neurovascular bundle along the inferior surface of the pubis, excision of bone must be limited to the midline.

    4. *Rerouting the urethra around the corporal body:* As a final maneuver, the urethra can be laterally rerouted around the corporal body and through the tunnel created by the inferior pubectomy (Fig. 12.3F). A tunnel is created in the soft tissue around the corporal body, taking care to stay away from the corporal body, thereby preventing damage to the neurovascular bundle close to its surface. This supracrural rerouting achieves at least a further centimeter of urethral lengthening and is required in about 15% of cases. It is difficult to predict preoperatively which patients require these final two maneuvers since urethrograms only estimate the length of the distraction defect in one radiographic plane and give little information about associated spongiofibrosis and urethral elasticity. Subsequent transurethral instrumentation or insertion of a penile prosthesis has not been adversely affected by the new course of the urethra.

THE ANASTOMOSIS

A long nasal speculum is inserted retrogradely into the prostatic urethra and under direct vision a mucosa-to-mucosa bulboprostatic anastomosis is performed using interrupted 3-0 polyglycolic acid sutures. The verumontanum is an important landmark and identification of the prostatic urethral mucosa is of utmost importance. Using needles bent into a J-shape (Fig. 12.4), each

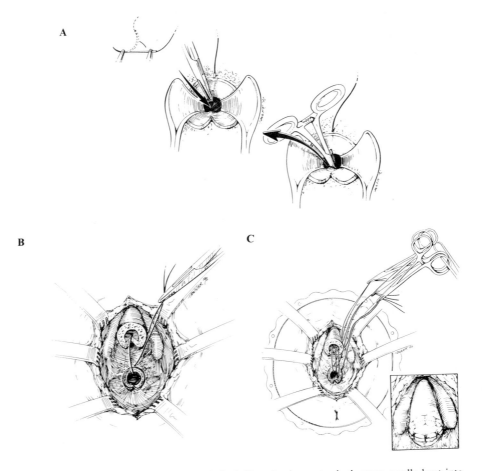

Fig. 12.4 **A** Bulboprostatic anastomosis is facilitated using a standard suture needle bent into a J-shape. The needle is advanced through the prostatic urethral edge and the needle tip retrieved in the prostatic lumen. The needle is advanced through the bladder neck to clear the needle, and then withdrawn. **B** Suture placement is commenced with the 12 o'clock suture in the prostatic urethra. **C** Sequential sutures are then placed in a clockwise direction around the prostatic urethral opening but are not tied. Hemostats placed on the end of each suture are stacked sequentially on an Allis clamp. After approximately eight sutures have been placed they are then individually tied, commencing with the 12 o'clock suture and proceeding clockwise. A catheter is inserted following suture placement and typing.

suture is inserted before being individually tied. The needles are advanced through the prostatic urethral edge from outside to inside; the point of the needle is retrieved within the prostatic urethra and advanced until clear; and then removed. Approximately eight sutures are inserted, commencing at the 12 o'clock position and proceeding clockwise before being tied individually in the same order as they were inserted.

A 16F fenestrated silicone catheter is inserted after the anastomosis is complete, along with a suprapubic cystostomy tube. A periurethral Jackson-Pratt drain is inserted for wound drainage and in most cases is removed on the third postoperative day.

Urethral stenting with an indwelling Foley catheter is required for approximately 2–3 weeks, and is only removed after a retrograde urethrogram around the catheter proves no extravasation. The suprapubic catheter is usually removed on the same day after a successful trial of voiding. We routinely repeat the retrograde urethrogram 3 and 12 months postoperatively.

RESULTS

This one-stage anastomotic perineal repair is very versatile and can be used to treat the majority of postpelvic fracture posterior urethral distraction defects. In a series of 114 cases, one of these authors experienced a surgical cure rate of 95% as determined by a retrograde urethrogram 12 months postoperatively.[32] Six patients required further surgery for restenosis; 3 were managed endoscopically and 3 required open surgery. Overall, 38% of these patients remained potent in the long term, and potency was unaffected by this surgical repair. In approximately 5% of patients, complicating factors render this one-stage repair either inappropriate or too difficult, and these cases are probably best managed by a combined abdominoperineal transpubic repair.[29] In these authors' experience the leading indications for a combined approach are the presence of fistulous tracts involving the bladder base and prostatic urethra; periurethral epithelialized cavities, and the inability to place the patient in the exaggerated lithotomy position because of associated orthopedic injuries. Staged substitution urethroplasty is only rarely indicated in cases in which the anterior urethra is also diseased or injured so that the urethra cannot be mobilized as a distally based flap.

SUMMARY

Injuries of the posterior urethra associated with pelvic fractures have the potential to cause significant long-term patient morbidity. Although controversies in management exist, it is universally accepted that for optimal results one requires sound judgment as well as surgical experience and expertise.

REFERENCES

1   Glass RE, Flynn JT, King JB et al. Urethral injury and fractured pelvis. Br J Urol 1978; 50: 578
2   Cass AS, Godee CJ. Urethral injury due to external trauma. Urology 1978; 11: 607
3   Gosling JA. The structure of the bladder and urethra in relation to function. Urol Clin North Am 1979; 6: 31
4   Turner-Warwick R. Clinical urodynamics. Urol Clin North Am 1979; 13: 30
5   Turner-Warwick R. Urethral stricture surgery. In: Mundy AR ed. Current operative surgery: urology. London: Bailliere Tindall, 1988: pp 160–218
6   Turner-Warwick R. A personal view of the management of traumatic posterior urethral strictures. Urol Clin North Am 1977; 4: 111
7   Pokorny M, Portes JE, Price JM. Urologic injuries associated with pelvic trauma. J Urol 1979; 121: 1455
8   Turner-Warwick R. Prevention of complications resulting from pelvic fracture urethral injuries and from their surgical management. Urol Clin North Am 1989; 16: 335
9   McAninch JW. Traumatic injuries to the urethra. J Trauma 1981; 21: 4
10 Hand JR. The use of catheter in the management of acute disruption of the membranous urethra. In: Scott R, Gordon HL, Scott FB, Carlton CE, Beach PD, eds. Current controversies in urologic management. Philadelphia: WB Saunders, 1972: p 131
11 Turner-Warwick R. A personal view of the immediate management of pelvic fracture urethral injuries. Urol Clin North Am 1977; 4: 81
12 Coffield KS, Weems WL. Experience with management of posterior urethral injury associated with pelvic fracture. J Urol 1977; 117: 722
13 Turner-Warwick R. Three approaches to the management of acute disruption of the membranous urethra. In: Scott R, Gordon HL, Scott FB, Carlton CE, Beach PD, eds. Current controversies in urologic management. Philadelphia: WB Saunders, 1972: p 144
14 Malek RS, O'Dea MJ, Kelalis PP. Management of ruptured posterior urethra in childhood. J Urol 1977; 117: 105
15 Follis HW, Koch MO, McDougal WS. Immediate management of prostatomembranous urethral disruptions. J Urol 1992; 147: 1259
16 Patterson DE, Barrett DM, Myers RP et al. Primary realignment of posterior urethral injuries. J Urol 1992; 129: 513
17 Gelbard MK, Heyman AM, Weintraub P. A technique for immediate realignment and cathetherization of the disrupted prostatomembranous urethra. J Urol 1989; 142: 52
18 Morehouse DD, Belitsky P, MacKinnon K. Rupture of the posterior urethra. J Urol 1972; 107: 255
19 Webster GD, Mathes GL, Selli C. Prostatomembranous urethral injuries: a review of the literature and a rational approach to their management. J Urol 1983; 130: 898
20 Herschorn S, Thijssen A, Radomski SB. The value of immediate or early catheterization of the traumatized posterior urethra. J Urol 1992; 148: 70
21 Mitchell JP. Injuries to the urethra. Br J Urol 1968; 40: 649
22 Mundy AR. The role of delayed primary repair in the acute management of pelvic fracture injuries of the urethra. Br J Urol 1991; 68: 273
23 Cohen JK, Berg G, Carl GH et al. Primary endoscopic realignment following posterior urethral disruption. J Urol 1991; 146: 1548
24 Gonzalez R, Chiou RK, Hekmat K et al. Endoscopic re-establishment of urethral continuity after traumatic disruption of the membranous urethra. J Urol 1983; 130: 785
25 Chiou RK, Gonzalez R, Ortlip S et al. Endoscopic treatment of posterior urethral obliteration: long term followup and comparison with transpubic urethroplasty. J Urol 1988; 140: 508
26 Fishman IJ, Hirsch IH, Toombs BD. Urological reconstruction of posterior urethral disruption. J Urol 1987; 137: 283
27 Yasuda K, Yamanishi T, Isaka S et al. Endoscopic re-establishment of membranous urethral disruption. J Urol 1991; 145: 977
28 Marshall FF, Chang R, Gearhart JP. Endoscopic reconstruction of traumatic membranous urethral transection. J Urol 1987; 138: 306
29 Webster GD. The management of complex posterior urethral strictures. In: Problems in urology. Paed Urol 1987; 1: 226–247

30 Webster GD, Sihelnik S. The management of strictures of the membranous urethra. J
    Urol 1985; 134: 469
31 Webster GD. Perineal repair of membranous urethral stricture. Urol Clin North Am
    1989; 16: 2
32 Webster GD, Mark SD. Delayed perineal urethroplasty for pelvic fracture urethral
    distraction defects. J Urol 1993; (In press)
33 Webster GD, Kirby R, King LR, Goldwasser G (eds) Reconstructive urology. Oxford:
    Blackwell Scientific Publications, 1993

13

Testicular cancer: reducing the toxicity of treatment of germ cell tumours

A. Horwich   W. F. Hendry

Considerable progress has been made over the last two decades in the management of patients with testicular cancer, so that at present more than 90% of men can expect to be cured. This high cure rate together with the relatively young age of presentation places a particular burden on the management policy to avoid toxicity, especially longer-term toxicities. This must not be at the expense of treatment efficacy and therefore any reduction in treatment requires extremely careful evaluation. This chapter will review approaches to toxicity reduction in the management of patients with either seminoma or non-seminoma.

SURVEILLANCE

Role

Surveillance has become the standard management of patients with stage I non-seminoma of the testis in the UK[1,2] and is gaining acceptance in many countries in Europe, and also in the USA. It is known that approximately one-third of patients will relapse, but with an active surveillance policy it is expected that relapse will occur with a disease extent which can easily be cured with combination chemotherapy and it has also been shown that surveillance achieves the same overall survival as the alternative management policies in stage I non-seminoma, namely, retroperitoneal lymph node dissection, adjuvant radiotherapy (historical) or adjuvant chemotherapy (experimental).[3] The timing of recurrence is very predominantly within the first 18 months following orchidectomy.

Toxicity of surveillance

Since surveillance itself represents an attempt to reduce treatment, reserving chemotherapy for those in whom the need has been demonstrated by progression of the disease, it may reasonably be considered that surveillance would represent the ultimate in reduction of treatment toxicity, especially in those destined to remain relapse-free. However, it should be remembered that the policy allows one-third of patients to progress and these patients then require standard chemotherapy (see below). Furthermore, the policy itself carries some toxicity, for example in the frequency of outpatient visits, tumour marker estimates and computed tomography (CT) scans of thorax and abdomen required for safe monitoring. Some patients find the lack of treatment together with the possibility of progression stressful, and some are unreliable in attendance.

Approaches to reducing toxicity of surveillance

Selective surveillance

A prognostic factor analysis based on the primary tumour histology has revealed that the risk of recurrence can be predicted, with each of the following factors having independent significance.[2]

1. Invasion of lymphatics.
2. Invasion of blood vessels.
3. Presence of undifferentiated cells
4. Absence of yolk sac elements.

A simplified prognostic index can be constructed by scoring each of these factors with a 0 or + 1, and this index has now been tested in a prospective multicentre evaluation of surveillance.[4] The patient with three or four risk factors has a 50% chance of recurrence within 2 years, whereas the risk is only 25% in patients with fewer histological risk factors. Reanalysis of 900 patients managed by surveillance and registered in the Medical Research Council Trials Office indicates a simplified risk factor index can be based entirely on vascular invasion (either lymphatic or blood vessel). If this is present then the risk of recurrence is 45% and if this is absent the risk is 20%.

The identification of patients with a high risk of recurrence allows a more selective policy of surveillance, reserving it for those with a very low probability of relapse and treating the high-risk patients with chemotherapy following orchidectomy. At present the Medical Research Council Testicular Tumour Working Party is evaluating the use of only two cycles of adjuvant chemotherapy in this setting, and the preliminary results on 66 patients would suggest that this approach will prevent recurrence.[5]

Reducing the intensity of surveillance

Testicular cancer can be a very rapidly proliferating tumour and it is important for a safe surveillance policy that patients are monitored frequently, especially with respect to serum tumour markers and chest X-ray. However, the need for frequent CT scanning of thorax and abdomen has been questioned. In the Medical Research Council studies different centres used CT scanning at different frequency and a retrospective analysis has been performed of the impact of CT scanning frequencies on stage at recurrence.

There was little impact on either stage or on prognosis when comparing one or two scans per year, three or four scans per year, or more than four scans per year, and indeed the only detectable effect was on the size of a retroperitoneal node mass which was on average 2 cm smaller in the patients scanned at least three times per year than in the patients scanned less often. On the basis of this study it seems reasonable to recommend only three or four CT scans per year in the first year of surveillance.

SURGERY

Role of surgery

The surgeon can reduce the toxicity of treatment of testicular tumours in many ways. By early and accurate diagnosis the need for adjuvant treatment is minimized. With a careful surgical technique operative complications should be few. Potential toxicity to the man's reproductive system can be circumvented by timely referral for seminal analysis and sperm cryopreservation. Furthermore, those patients likely to develop second cancers of the contralateral testicle can now be identified and the risk eliminated without the need for second orchidectomy.

The urologist's role was once thought to be rather dull: orchidectomy and referral. The modern management of testicular tumours requires much more active involvement from the time of first presentation, during initial assessment, at primary surgery and in collaborative management of advanced disease. Most young men presenting with testicular tumours expect to be able to become fathers;[6] the person who also has much to gain from adequate testicular function—the female partner—must be kept well-informed, and involved in management, since she has considerable vested interest in minimizing toxicity.

Early diagnosis

The most important variables affecting the outcome of treatment for testicular tumours are tumour volume and serum marker levels at presentation, and these correlate directly with delay from first symptom to start of treatment. For example, Bosl et al[7] showed that median patient-plus-physician delay for stage I tumours was 75 days, for stage 2 was 101 days, and for stage 3 was 134 days—a highly significant correlation. Similarly, Wishnow et al[8] showed that 62% of 65 men undergoing orchidectomy within 1 month were stage I, compared to only 28% of 89 delaying for more than this time; only 1 of the former group died, compared to 11 of the latter. Amongst men with metastatic disease, data from a Medical Research Council study[9] showed that when the history was less than 6 months, 54% of patients had small-volume metastases and 65% low serum markers, compared to 39 and 51% respectively for those with a history of more than 6 months. Three-year survival figures in a follow-up Medical Research Council study for men with a history of less than 3 months was 87%, compared to 80% when the history was longer than this: the significant difference ($P = 0.04$) was associated with more advanced disease found with delay in diagnosis.[10] Part of the problem is delay by the patient in seeking medical advice: over 80% wait for more than 1 month, over 50% for more than 3 months;[11] and part is due to failure to establish the correct diagnosis once the man reaches the doctor: this was estimated at only 43% by Ekman.[12]

There are several reasons why the diagnosis of testicular tumours is treacherous, not least because the man himself tends to make light of his disease—we often see men brought to the clinic by their female partners protesting that they feel little wrong. A history of trauma is often given by men with testicular tumours, either recent or remote, and this should not distract attention from the true underlying condition—it is probably true that in some cases the man never felt the tumour until he banged the affected testicle. In other cases pain may draw attention to the disorder in the testicle; although most tumours are painless, some present with severe discomfort, and may be tender on examination. This will often lead to misdiagnosis and delay while the condition is treated as inflammatory.[13] Special care is needed in dealing with testes known to be a high risk of neoplasia, especially after previous orchidopexy[14] or affecting an atrophic testis.[15] Ultrasound scanning may clarify the situation, for example with impalpable intratesticular tumours,[16] though the error rate for both false-positive and false-negative results is around 10%.[17] Testicular abscess is particularly difficult to differentiate from tumour clinically, but can be distinguished by ultrasonography.[18]

Surgical technique

Surgical exploration remains the most accurate way to establish the diagnosis of testicular tumour, and the surgeon will not hesitate to operate on a suspicious lump, irrespective of the history or findings on ultrasound scan. The surgery can be done on a day-care basis with modern anaesthetic techniques. A groin incision is generally recommended, to minimize the possibility of scrotal contamination with tumour, although three studies have shown no increase in local or systemic recurrence rates after scrotal orchidectomy.[19-21] Nevertheless, a groin incision allows a cleaner removal of the tumour with the testicle and cord intact, and it is easy to insert a prosthesis at the same time with minimal risk of it sloughing through the scrotal skin. Careful haemostasis will eliminate the risk of haematoma formation, and antibiotic cover is recommended, especially if a prosthesis is inserted. Wound infection not only increases local discomfort and jeopardizes the prosthesis; it may also hold up further treatment with radiotherapy or chemotherapy which may be urgently needed for the young man with advanced disease. Care should be taken not to encircle the ilioinguinal nerve when closing the external oblique aponeurosis: many patients continue to complain of discomfort in this area long after other treatments are completed and forgotten.

Most testicular tumour patients are young, and most adapt well psychologically to their disease, ultimately attaining average or better than average sexual relations.[22] However, loss of a testicle is associated with a perceived reduction in manhood,[23] and provision of a prosthesis is associated with a high level of satisfaction in most men.[24] Occasionally, benign tumours may be encountered, such as adenomatoid tumours[25] or epidermoid cysts,[26] and there may be a case for local excision with testis preservation in carefully selected cases.[27]

Before referring the patient to the radiotherapist/medical oncologist for further assessment and treatment, thought should be given to the question of contralateral testicular biopsy. This is also the time to give consideration to seminal analysis and possible sperm cryopreservation. Both matters should be fully discussed with the patient and his next of kin.

Contralateral testicular biopsy

Bilateral testicular tumours occur in 3–5% cases.[28–30] There is good evidence that carcinoma-in-situ exists in the contralateral testis for a number of years before the overt disease develops, and its presence can be detected by testicular biopsy.[31] Follow-up studies indicate that at least half of such men will ultimately develop tumours, and that this progression can be prevented by a short course of local radiotherapy (20 Gy[32]). This raises the question of who should be advised to have a biopsy, and when it should be done. Certain well-defined risk factors have been defined: cryptorchidism, testicular atrophy and history of infertility.[33] Analysis of our experience at the Royal Marsden Hospital with 1219 patients treated between 1962 and 1984 indicated that 65% of 26 assessable men who developed second tumours had one or more of these risk factors.[34] Men with occult primary germ-cell tumours[35] also have a high incidence of carcinoma-in-situ. We therefore recommend that patients with such a history should undergo testicular biopsy, and we have found that most readily agree once it has been explained to them that this small procedure will indicate if they are likely to lose their remaining testicle to the same disease, and that such loss can be prevented. Sterility inevitably follows local radiotherapy, and so seminal analysis and cryopreservation if possible should precede treatment, although most have pre-existing impaired spermatogenesis and hence have little to lose whilst preserving Leydig cell function. The exact timing of the biopsy is probably not important, and there is a good case for getting it done as soon as convenient in high-risk cases; in Denmark it is usually done at the time of initial orchidectomy, which saves the need for a second anaesthetic.

The surgical procedure takes only minutes, and is usually done by a simple stab with a sharp pointed scalpel blade, a 3–4 mm piece of testicular tissue being extruded by squeezing the testicle. The resulting defect is closed with a fine catgut stitch. Care must be taken with small testes, especially if there is fibrosis after previous orchidopexy. Reinberg et al[36] reported that 28% of such men could not tolerate the procedure under local anaesthetic, and observed an infection rate of 1.5%; it is our practice to do this small procedure under general anaesthetic as a day-case, taking great care with haemostasis. The patient is seen, with his female partner if appropriate, in the outpatient clinic a week later to discuss the results.

Seminal analysis and cryopreservation

Many men with testicular tumours are infertile,[37] but it is not always clear whether this antedated the development of the tumour, or was due to the tumour itself or resulted from its treatment.[38] Certainly fertility can be preserved in some patients provided treatment is carried out carefully[39] and there is nothing wrong with the children produced by these men.[40] On the other hand, the majority of men subjected to bilateral para-aortic lymphadenectomy became infertile and noted decrease in libido and sexual performance.[41]

At presentation, only one-quarter of men have semen quality good enough to permit cryopreservation.[42] One-quarter have severe irreversible impairment of spermatogenesis demonstrable on testicular biopsy.[43] Amongst the remainder, there is the potential for recovery of normal spermatogenesis, even after chemotherapy: indeed, in our experience, return to normal was seen in 35% of those starting with initially poor sperm counts, but in only 25% of those with good initial counts.[42] It is, therefore, very important to limit toxicity of treatment in these young men, and to offer cryopreservation to those in whom treatment is likely to lead to irreversible damage.[44–46] Sadly, this service is severely under-resourced in this country at the present time.[47]

Para-aortic lymphadenectomy

The principal cause of permanent damage to sexual function, with long-term psychosocial problems, is retroperitoneal para-aortic lymphadenectomy.[48] Compared to married healthy men, testicular tumour patients after lymphadenectomy showed less sexual activity, lower desire, more erectile dysfunction, more difficulty achieving orgasm and reduced orgasmic intensity; 82% had reduced semen volume amongst 121 patients studied.[49] The problem is due to interruption of the lumbar sympathetic outflow, and occurs either at the level of the lumbar sympathetic ganglia or at the presacral hypogastric plexus, which lies just below the bifurcation of the aorta.[50] Study of 101 patients after bilateral lymphadenectomy by Nijmau et al[51] showed that ejaculation was normal in only 12 postoperatively. Amongst the remainder, ejaculation was retrograde in 55 and there was no emission in 20; 12 had difficulty with orgasm and 6 had erectile dysfunction.

As a result of these difficulties, a nerve-sparing technique of lymphadenec-tomy was devised,[52] which adds considerably to the operative time, but does preserve ejaculation in most patients.[53,54] None the less, it is hard to understand why surgeons persist with this procedure for stage I disease, when equally good results can be obtained by surveillance.

A residual mass may be found in the retroperitoneal lymph nodes after completion of chemotherapy in up to 25% of patients.[55] Analysis of 231 such cases treated at the Royal Marsden Hospital between 1976 and 1990 by retroperitoneal lymphadenectomy showed that there was residual undifferen-tiated teratoma in 21%. Multivariate analysis showed that completeness of surgical excision, pathology of excised mass, timing of surgery after chemo-therapy and year of treatment were independent prognostic variables. Para-aortic lymphadenectomy in this setting thus provides both therapeutic benefit and information of prognostic value in planning future treatment.[56] Operative mortality was low at 1%, but 12.5% of patients lost the ipsilateral kidney which was often poorly functioning. Analysis of ejaculatory function in 186 of these men showed that 22% lost ejaculation, but this was significantly more likely to occur if the dissection was bilateral (45%) or if the mass was very large (greater than 8 cm diameter: 58%). Careful attention to nerve-sparing operative technique led to a reduction in the incidence of loss of ejaculation from 36% before 1984 to 16% since then.[57]

Loss of ejaculation after para-aortic lymphadenectomy may recover spon-taneously but is likely to be permanent in the majority of cases. Drug therapy such as imipramine 25 mg twice daily may help to restore antegrade ejaculation,[58] or electroejaculation may be successful: Ohl et al[59] obtained more than 10 million motile spermatozoa from 21 of 24 men with loss of ejaculation after lymphadenectomy, and 7 pregnancies were produced by artificial insemination.

RADIOTHERAPY

Role of radiotherapy

Radiotherapy is now rarely used in the management of non-seminoma. It is, however, the appropriate management for adjuvant treatment of stage I seminoma following orchidectomy and also for a small volume of stage II seminoma. In stage I seminoma radiotherapy is used to treat the possibility of subclinical metastases in retroperitoneal and ipsilateral pelvic lymph nodes. The conventional dose is 30 Gy in 15 fractions over 3 weeks using equally weighted anterior and posterior portals and treating both fields daily. The Royal Marsden Hospital experience[60] is similar to that from other centres and the very great majority of patients do not relapse.

In stage II seminoma the risk of recurrence after radiotherapy is related to the volume of the abdominal lymph nodes. The analysis by Gregory & Peckham[61] suggested that for node metastases more than 5 cm in transverse diameter the recurrence rate was more than 25%; they concluded that these patients should therefore be treated initially with chemotherapy. Others have reported excellent results with initial radiotherapy for masses up to 10 cm in diameter, especially in patients carefully staged in the modern era with CT scanning.[62] Following radiotherapy confined to retroperitoneal and pelvic nodes, patients who relapse can be treated with combination chemotherapy with a high success rate.[63]

Toxicity of radiotherapy

The doses of radiation required to treat seminoma are relatively low. Acute toxicity is usually confined to mild gastrointestinal side-effects in about half of treated patients. Later toxicities may include peptic ulceration in about 5% of patients,[64] though the risk of this is mainly in patients with previous ulceration or with a history of abdominal surgery.

With any radiotherapeutic treatment there is scatter of radiation to the contralateral testis. With standard dose and fields used for seminoma the dose is sufficient to reduce the sperm count transiently but should not cause infertility. In view of the possibility of genotoxicity, patients are advised to avoid conception for 1 year after treatment.

There is also concern over the possibility of radiation carcinogenesis or leukaemogenesis. There is some controversy over this issue. The review from five Scottish Radiotherapy Centres by Hay et al[65] reported a slight excess risk of second cancers in patients undergoing treatment for stage I testicular cancer with radiotherapy. However, the risk was just as high for sites outside the radiation fields as within the radiation fields. Fossa et al[66] found a significant excess risk of cancers only in patients who had both infradiaphragmatic and supradiaphragmatic radiotherapy. Our studies are based on patients registered in the South Thames Cancer Registry in an analysis of 859 patients treated with radiotherapy for stage I seminoma between 1961 and 1985.[67] There were no overall excess deaths from causes other than testicular cancer, and also there was no overall significant excess of non-testicular malignancies amongst the causes of death. However, for leukaemia there was a significant excess (observed/expected = 5.4).

Reducing the toxicity of radiotherapy

There are two main approaches to reducing radiation toxicity. The first consideration is whether the extent of the radiation field can be reduced. The first-station lymph nodes for metastatic spread from the testis are in the para-aortic region and it has been suggested that the pelvic component of the standard radiation field may not be required unless the patient has previously had inguinal surgery which may distort the usual spread pattern.[68] The Medical Research Council is currently performing a prospective randomized trial comparing standard para-aortic plus pelvic radiotherapy with a reduced field confined to the para-aortic region. This will have the advantage of considerably reducing the dose to pelvic bone marrow and also reducing the scatter dose to the contralateral testis.

The second approach to reducing radiation toxicity is to reduce the radiation dose. Though the conventional treatment of stage I seminoma at the Royal Marsden Hospital has for the last 30 years been a dose of 30 Gy in 15–20 fractions over 3–4 weeks, the standard dose at Princess Margaret Hospital in Toronto has been approximately 25 Gy in 20 fractions over 4 weeks, and at the Institute Gustave-Roussy in Paris the standard dose has been 22 Gy in 11 fractions over 2½ weeks. Lower doses have not led to infield recurrence and, though this has not been tested in prospective randomized trials, it seems likely that doses of the order of 22–25 Gy will prove sufficient. It will be, however, difficult to prove reduction in treatment toxicity with this relatively modest reduction of dose.

There are very few data on the dose required to eradicate carcinoma-in-situ for the contralateral testis. Doses of 20 Gy in 10 fractions over 2 weeks appear adequate to prevent recurrence of lesion;[32] however, follow-up hormone studies have revealed some elevation of pituitary gonadotrophins. Even though this has not yet been associated with a fall in serum testosterone to below the normal range, there is some concern that this may be a late effect. Prospective studies will therefore evaluate reduced radiation doses in the treatment of carcinoma-in-situ.

CHEMOTHERAPY

Role

Combination chemotherapy based on platinum has dramatically improved the prognosis of patients with metastatic non-seminoma and of patients with advanced metastatic seminoma.[69] Combination chemotherapy is standard management for patients with stage III or IV testicular cancer. In the UK the stage I marker-positive and all stage II non-seminomas are treated initially with chemotherapy and following chemotherapy only those with residual masses have a lymphadenectomy.

There is a good prognosis for all patients with metastatic germ cell tumours. A prognostic factor analysis has recently been performed by the Medical Research Council based on 895 patients treated between 1982 and 1986.[10] This showed that the overall 3-year survival probability was 85% and it is likely that this figure approximates to cure. The analysis found that the prognosis was influenced adversely by increasing bulk of disease and by increasing concentration of tumour markers. The multivariate analysis showed that a simple prognostic index could be constructed from the four independent significance factors:

1. More than 20 lung metastases.
2. Mediastinal mass more than 5 cm in diameter.

3. Presence of bone, liver or central nervous system metastasis.
4. Presence of high tumour markers (alpha-fetoprotein $\geqslant 1000$ u/l or human chorionic gonadotrophin $\geqslant 10\,000$ u/l).

Recently a detailed analysis was performed of the success of primary chemotherapy following orchidectomy in stage IIA and IIB metastatic non-seminomas. Since this analysis was confined to stages of non-seminoma with retroperitoneal node metastasis less than 5 cm in diameter, the results can be compared with those of initial lymphadenectomy in these stages. The conclusion was that primary chemotherapy led to an extremely high cure rate, but that only approximately 30% of patients would come to lymphadenectomy.[70]

The success rate of chemotherapy is equally high when used for advanced seminoma.[63] When bulky metastatic disease is treated a residual mass is common, but often composed of fibrotic tissue difficult to resect. The usual practice is therefore to monitor closely a residual mass and to perform a CT-guided biopsy of those masses that do not appear to continue to regress following the end of chemotherapy. Alternatively, especially when single-agent chemotherapy has been used for advanced seminoma, it may be reasonable to incorporate adjuvant radiotherapy following chemotherapy.[71]

Toxicity of chemotherapy

The pattern of toxicity depends upon the choice of drugs, current drug doses and number of cycles of chemotherapy influencing the cumulative drug dose.[72]

The standard BEP schedule (bleomycin, etoposide, cisplatin) is usually administered for four cycles, beginning a new cycle every 3 weeks.[73] The main acute side-effects are nausea and vomiting, especially during the first few days of chemotherapy when cisplatin is being administered daily. This can usually be counteracted by the combination of dexamethasone and metoclopramide, but in resistant cases ondansetron may be helpful. Alopecia secondary to etoposide is complete and usually begins about 9–10 days following initiation of chemotherapy; this virtually always reverses completely after completion of treatment. The combination is moderately myelosuppressive with a nadir from 10 to 14 days following start of chemotherapy. It is uncommon for the total white blood count to fall below 1.0×10^9 l or for the platelet count to fall below 100×10^9 l. Patients should be warned to report directly to the oncologist any episodes of fever, spontaneous bruising or bleeding.

Cisplatin also causes renal tubular damage and on average a complete course of chemotherapy incorporating three or four cycles leads to approximately a 25% reduction in glomerular filtration rate.[74] Cisplatin also causes a dose-dependent high-tone hearing loss and idiosyncratic sensory peripheral neuropathy. Bleomycin is usually well-tolerated but causes a flu-like reaction, which can be prevented by the simultaneous administration of low doses of hydrocortisone. Some 10–20% of patients suffer skin reactions to bleomycin with inflammatory subcutaneous nodals, especially at the site of mild trauma such as the palms of the hands. It causes pigmentation at sites of skin inflammation, and Raynaud's phenomenon which often appears following the completion of chemotherapy and may be very long-lasting. The most worrisome side-effect of standard doses of bleomycin chemotherapy is pneumonitis. Mild symptoms and radiological changes are seen in approximately 20% of patients; however, 1–2% of patients treated to a total accumulative dose of 360 units experience irreversible lung fibrosis which is fatal.

Combination chemotherapy also causes impairment of spermatogenesis, though for the very great majority of patients who have a normal sperm count before starting, this form of chemotherapy allows a full recovery to normal fertility. Genotoxicity is theoretically possible; however, a significant risk to the offspring of treated fathers has not been demonstrated.[40]

Approaches to reducing chemotherapy toxicity

Reduction of drug dose

In the early days of successful germ-cell tumour chemotherapy, the standard regimen incorporated platinum, vinblastine and bleomycin (PVB) and the vinblastine dose was high, at 0.2 mg/kg on each of the first 2 days. This led to bowel toxicity, ileus and profound bone marrow suppression. The dose of vinblastine was subsequently reduced to 0.15 mg/kg on each of the first 2 days with no loss of efficacy.[75] Subsequently the combination of PVB has been compared with BEP.[76] It was apparent that the BEP schedule was less toxic both in terms of bone marrow suppression and in terms of abdominal cramp. Furthermore, BEP was more effective in patients with advanced stages of metastatic non-seminoma and has therefore become the standard regimen. Investigation of the dose of cisplatin strongly suggested that each cycle requires a minimum of 100 mg/m^2.[77] There is retrospective evidence favouring the maintenance of dose levels of both etoposide[78] and of carboplatin.[79,80]

Drug deletion

The major target for this approach has been bleomycin because of the unpredictable and potentially fatal lung fibrosis found in 1–2% of patients having standard doses. It seems clear that for the best-prognosis group of metastatic non-seminoma, if patients are treated with four cycles of chemotherapy, a combination of etoposide and platinum (EP) is not significantly less effective than the combination of BEP.[81] On the other hand, if only three cycles of chemotherapy are used, the EP combination was distinctly inferior to the combination of BEP[82] and this was also true if patients with a slightly worse prognosis were included in the treatment series.[83] It therefore seems reasonable to maintain the place of bleomycin in standard chemotherapy, but to consider modification of the total dose either in relation to the number of cycles or the number of injections of bleomycin within each cycle. Current Medical Research Council trials are based on the dose of bleomycin at 30 units per cycle, i.e. 30 units once every 3 weeks. The total dose should be thus considerably less than the threshold for pneumonitis.

Drug analogues

Because of the side-effects of cisplatin, an analogue carboplatin has entered clinical practice in the treatment of both seminoma[79] and non-seminoma.[84] At standard doses this drug does not cause renal tubular damage, neuropathy or ototoxicity; however, it has more bone marrow toxicity than cisplatin and also since the main route of excretion is renal, it is appropriate to modify the dose in the light of accurate assessment of renal function.[80] In treatment of advanced seminoma approximately 75% of patients have prolonged progression-free remission after single-agent carboplatin and because a high proportion of these can be salvaged after recurrence with combination chemotherapy, the overall survival in patients initially treated with single-agent carboplatin is equivalent to those initially treated with combination chemotherapy. At present a Medical Research Council trial is comparing these management policies.

In the treatment of metastatic non-seminoma, combination chemotherapy incorporating carboplatin has been reported to be extremely effective.[84] However, a randomized trial in 265 good-risk metastatic germ-cell tumour patients compared the combination of etoposide + cisplatin given every 3 weeks with the combination of etoposide + carboplatin given every 4 weeks and found the carboplatin combination was inferior.[85] It is unclear whether the loss of efficacy was due to the 4 weeks' cycling or due the replacement of cisplatin with carboplatin. The Medical Research Council Testicular Tumour Working Party is currently pursuing a randomized trial comparing the combination of bleomycin, etoposide and cisplatin with bleomycin, etoposide and carboplatin, with both schedules being administered every 3 weeks. Until this has been completed an analysed cisplatin-based chemotherapy should be regarded as standard.

CONCLUSIONS

The concentration of patients with germ-cell tumours within specialized centres has greatly facilitated careful evaluation of treatment advances, and this review has summarized the consequent reduction in treatment toxicity which can now be offered to benefit patients. For the great majority of patients with germ-cell tumours this will mean that they can receive appropriate curative therapy with minimal short-term and long-term toxicity.

REFERENCES

1   Peckham MJ, Barrett A, Husband JE, Hendry WF. Orchidectomy alone in testicular stage I non-seminomatous germ-cell tumours. Lancet 1982; ii: 678–680
2   Freedman LS, Parkinson MC, Jones WG et al. Histopathology in the prediction of relapse of patients with stage I testicular teratoma treated by orchidectomy alone. Lancent 1987; ii: 294–298
3   Horwich A. Editorial: current issues in the management of clinical stage I testicular teratoma. Eur J Cancer 1993; 29A: 933–934
4   Read G, Stenning SP, Cullen MH et al. Medical Research Council prospective study of surveillance for stage I testicular teratoma. J Clin Oncol 1992; 10: 1762–1768
5   Cullen MH, Stenning S, Fossa SD, Horwich A, Kaye SB, MRC Testicular Teratoma Working Party. Short course adjuvant chemotherapy in high risk stage I non-seminoma germ cell tumours of the testis (NSGCTT): preliminary report of an MRC study. Br J Cancer 1992; 65 (suppl XVI): abstract 8 p. 8
6   Aass N, Fossa SD. Paternity in young patients with testicular cancer—expectations and experience. Progr Clin Biol Res 1988; 269: 481–491
7   Bosl GJ, Vogelzang NJ, Goldman A et al. Impact of delay in diagnosis on clinical stage of testicular cancer. Lancet 1981; ii: 970–973
8   Wishnow KI, Johnson DE, Preston WL, Tenney DM, Brown BW. Prompt orchiectomy reduces morbidity and mortality from testicular carcinoma. Br J Urol 1990; 65: 629–633
9   MRC Working Party on Testicular Teratoma. Prognostic factors in advanced non-seminomatous germ cell testicular tumours: results of a multicentre study. Lancet 1985; i: 8–11
10 Mead GM, Stenning SP, Parkinson MC et al. The second Medical Research Council study of prognostic factors in nonseminomatous germ cell tumours. J Clin Oncol 1992; 10: 85–94
11 Thompson IM, Wear J, Almond C, Schewe EJ, Sala J. An analytical survey of 178 testicular tumours. J Urol 1961; 85: 173–179
12 Ekman P. Delay in the diagnosis of testicular cancer. Larartidningen 1980; 77: 4275–4277
13 Sandeman TF. Symptoms and early management of germinal tumours of the testis. Med J Aust 1979; 2: 281–284
14 Gehring GC, Rodriguez FR, Woodhead DM. Malignant degeneration of cryptorchid testes following orchiopexy. J Urol 1974; 112: 354–356
15 Hausfeld KF, Schrandt D. Malignancy of the testis following atrophy: report of three cases. J Urol 1965; 94: 69–72
16 Casapo Z, Bornhof C, Giedl J. Impalpable testicular tumours diagnosed by scrotal ultrasonography. Urology 1988; 32: 549–552
17 Lightner DJ, Grund F, Lange PH. Noninvasive scrotal imaging techniques. In: McCullough DL, ed. Difficult diagnosis in urology. New York: Churchill Livingstone, 1989: pp 249–258
18 Mevorach RA, Lerner RM, Dvoretsky PM, Rabinowitz R. Testicular abscess: diagnosis by ultrasonography. J Urol 1986; 136: 1213–1216
19 Kennedy CL, Hendry WF, Peckham MJ. The significance of scrotal interference in stage I testicular cancer managed by orchiectomy and surveillance. Br J Urol 1986; 58: 705–708
20 Ozen H, Altug N, Bakkaloglu MA, Remzi D. Significance of scrotal violation in the prognosis of patients with testicular tumors. Br J Urol 1988; 62: 267–270
21 Giguere JK, Stablein DM, Spaulding JT, McLeod DG, Paulson DF, Weiss RB. The clinical significance of nonconventional orchidectomy approaches in testicular cancer: a report from the Testicular Cancer Intergroup Study. J Urol 1988; 139: 1225–1228
22 Cassileth B, Stanfeld A. Psychological preparation of the patient and family. Cancer

1987; 60; 547–552

23   Blackmore C. The impact of orchidectomy upon the sexuality of the man with testicular cancer. Cancer Nurs 1988; 11: 33–40

24   Lynch MJ, Pryor JP. Testicular prosthesis: the patient's perception. Br J Urol 1992: 70: 420–422

25   Upton JD, Das S. Benign intrascrotal neoplasms. J Urol 1986; 135: 504–506

26   Malek RS, Rosen JS, Farrow GM. Epidermoid cyst of the testis: a critical analysis. Br J Urol 1985; 58: 55–59

27   Kressell K, Schnell D, Thon WF, Heymer B, Hartmann M, Altwein SE. Benign testicular tumours: a case for testis preservation? Eur Urol 1988; 15: 200–204

28   Sokal M, Peckham MJ, Hendry WF. Bilateral germ cell tumours of the testis. Br J Urol 1980; 52: 158–162

29   Scheiber K, Ackermann D, Studer UE. Bilateral testicular germ cell tumors: a report of 20 cases. J Urol 1987; 138: 73–76

30   Thompson J, Williams CJ, Whitehouse JMA, Mead GM. Bilateral testicular germ cell tumours: an increasing incidence and prevention by chemotherapy. Br J Urol 1988; 62: 374–376

31   Skakkebaek NE. Possible carcinoma-in-situ of the testis. Lancet 1972; ii: 516–517

32   Von der Maase H, Giwercman A, Muller J, Skakkebaek NE. Management of carcinoma in situ of the testis. Int J Androl 1987; 10: 209–220

33   Berthelsen JG, Skakkebaek NE, Von der Maase H, Sorensen BL. Screening for carcinoma in situ of the contralateral testis in patients with germinal testicular cancer. Br Med J 1982; 285: 1683–1686

34   Fordham MVP, Mason MD, Blackmore C, Hendry WF, Horwich A. Management of the contralateral testis in patients with testicular germ cell cancer. Br J Urol 1990; 65: 290–293

35   Powell S, Hendry WF, Peckham MJ. Occult germ-cell testicular tumours. Br J Urol 1983; 55: 440–444

36   Reinberg Y, Manivel JC, Fraley EE. Carcinoma in situ of the testis. J Urol 1989; 142: 243–247

37   Jewett MAS, Thachil JV, Harris JF. Exocrine function of testis with germinal testicular tumour. Br Med J 1983; 286: 1849–1850

38   Schilsky RL. Infertility in patients with testicular cancer: testis, tumour or treatment? J Natl Cancer Inst 1989; 81: 1204–1205

39   Smithers DW, Wallace DM, Austin DE. Fertility after unilateral orchidectomy and radiotherapy for patients with malignant tumours of the testis. Br Med J 1973; 4: 77–79

40   Senturia YD, Peckham CS, Peckham MJ. Children fathered by men treated for testicular cancer. Lancet 1985: ii: 766–769

41   Bracken RB, Johnson DE. Sexual function and fecundity after treatment for testicular tumours. Urology 1976; 7: 35–38

42   Hendry WF, Stedronska, J, Jones CR, Blackmore AA, Barrett A, Peckham MJ. Semen analysis in testicular cancer and Hodgkin's disease: pre- and post-treatment findings and implications for cryopreservation. Br J Urol 1983; 55: 769–773

43   Berthelsen JG, Skakkebaek NE. Gonadal function in men with testis cancer. Fertil Steril 1983; 39: 68–75

44   Scammell GE, White N, Stedronska J, Hendry WF, Edmonds DK, Jeffcoate SL. Cryopreservation of semen in men with testicular tumour or Hodgkin's disease: results of artificial insemination of their partners. Lancet 1985; ii: 31–32

45   Bracken RB, Smith KD. Is semen cryopreservation helpful in testicular cancer? Urology 1980; 15: 581–583

46   Rhodes EA, Hoffman DJ, Kaempfer SH. Ten years of experience with semen cryopreservation by cancer patients: follow-up and clinical considerations. Fertil Steril 1985; 44: 512–516

47   Milligan DW, Hughes R, Lindsay KS. Semen cryopreservation in men undergoing cancer chemotherapy—a UK survey. Br J Cancer 1989; 60: 966–967

48   Tamburini M, Filiberti A, Barbieri A et al. Psychological aspects of testis cancer therapy: a prospective study. J Urol 1989; 142: 1487–1490

49   Schover LR, Von Eschenbach AC. Sexual and marital relationships after treatment for non-seminomatous testicular cancer. Urology 1985; 25: 251–255

50   Leiter E, Brendler H. Loss of ejaculation following bilateral retroperitoneal lymphadenectomy. J Urol 1967; 98: 375-378

51   Nijman JM, Koops HS, Oldhoff J, Kremer J, Jager S. Sexual function after bilateral retroperitoneal lymph node dissection for nonseminomatous testicular cancer. Arch Androl 1987; 18: 255-267

52   Jewett MAS, Kong YS, Goldberg SD et al. Retroperitoneal lymphadenectomy for testis tumor with nerve sparing for ejaculation. J Urol 1988; 139: 1220-1224

53   Jewett MAS. Nerve sparing technique for retroperitoneal lymphadenectomy in testis cancer. Urol Clin North Am 1990; 17: 449-456

54   Richie JP. Clinical stage I testicular cancer: the role of modified retroperitoneal lymphadenectomy. J Urol 1990; 144: 1160-1163

55   Tait D, Peckham MJ, Hendry WF, Goldstraw P. Post-chemotherapy surgery in advanced non-seminoma germ cell tumours: the significance of histology with particular reference to differentiated (mature) teratoma. Br J Cancer 1984; 50: 601-609

56   Hendry WF, A'Hern RP, Hetherington JW, Peckham MJ, Dearnaley DP, Horwich A. Paraaortic lymphadenectomy after chemotherapy for metastatic non seminomatous germ cell tumours: prognostic value and therapeutic benefit. Br J Urol 1993; 71: 208-213

57   Jones DR, Norman AR, Horwich A, Hendry WF. Ejaculatory dysfunction after retroperitoneal lymphadenectomy. Eur Urol 1993; 23: 169-171

58   Nijman JM, Jager S, Boer PW, Kremer J, Oldhoff J, Koops HS. The treatment of ejaculation disorders after retroperitoneal lymph node dissection. Cancer 1982: 50: 2967-2971

59   Ohl DA, Denil J, Bennett CJ, Randolph JF, Menge AC, McCabe M. Electroejaculation following retroperitoneal lymphadenectomy. J Urol 1991; 145: 980-983

60   Hamilton CR, Horwich A, Easton D, Peckham MJ. Radiotherapy for stage I seminoma testis: results of treatment and complications. Radiother Oncol 1986; 6: 115-120

61   Gregory C, Peckham MJ. Results of radiotherapy for stage II testicular seminoma. Radiother Oncol 1986; 6: 285-292

62   Thomas G. Management of metastatic seminoma: role of radiotherapy. In: Horwich A, ed. Testicular cancer—clinical investigation and management. London: Chapman & Hall, 1991: pp 117-128

63   Horwich A, Dearnaley DP. Treatment of seminoma. Semin Oncol 1992; 19: 171-180

64   Hamilton CR, Horwich A, Bliss JM, Peckham MJ. Gastrointestinal morbidity of adjuvant radiotherapy in stage I malignant teratoma of the testis. Radiother Oncol 1987: 10: 85-90

65   Hay JH, Duncan W, Kerr GR. Subsequent malignancies in patients irradiated for testicular tumours. Br J Radiol 1984; 57: 597-602

66   Fossa S, Kreuser ED, Roth GJ et al. Long-term side effects after treatment of testicular cancer. In: Newland DWW, Jones WG eds. EORTC Genitourinary Group monograph 7: Prostate cancer and testicular cancer. New York: Wiley-Liss, 1990: pp 321-330

67   Horwich A, Bell J. Late mortality after radiotherapy for stage I seminoma of the testis. Eur J Cancer 1991; 27 (suppl 2): abstract p. S109

68   Mason MD, Featherstone J, Olliff J, Horwich A. Inguinal iliac lymph node involvement in germ cell tumours of the testis: implications of radiological investigation and for therapy. Clin Oncol 1991; 3: 147-150

69   Horwich A. Current controversies in the management of testicular cancer. Eur J Cancer 1991; 27: 322-326

70   Horwich A, Dearnaley DP, Norman A, Hendry WF. Primary chemotherapy for stage II low volume non seminomatous germ cell tumours of the testis. Proc Am Soc Clin Oncol 1992; 11: abstract p. 197

71   Horwich A, Dearnaley DP, A'Hern R et al. The activity of single-agent carboplatin in advanced seminoma. Eur J Cancer 1992; 28A: 1307-1310

72   Vogelzang NJ. The acute and chronic toxicities of chemotherapy for metastatic testicular cancer. In: Horwich A, ed. Testicular cancer—clinical investigation and management. London: Chapman & Hall, 1991: pp 331-351

73   Dearnaley DP, Horwich A, A'Hern R et al. Combination chemotherapy with bleomycin, etoposide and cisplatin (BEP) for metastatic testicular teratoma: long-term follow-up. Eur J Cancer 1991; 27: 684-691

74   Barton C, Duchesne G, Williams M, Fisher C, Horwich A. The impact of

hydronephrosis on renal function in patients treated with platinum-based chemotherapy for metastatic non-seminomatous germ cell tumours. Cancer 1988; 62: 1439–1443

75 Einhorn LH,Williams SD. Chemotherapy of disseminated testicular cancer: a random prospective study. Cancer 1980; 46: 1339–1344

76 Williams SD, Birch R, Einhorn LH, Irwin L, Greco FA, Loehrer PJ. Treatment of disseminated germ-cell tumors with cisplatin, bleomycin and either vinblastine or etoposide. N Engl J Med 1987; 316: 1435–1440

77 Samson MK, Rivkin SE, Jones SE et al. Dose-response and dose-survival advantage for high versus low-dose cisplatin combined with vinblastine and bleomycin in disseminated testicular cancer. A Southwest Oncology Group Study. Cancer 1984; 53: 1029–1035

78 Brada M, Horwich A, Peckham MJ. Treatment of favourable prognosis non seminomatous testicular germ cell tumours with etoposide, cisplatin and reduced dose of bleomycin. Cancer Treat Rep 1987; 7: 655–656

79 Horwich A, Dearnaley DP, Duchesne GM, Williams M, Brada M, Peckham MJ. Simple non-toxic treatment of advanced metastatic seminoma with carboplatin. J Clin Oncol 1989; 7: 1150–1156

80 Childs WJ, Nicholls EJ, Horwich A. The optimization of carboplatin dose in carboplatin, etoposide and bleomycin combination chemotherapy for good prognosis metastatic nonseminomatous germ cell tumours of the testis. Ann Oncol 1992; 3: 291–296

81 Stoter G, Kaye S, Sleyfer D et al. Preliminary results of BEP (bleomycin, etoposide, cisplatin) versus an alternating regimen of BEP and PVB (cisplatin, vinblastine, bleomycin) in high volume metastatic (HVM) testicular non-seminomas. Proc Am Soc Clin Oncol 1986; 5: abstract p. 106

82 Loehrer PJ, Elson P, Johnson DH, Williams AN, Trump DL, Einhorn LH. A randomized trial of cisplatin (P) plus etoposide (E) with or without bleomycin (B) in favourable prognosis disseminated germ cell tumors (GCT): an ECOG study. Proc Am Soc Clin Oncol 1991; 10: abstract p. 169

83 Peckham MJ, Horwich A, Blackmore C, Hendry WF. Etoposide and cisplatin with or without bleomycin as first-line chemotherapy in patients with small-volume metastases of testicular nonseminoma. Cancer Treat Rep 1985; 69: 483–488

84 Horwich A, Dearnaley DP, Nicholls J, Jay G, Mason M, Harland S. Effectiveness of carboplatin, etoposide, bleomycin (CEB), combination chemotherapy good prognosis metastatic testicular non seminomatous germ cell tumours. J Clin Oncol 1991; 9: 62–69

85 Bajorin DF, Sarosdy MF, Bosl GJ, Mazumdar M. Good-risk germ cell tumor (GCT): a randomized trial of etoposide + carboplatin (EC) vs etoposide + cisplatin (EP). Proc Am Soc Clin Oncol 1992; 11: abstract p. 203

14

Penile revascularization

J. Lumley

The increased awareness and recognition of impotence problems by the medical profession over the last decade has led to improved evaluation techniques, and the introduction of a number of effective treatment regimes. These studies have shown that in approximately 90% of cases there is a demonstrable organic cause of impotence and a large number of patients can benefit from intracavernous self-injection of vasoactive agents.

Less than 5% of patients presenting in an impotence clinic have focal arterial disease. However, it is important to identify those that do, since their problems may be amenable to effective therapy. These measures can avoid the inconveniences of intracavernous self-injection or the potential complications of prosthetic devices. The outcome depends on patient selection, the choice of bypass procedure and the skill with which the treatment is undertaken.

AETIOLOGY

Erection is dependent on an adequate pressure within the corpora cavernosa and this is to a large extent related to the integrity of a normal arterial supply. The arterial input may be compromised by disease at any site from the aorta to the penile vessels. In 1923 Leriche[1] first described impotence in patients with occlusive disease of the lower aorta and iliac arteries. The syndrome also included buttock pain and lower limb claudication.

The angle of erection declines with age, as noted in the Kinsey report.[2] However, no equivalent population survey has been undertaken to determine whether these changes are likely to be due to peripheral arterial disease or other defects in the erectile mechanism. Specific questionnaires in a peripheral vascular clinic have yielded an incidence of between 21 and 73%. This wide range may be related to the depth of questioning or the definition of impotence, both by the questioner and the patient. Older patients vary considerably with respect to their expectation of potency.

The vast majority of large vessel disease causing impotence is atheromatous in origin. Common and internal iliac artery disease has to be severe and bilateral to produce impotence. In the presence of widespread aortoiliac stenotic disease, flow in the pudendal arteries can be reduced on exercise, be this lower limb or specifically of the gluteal muscles, the so-called pelvic steal syndrome.[3]

Arterial surgery of large vessel disease can improve impotence but it can also precipitate this symptom by a number of mechanisms. Dissection of iliac vessels involving the presacral region can damage the pelvic parasympathetic plexuses controlling erection. Bilateral lumbar sympathectomy produces retrograde ejaculation and these factors must be taken into account in large vessel surgery. In this group of patients, embolism of debris into the pudendal vessels may also produce impotence, the so-called trash pelvis. Such debris can accumulate in the arterial lumen during endarterectomy and other forms of reconstructive surgery and then be flushed into the pelvic arterial tree on reperfusion.

Arterial bypass from the aorta to the external iliac or femoral vessels can exclude the internal iliac arteries. End-to-side anastomosis of the graft on to the aorta or distal vessels may mean that the internal iliac arteries are still perfused antegradely or retrogradely, provided the internal iliac and its peripheral branches are not totally occluded. Much of the evidence in relation to impotence with large vessel surgery is anecdotal, but Queral et al[4] studied the haemodynamics of pelvic flow after 38 aortoiliac reconstructions. The high (71%) preoperative impotence level emphasized the magnitude of the problem, which is uncovered by detailed history-taking in this group of patients. The varied response to surgery was also documented by these workers, in that the penile arterial pressures were increased in 37% of patients and reduced in 21% after surgery.

A recent study by Gossetti et al[5] demonstrated impotence in 148 of 386 patients undergoing aortoiliac or aortofemoral reconstruction for peripheral vascular disease. Thirty-seven of these patients were diabetic. These workers noted only a 20.7% improvement of impotence by conventional lower limb reconstructive techniques but in the region of 75% improvement if the bypass was to the distal common iliac bifurcation or if an internal iliac artery was revascularized by implantation on to a limb of a graft or by an additional vein bypass. Only 5 of the diabetic patients in the series showed improvement of symptoms.

The dramatic reduction in surgery for aortoiliac occlusive disease, due to the widespread use of percutaneous transluminal angioplasty, makes it more difficult currently to assess the relative value of different surgical approaches; these factors are considered again later in the chapter.

Bilateral internal iliac artery disconnection, such as in bilateral renal transplantation, may give rise to impotence. However, this is unpredictable since brachiopenile arterial pressure indices were not reduced in 55% of patients in this group. Disease of the pudendal and penile arteries is not routinely looked for in the assessment of lower limb peripheral vascular disease and the incidence of coexistent proximal and distal disease is poorly documented.

Bilateral focal pudendal and penile vascular disease is not infrequently encountered in an impotence clinic. The aetiology of these lesions is usually assumed to be atheromatous in nature, although patients are often in the third and fourth decade, and may have no marked associated proximal disease. The lesions are usually bilateral and symmetrical and particularly involve the distal pudendal arteries. These vessels and other collateral pelvic arteries may be damaged in severe pelvic fractures, with impotence becoming apparent as a late sequela of these events. Impotence has also been reported in cyclists; the saddle presumably presses on the internal pudendal arteries in the pudendal canals.

Hauri[6] found an incidence of 30–40% of impotence after rectal surgery and considered that this could be reduced if more attention was given to the preservation of neural structures and small vessels around the pelvis.

ASSESSMENT

Assessment of patients with arterial impotence, as with all forms of impotence, commences with a detailed history and examination. It is important to establish whether a patient has ever had normal erectile function as this is closely linked with his expectations of any therapeutic measures. Arterial impotence is suggested by the slow onset of tumescence and failure to reach rigidity. Progression of the arterial disease is accompanied by decreasing potency until erection disappears completely. This contrasts with venous impotence in which erections usually develop promptly but do not reach full rigidity or rapidly disappear. However, these problems may coexist and there may be superadded neuropathic disease, such as in the diabetic patient.

The preservation of normal early morning erections suggests that there is no significant vascular disease. Similarly, intermittent problems are unlikely to be vascular-mediated. The history should include a full vascular survey, encompassing lower limb symptoms of intermittent claudication or rest pain, angina or myocardial infarction and cerebrovascular symptoms, such as transient ischaemic attacks and strokes. Note all risk factors, such as hypertension, smoking and diabetes. Examination includes a thorough assessment of the genitalia and lumbosacral nervous system. Cardiovascular examination pays particular attention to lower limb pulses and the nutrition of the feet. Bruits are sought over the carotid and subclavian vessels in the neck, the abdominal aorta and iliac vessels in the abdomen and the femoral arteries along the length of each thigh. It is sometimes difficult to feel a penile pulse in a normal individual and the presence or absence of this sign is not a good diagnostic indicator.

It is our practice to undertake an endocrine screen on patients with impotence although it rarely identifies unsuspected abnormalities. Of prime importance is to check for glycosuria and a raised blood sugar. The screen includes testosterone, prolactin, follicle-stimulating hormone and luteinizing hormone. Our next screening test is an intracorporeal injection of 30–60 mg papaverine, the dosage depending on the degree of impotence reported. A normal response is interpreted as there being competent arterial and venous systems and no further vascular investigations are undertaken.

If the response to papaverine is reduced or short-lived, further studies are undertaken. Our initial research programme included sleep laboratory testing and visual erotic stimulation. While these were valuable in establishing the baselines against which to assess other investigations, they were not of sufficient discriminatory value to include as routine studies. Similarly, isotope penile blood flow techniques were initially developed and found of value in diagnosing large vessel abnormalities but were less discriminatory for small vessel disease. The technique used in these investigations was deconvolution analysis of penile artery isotope transit times.

Ultrasound has revolutionized the non-invasive assessment of peripheral vascular disease; this has included its use in vasculogenic impotence. Abelson[7] was one of the first to measure penile blood pressure in impotent patients. A more valuable measure is the penile/brachial pressure index, since this takes the systemic pressure into the equation.[8] Indices below 0.6 are a useful indicator of severe arterial disease. However, values between 0.6 and 0.9 are less sensitive or specific in the diagnosis of arterial impotence.[9]

The superficial dorsal arteries of the penis can be assessed easily with a hand-held Doppler probe, but flow in the deeper arteries is difficult to identify with this instrument. In recent years, attention has been directed at Duplex scanning of penile arteries.[10] The Duplex instrument provides a means of assessing the deep arteries as well as the dorsal artery and is currently the only reliable non-invasive measure for assessing flows in these vessels.[11] The Duplex instrument also enables wave form analysis of all penile vessels,[12] providing information on arterial flow.

Gehl et al[13] compared colour-coded Dopper sonography with continuous-wave Doppler in postoperative evaluation of revascularization procedures. Strength and direction of flow could be assessed and differentiation made between arteries and vein, and deep and superficial vessels. Both techniques were effective in demonstrating anastomotic patency but the deep vasculature was more clearly demonstrated using colour-coded techniques.

Pickard et al,[14] using colour Duplex ultrasonography to assess mean peak systemic velocity of the deep penile artery at rest, and after papaverine-induced tumescence, found that the flow of less than 20 cm/s was diagnostic of inadequate arterial inflow.

The combination of an intracorporeal injection of papaverine and ultrasonic assessment provides an indication of the presence of arterial disease and enables the decision to be made as to the necessity of progressing to angiography. The latter not only provides supportive evidence of arterial disease but also identifies the site of any lesions, and enables the planning of a treatment regime. If there is a suggestion of a venous component to a patient's impotence, preliminary venous studies are advisable. This usually takes the form of cavernosometry and cavernosography.

ANGIOGRAPHY

Arteriography is undertaken in patients in whom arterial disease has been identified by non-invasive studies and who would consider undergoing reconstructive arterial surgery. It should not be carried out without valid reason, since it can produce focal vascular and systemic complications. If the history and clinical findings are suggestive of major aortoiliac disease, the study is primarily to visualize these large vessels. The usual procedure is a retrograde femoral aortogram or, in severe occlusive disease, an intravenous digital subtraction arteriogram. The latter is preferred to translumbar or transbrachial catheterization.

In most impotent patients being considered for reconstructive surgery, the lesions are more distally sited and selective demonstration of the internal iliac tree is required. Even in these patients, a preliminary flush aortogram is advised to identify coexistent large vessel disease.

The penile arteries are not visualized on routine aortography and cannulation of the internal pudendal arteries can be technically difficult and is prone to artefact. Initial studies[3,15] were undertaken under general anaesthesia to overcome some of the problems of spasm. However, improvements and modifications have made it possible to undertake the procedure under local anaesthetic.[16] Bilateral disease is present in these patients and views are required of both internal pudendal arteries. Conversely, if the first side examined shows a completely normal study, there is little to be gained from proceeding to investigation of the second side. Cannulation is usually via the femoral artery in the groin and it may be possible to cannulate both internal iliac and internal pudendal ateries through a single access site. As with pharmococavernosography, improved results are obtained by preliminary intracorporeal injection of 40 mg papaverine.[17] The procedure has been further facilitated by improvements in catheter and guidewire design, primarily due to developments in the coronary artery field. The amount of contrast medium can be reduced using digital subtraction techniques: low osmolality contrast agents further reduce pain and associated spasm.

Positioning of the patient is important. The penis is placed horizontally across the contralateral thigh; views are taken anteroposteriorly after tilting the pelvis to 45°. In the latter view, the internal pudendal artery crosses the head of the femur but its branches are not overlain by bony structures and abnormalities are more clearly demonstrated. Contrast (20–30 ml) is required to demonstrate the iliac and 10 ml for the internal pudendal arteries. Typical injection rates are 3 ml/s; the timing and number of films depend on the blood flow rate and available apparatus. Decisions on surgical management can only be made after the bilateral anatomy and any abnormalities of the pudendal arteries have been demonstrated.

Absence of a dorsal or deep artery on one side does not in itself constitute the cause of arterial impotence, since congenital anomalies are common. However, bilateral focal occlusive or stenotic lesions in the internal pudendal artery, or the deep or dorsal arteries, and the presence of collateral vessels, are suggestive of arteriogenic causes of impotence.

SURGICAL PROCEDURES

Although the relation of arterial disease to impotence has been recognized since Leriche's original report,[1] the surgical management of these lesions was slow to follow. The problems and unpredictability of aortoiliac reconstruction have already been referred to and, when appropriate, percutaneous transluminal angioplasty presents a much more satisfactory alternative for large vessel occlusive disease. Common, external and internal iliac stenoses can be effectively catheterized and dilated with minimal morbidity and without the risk of pelvic denervation.

The incidence of distal embolization after angioplasty is surprisingly low, in view of the unstable surfaces observed at operation. In our experience it has also been possible to negotiate and successfully dilate just over half the occluded common iliac arteries currently encountered in peripheral lower limb disease. Selective cannulation and dilatation of the distal internal iliac arteries are more difficult, and occlusive lesions in the pudendal artery and its penile branches do not currently lend themselves to this technique. In view of this, some form of bypass has to be considered.

One of the first reported operative procedures was direct surgery to the pudendal artery, using a vein bypass from the femoral artery.[18] Subsequent reports for most of the next decade were towards revascularization of the corpora cavernosa. Michal's group was again actively involved in these procedures. Vein grafting from a femoral artery to a window in the tunica albuginia was an early procedure of choice. The main complication of this approach was a high incidence of priapism. A smaller bypass vessel was therefore considered necessary: the inferior epigastric became the donor vessel of choice.

Michal et al[19] reported initial success with the latter procedure; however, long-term follow-up of bypass procedures to the corpora cavernosa were unsatisfactory. Hawatmeh et al[20] demonstrated a high incidence of fibrous thickening of the septum and, to a lesser extent, the cavernous tissue following long saphenous vein, femoral-to-cavernous bypass. They considered these effects were due to the high pressure within the intracavernous tissue. Metz & Frimodt-Moller[21] assessed the long-term results in 9 patients in whom they had undertaken epigastric-to-cavernous anastomoses. Only two of the anastomoses were patent, these being at 12 and 24 months following surgery. This team considered the operation to be an unsatisfactory procedure in the management of arterial impotence.

A novel alternative approach was introduced by Virag et al,[22] who reported improvement of erectile function after arterializing the deep dorsal vein. Furlow[23] modified the approach by proximal ligation of the arterialized segment, together with ligation of the circumflex veins, but leaving the perforator veins intact. Virag later extended the latter modification by arterializing the corpora cavernosa from the arterialized segment of vein, by a side-to-side anastomosis to a window in the tunica albuginea. This Virag V procedure was accompanied by less priapism than a femorocavernous vein bypass.

One of the problems of venous arterialization is hypervascularization and hypersensitivity of the glands. Wilms et al[24] had reported a patient with hypervascularization and glans ischaemia after combined venous arterialization and venous leak surgery. Bypass in this patient required embolization to reverse the problem.

Hauri et al[25] have recently postulated that venous disease is due primarily to impairment of cavernous tissue and that this is present in 90% of patients with arterial disease. They suggest that arterial revascularization should be combined with mechanical penis banding in these patients.

Current trends have returned to Michal's original principle of revascularizing the arteries normally supplying penile blood flow, i.e. the internal pudendal and the deep and dorsal penile arteries. On physiological grounds the deep artery is the most appropriate vessel to revascularize, since it feeds directly into the cavernous vascular plexuses, and is most likely to re-establish normal erection. The deep artery, however, is relatively inaccessible. The terminal portion of the internal pudental artery is deeply placed in the perineum and there is no convenient adjacent artery for bypass. A vein bypass is therefore required and the denervated free graft has less satisfactory characteristics in terms of size and physiological control compared with a natural artery.

The deep artery of the penis can be exposed in the corpora cavernosa at the base of the penis (Fig. 14.1) The tunica albuginea is incised and a blunt nerve hook is swept transversely from lateral to medial, gently lifting out the deep artery. The artery is medially placed within the corpora cavernosa and can be stretched to the dorsal surface for end-to-side anastomosis with a donor vessel. The procedure has a number of disadvantages. The tunica is opened and has to be left unsutured, at least in part, to allow passage of the donor vessel. Locating the deep artery can be difficult: it is variable in size and may be congenitally absent, resulting in technical problems; re-establishment of normal flow may be unsuccessful. Dissection invariably involves local destruction of cavernous tissue and the tumescence mechanisms at this site.

These comments are based on the disappointing personal experiences of the author, since the technical details and results of this procedure are poorly documented in the literature. Generally they have been incorporated in an overview of the surgical practice of individual surgeons, and specific technical details and results are not available.

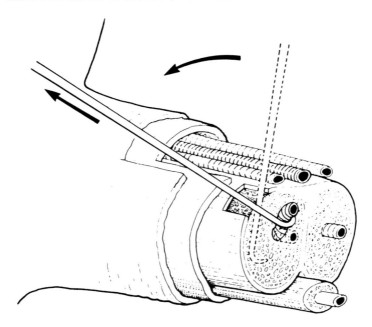

Fig. 14.1   Dissection of the deep (cavernosal) artery of the penis. The tunica albuginea is divided longitudinally on one side of the midline, at the base of the penis. A blunt hook is inserted into the lateral aspect of the corpus cavernosum. The hook is then gently swept medially to engage the deep artery, which is lifted to the surface for anastomosis. Reproduced with permission from Kirby RS, Carson C, Webster GD eds. Impotence—diagnosis and management of male erectile dysfunction. Oxford: Butterworth-Heinemann, 1992

The dorsal penile arteries are more readily accessible for surgical bypass than the deep. However, they carry physiological disadvantages, as their terminal supply is predominantly to the glans penis. They do have branches to the corpora cavernosa but these are ill-defined and inconsistent, and probably are of little importance in normal erection. The justification for their use in revascularization is therefore based on retrograde flow to the origin of the vessels and thence to the deep penile artery. This in turn is dependent on normal vessels back to and including the bifurcation of the internal pudendal artery, and the presence of a normal deep penile artery on the side of anastomosis. These features may have been demonstrated radiologically, the artery filling via collaterals beyond proximal disease; however, occasionally this information is not available until per- and postoperative assessment.

Goldstein[26] advocated end-to-end anastomosis of the inferior epigastric to the proximal cut end of one or both dorsal penile arteries (Fig. 14.2). This serves to ensure maximum retrograde flow in the dorsal arteries and from thence to the deep penile arteries. Turpitko et al[27] described a technique whereby the end of a vein bypass can be anastomosed to both ends of the

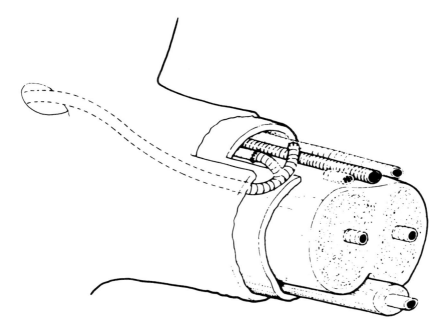

Fig. 14.2   Inferior epigastric to bilateral dorsal artery anastomoses. The cut end of the inferior epigastric artery has been anastomosed end to side onto the left dorsal artery of the penis. A large muscular branch of the donor artery has been anastomosed end to end onto the proximal right dorsal artery of the penis because of distal occlusion of the latter vessel. Reproduced with permission from Kirby RS, Carson C, Webster GD eds. Impotence— diagnosis and management of male erectile dysfunction. Oxford: Butterworth-Heinemann, 1992

divided dorsal penile artery. Longitudinal division of the end of the vein along two diametrically opposite points and sewing the ends of the two flaps together leaves an opening on each side for anastomosis of the cut arterial ends. This could also be applicable to an arterial bypass when technical difficulties are encountered with an end-to-side anastomosis.

The flow in a vessel is dependent on the pressure gradient across a vascular bed. Microanastomoses are therefore more likely to remain patent if the donor artery, providing blood at systemic pressure, is anastomosed to a vessel with a low peripheral resistance. Resistance in the cavernous plexus falls during the initial phase of erection but is high during full tumescence and may also be relatively high in the resting phase. The concept of shunt vessels, as proposed by Wagner et al,[28] does provide a physiological means of lowering peripheral resistance, although the mechanism remains uncertain. To overcome potential peripheral resistance problems, a useful addition to the dorsal artery revascularization procedure is a concomitant arteriovenous fistula, as proposed by Hauri.[29]

TECHNICAL CONSIDERATIONS

The author favours revascularization through an inferior epigastric to dorsal penile artery anastomosis. This is usually an end-to-side anastomosis on to the penile vessel with an additional side-to-side anastomosis to the second dorsal artery, if two satisfactory vessels are located. A concomitant arteriovenous fistula is fashioned to the deep dorsal vein of the penis.

THE INFERIOR EPIGASTRIC ARTERY AS A DONOR VESSEL

The inferior epigastric artery has to be mobilized from the deep inguinal ring to the level of the umbilicus to provide an adequate length for bypass. At the latter site, the major component of the artery enters the deep surface of the rectus abdominis muscle; its continuation for anastomosis to the superior epigastric artery is smaller and less suitable for anastomosis.

The vessel is exposed by a longitudinal lower abdominal incision, on to and then through the rectus sheath. A paramedian incision allows exposure of the inferior epigastric artery, but the rectus muscle requires a good deal of lateral retraction and the proximal dissection of the vessel has to pass deep to the muscle and then beyond its lateral edge. A lateral pararectal incision is therefore more convenient. The rectus sheath is incised near the lateral border of the rectus muscle and the muscle retracted medially (Fig. 14.3). The lower thoracic nerves supplying the rectus abdominis muscle are often ill-defined but when identified must be carefully preserved. The inferior epigastric artery is mobilized together with its venae comitantes. Separating the artery from these one or two veins is difficult and carries the potential of arterial damage; it is unnecessary. Small branches can be coagulated with a bipolar instrument away from the main vessel. Two or three larger branches passing to the deep surface of the rectus abdominis muscle are best ligated with a 6/0 tie. The large branch entering the muscle at the level of the umbilicus is identified but only ligated and divided with the main vessel when it is needed for bypass.

The proximal end of the inferior epigastric artery dissection passes to within a centimetre of the deep ring, beneath the conjoined tendon. No attempt is made to define its origin, since this is usually surrounded by fatty tissue and the vessel can be easily damaged at this site. While the penile dissection is being undertaken, the inferior epigastric artery is left in continuity. The vessel is kept moist and a few drops of papaverine or an alpha-blocking agent may be placed on it to relieve any spasm. When ready for anastomosis the distal vessel is transected at approximately the level of the umbilicus, preserving the last perforating rectus muscle branch as this may be larger than the main trunk, or two ends may be needed for revascularization.

The route to the dorsum of the penis is through the superficial inguinal ring. Gentle blunt dissection is used to fashion a pathway from the abdominal wound through to the incision over the base of the penis, in a deep subcutaneous plane. In closing the abdominal incision care must be taken not

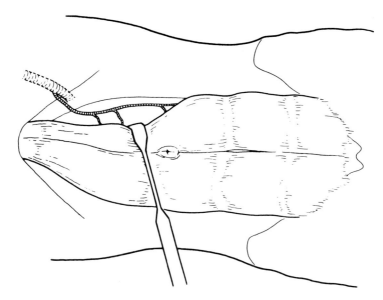

Fig. 14.3 Exposure of the inferior epigastric artery. The skin, superficial abdominal fascial layers and the anterior rectus sheath have been divided along the lateral border of the right rectus muscle. After distal division of the artery, the cut end is passed anterior to the conjoint tendon and through the superfical inguinal ring to the root of the penis. Reproduced with permission from Kirby RS, Carson C, Webster GD eds. Impotence—diagnosis and management of male erectile dysfunction. Oxford: Butterworth-Heinemann, 1992

to damage the pedicle when suturing the lower extremity of the divided anterior rectus sheath. Usually bleeding is minimal at the time of closure and in this case it is unnecessary to drain the wound.

EXPOSURE OF DORSAL PENILE VESSELS

The incision at the base of the penis is approximately 2.5 cm long and may be transverse or longitudinal. Even if the skin incision is transverse, the fascial incision and vessel dissection are longitudinal. Approximately 1 cm of at least one dorsal artery is required for satisfactory anastomosis and a similar length of deep dorsal vein when a fistula is being fashioned. The incision is deepened on to these vessels by a mixture of blunt and sharp dissection, particular attention being paid to preservation of neuronal and vascular structures. Magnification must be used during this procedure but two to four surgical loups are usually sufficient at this stage. A surprising number of fascial layers are encountered in the search for suitable vessels, but careful gentle dissection, starting from the midline and working first to the side of the abdominal incision and then to the contralateral side, is usually rewarded by the definition of a satisfactory length of dorsal penile artery on at least one side.

Normal dorsal penile arteries are to be expected in patients post pelvic trauma, post bilateral renal transplant or post rectal surgery. However, occasionally in the elderly patient, an occluded atheromatous dorsal vessel is present on one side and a stenosed artery on the other. Following these vessels proximally may allow the definition of a more normal segment which, on transection, produces a weak forward flow. End-to-end anastomosis is the procedure of choice in this situation, preferably using both dorsal arteries, possibly using the last rectus branch of the inferior epigastric artery to provide two end-to-end anastomoses.

When at least one normal dorsal penile artery is present, the author's preference is to undertake a single end-to-side anastomosis. With such a normal vessel it is also possible to incorporate the arteriovenous fistula within the single anastomosis (Fig. 14.4). The dorsal artery and vein are mobilized and brought alongside each other and subsequent manoeuvres are carried out under a dissecting microscope. At this stage the adequacy of the tunnel for the donor artery is checked and the inferior epigastric is drawn into the penile wound. A microvascular clip is applied to the divided artery and bleeding

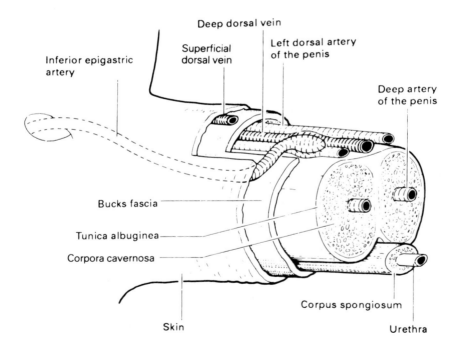

Fig. 14.4 The Hauri operation. The inferior epigastric artery is anastomosed over the site of a dorsal artery to deep dorsal vein arteriovenous fistula. Reproduced with permission from Kirby RS, Carson C, Webster GD eds. Impotence—diagnosis and management of male erectile dysfunction. Oxford: Butterworth-Heinemann, 1992

veins bipolar coagulated or ligated. Care is taken to ligate the distal cut ends, since a considerable haematoma can ensue if these ligatures come off.

Micro Mayfield clips are applied proximally and distally to the adjacent dorsal penile artery and vein. Adventitial strands and residual adherent tissues must be teased out and divided from the segments to ensure they are not pulled into the anastomosis during suture. Equal ellipses of adjacent walls are removed with curved microscissors, firmly picking up the centre of each ellipse with a forceps. The length of anastomosis is approximately 2 mm. Pulling up on a forceps allows the length of the incision to be carefully judged. Care must be taken not to remove more than a quarter of the circumference of either vessel since this will leave inadequate vessel wall for suture without producing a stenosis. Incisions can be made with a diamond knife or other microblades; however, the anastomosis is facilitated by removal of the ellipse.

The posterior adjacent walls of the incised artery and vein are sutured first. A 10/0 monofilament nylon suture is used. Although a continuous suture technique can be used, long loops cannot be visualized under the microscope and catch on adjacent tissues. This will exert excessive traction on the anastomosis or break the suture. An interrupted suture technique is therefore usually undertaken. The first stitch is placed in the middle of the back wall, the knot being tied on the outside of the lumen. Subsequent stitches are placed on either side of the first until the two corner sutures are in place.

The divided end of the inferior epigastric artery is now brought alongside the anastomosis. It is usually 1 mm in diameter and therefore will need to be divided slightly obliquely to match the length of the anastomosis. Excessive adventitia must be removed to expose at least 1 mm length of clearly dissected normal vessel end. The anastomosis is completed between the donor vessel and the dorsal penile vein on one side, and the dorsal penile artery on the other, using interrupted sutures. On completion of the anastomosis the microclips are first removed from the deep dorsal vein, and blood is allowed to flow across the anastomosis to check for obvious leaks. If these are absent or once they have been sutured, the clips are removed from the dorsal artery, haemostasis rechecked, and a swab placed over the anastomosis while the clamp is removed from the donor artery. The swab is left in place for 2–3 min. The clamp may require replacement to deal with a spurting leak but stitch holes should be gently covered until haemostasis is obtained.

Following this procedure there should be no stenoses and flow should be demonstrable in all limbs of the anastomosis. This may be tested by gently occluding each limb with a forceps and gently milking out the blood from the adjacent segment with a second forceps: on release of the first forceps the milked segment should refill across the anastomosis. If this is not so, gentle manipulation of the vessels and removal of all adventitial strands is necessary.

At all times the dissection must be kept moist with heparinized saline. Systemic heparinization is not required in these microanastomoses but debris must be washed away from the lumen before completion, using a stream of heparinized saline from a syringe and needle. The operator must be confident that the anastomosis and the fistula are patent before wound closure. If back-bleeding was present from the dorsal penile artery and pulsatile forward flow from the inferior epigastric artery prior to anastomosis, primary patency should be obtainable. Occlusion of the deep dorsal vein on the proximal side of the anastomosis may be seen to improve pulsation in the dorsal artery and it may be appropriate to ligate one limb of the fistula. If there is any doubt about patency, however, it is wise to omit this manoeuvre.

In the absence of a suitable dorsal penile artery, a Virag V procedure is recommended. In this a 2.5 cm length of deep dorsal vein is mobilized and an adjacent length of tunica albuginea over the dorsal aspect of one corpora cavernosa is freed of adherent tissue. The incision in the tunica is approximately 12 mm long, removing a 1.5 mm strip of the wall with a pointed scalpel or microknife. The segment of vein is occluded proximally and distally with microclips and an ellipse of venous wall of equivalent length, and adjacent to the tunica defect, is removed with curved microscissors. A fine probe is passed distally along the vein to destroy the two or three valve cusps along the length of the penis, but preserving the valve adjacent to the glans penis. A venocavernous anastomosis is undertaken using a 10/0 monofilament vascular suture. A cutting needle is appropriate to suture the thick tunica wall. The inferior epigastric artery is anastomosed end-to-side on to the vein, proximal to the first anastomosis. The proximal limb of the venous fistula can be ligated at a later stage once flow and an erectile pattern have been established.

Operative complications from these various procedures are minimal. The patient can leave hospital after 2–3 days and stitches can be removed after 8 or 9 days. Sexual activity is encouraged but intercourse delayed for 5–6 weeks.

OUTCOME

The results of these various procedures have been variously reported. The disappointing outcome of the vein bypasses and direct anastomoses to the corpora cavernosa have already been referred to. Other figures are complex, including many procedures and ill-defined lengths of follow-up. Important factors such as aetiology and age are often difficult to analyse. In our own series, procedures were initially undertaken on severe arteriopaths and results were disappointing. However, this may also have been linked to development of the techniques and choice of operative procedure. In our first reported 12 patients followed up over a period of 4 years, only 6 showed prolonged improvement.

The four most recent cases using the Hauri fistula technique, however, have all shown marked improvement of erectile status and anastomotic patency has been retained by the addition of the arteriovenous fistula.

Goldstein[26] reported the results of 130 procedures followed from 6 months to 5 years with a return of coitus rate of 54%. Classification into atherosclerotic, idiopathic and traumatic vasculogenic groups, the obtained return of coitus rate was respectively 24, 40 and 81% of patients. One may still question whether an overall 50% success for a revascularization procedure is an acceptable figure. However, penile prostheses are not an acceptable alternative for all patients and the long-term complication rate remains a problem. Of prime importance, therefore, is patient selection. Traumatic, and to a lesser extent, congenital anomalies of the internal pudendal artery are of prime importance, since in these patients return of erectile function can be expected.

The reliability of the techniques is partly dependent on experience, and the expertise of the clinical team managing the assessment. It is also essential to have the patients' full understanding with regard to possible failure and their having a realistic expectation of outcome. Retention of the natural mechanism of erection is a desirable aim, particularly as it does not damage the normal sensation of erection. Revascularization does not prevent subsequent implant insertion, whereas this is not true for the reverse situation. Further research should be directed towards the understanding of the natural physiological mechanism involved in the erectile response, selection of patients for operative procedures, methods of bringing a physiologically controlled alternative blood supply to the penis and the factors influencing the long-term patency of revascularization procedures.

KEY POINTS FOR CLINICAL PRACTICE

- Ninety per cent of impotence is organic in origin.
- Patients are screened with an intracavernous injection of a vasoactive agent (ICV).
- If a normal response is obtained after ICV, consider treatment using self-injection by this technique.
- If there is a poor response, undertake cavernosometry with or without ICV to identify venous leaks.
- If there is a poor response and no venous disorders, undertake arteriography with or without ICV to identify arterial stenotic or occlusive disease and plan a revascularization procedure.
- Ultrasound with or without ICV provides additional information on the anatomy and function of penile arteries and veins pre- and postoperatively. Their future development may further reduce the need for invasive diagnostic procedures.

REFERENCES

1   Leriche R. Des obliterans arterielles hautes comme cause d'une insuffisance circulatoire des membres inferieurs. Bull Soc Chir 1923; 49: 1404
2   Kinsey AC, Pomeroy W, Martin C. Age and sexual outlet. In: Kinsey AC, Pomeroy WB, Martin CE, eds, Sexual behaviour in the human male. Philadelphia: WB Saunders, 1948: pp 297–325
3   Michal V, Pospichal J, Blazkova J. Phalloarteriography in the diagnosis of erectile

impotence. World J Surg 1978; 2: 239–247

4　Queral LA, Whitehouse WM, Flinn WR et al. Pelvic haemodynamics after aortoiliac reconstruction. Surgery 1979; 86: 799–809

5　Gossetti B, Gattuso R, Irace L, Intrieri F, Venosi S, Benedetti-Valentini F. Aorto-iliac/femoral reconstructions in patients with vasculogenic impotence. Eur J Vasc Surg 1991; 5: 425–428

6　Hauri D. Potency problems in rectal surgery. Schweiz Rundschau Med Praxis 1990; 79: 823–828

7　Abelson D. Diagnostic value of the penile pulse and blood pressure: a Doppler study of impotence in diabetes. J Urol 1975; 113: 636–639

8　Kempczinski RF. Role of the vascular diagnostic laboratory in the evaluation of male impotence. Am J Surg 1979; 138: 278

9　Metz P, Bengtsson J. Penile blood pressure. Scand J Urol Nephrol 1981; 15: 161–164

10　Lue TF, Hricak H, Marich KW, Tanagho EA. Vasculogenic impotence evaluated by high resolution ultrasonography and pulsed Doppler spectrum analysis. Radiology 1985; 155: 777–781

11　Robinson LQ, Woodcock JP, Stephenson TP. Duplex scanning in suspected vasculogenic impotence: a worthwhile exercise? Br J Urol 1989; 63: 432–436

12　Shabshigh R, Fishman IJ. Evaluation of erectile impotence. Urology 1988; 32: 83–90

13　Gehl HB, Sikora R, Bohndorf K, Sohn M, Vorwerk D. Imaging of penile vascular anastomoses using colour-coded Doppler ultrasound: comparison with CW Doppler ultrasound and clinical aspects. Ultraschall Med 1990; 11: 155–160

14　Pickard RS, Oates CP, Sethia KK, Powell PH. The role of colour duplex ultrasonography in the diagnosis of vasculogenic impotence. Br J Urol 1991; 68: 537–540

15　Struyven J, Gregoir W, Giannakopoulos X, Wauters E. Selective pudendal arteriography. Eur Urol 1979; 5: 233–242

16　Delcour C, Katoto RM, Richoz B et al. Penile arteriography: technical improvements. Int J Impotence Res 1989; 1: 43–47

17　Bookstein JJ, Valji K, Parsons L, Kessler W. Pharmacoarteriography in the evaluation of impotence. J Urol 1987; 133: 39–41

18　Michal V, Kramer R, Bartak V. Femoropudendal bypass in the treatment of sexual impotence. J Cardiovasc Surg 1974; 15: 356

19　Michal V, Kramer R, Pospichal J, Hejhal L. Arterial epigastrico-cavernous anastomosis for the treatment of sexual impotence. World J Surg 1977; 1: 515–520

20　Hawatmeh JS, Houttuin E, Gregory JG et al. The diagnosis and management of vasculogenic impotence. J Urol 1982; 127: 910–914

21　Metz P, Frimodt-Moller C. Epigastricocavernous anastomosis in the treatment of arteriogenic impotence. Scand J Urol Nephrol 1983; 17: 271–275

22　Virag R, Zwang G, Dermange H, Legman M. Vasculogenic impotence: a review of 92 cases with 54 surgical operations. J Vasc Surg 1981; 15: 9–17

23　Furlow WL. Therapy of impotence. In: Krane RJS, ed. Clinical neuro-urology. Boston: Little, Brown, 1979: pp 213–218

24　Wilms G, Oyen R, Claes L, Boeckx W, Baert AL, Baert L. Glans ischemia after penis revascularization: therapeutic embolization. Cardiovasc Intervent Radiol 1990; 13: 304–305

25　Hauri D, Alund G, Spycher M, Fehr JL, Muhlebach P. Venous leakage—a new therapeutic concept. Urologe [Ausg A] 1991; 30: 267–271

26　Goldstein I. Arterial revascularization procedures. Semin Urol 1986; 4: 252–258

27　Turpitko SA, Mamedov DM, Uchkin IG. A new method of surgical treatment of vasculogenic impotence. Grudn Serdechno-sosudistaia Khir 1990; 8: 45–47

28　Wagner G, Willis EA, Bro-Pasmussen F, Nielsen MH. New theory on the mechanism of erection involving hitherto undescribed vessels. Lancet 1982; i: 416–418

29　Hauri D. Anastomose des arterielle epigastrica inferiore mit der arterielle dorsalis penis und zusatzlieben AV-Shunt zur V dorsalis penis produnda. Proceedings of the Leiden Urological Foundation Symposium on Controversy in Diagnosis and Treatment of Erectile Impotence. 1985; 12

Index